Anthropology in Public Health

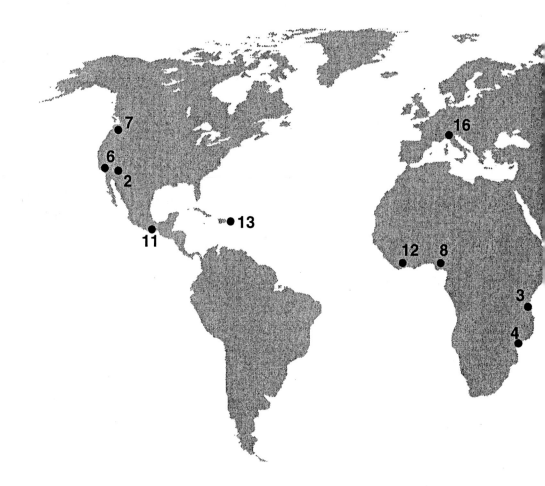

Locations of studies, by chapter number.

ANTHROPOLOGY IN PUBLIC HEALTH

Bridging Differences in Culture and Society

Edited by

ROBERT A. HAHN, Ph.D., M.P.H.

U.S. Centers for Disease Control and Prevention

With the Assistance of
KATE W. HARRIS

5

15

14

9

10

New York   Oxford
OXFORD UNIVERSITY PRESS
1999

Oxford University Press

Oxford   New York
Athens   Auckland   Bangkok   Bogotá   Buenos Aires   Calcutta
Cape Town   Chennai   Dar es Salaam   Delhi   Florence   Hong Kong   Istanbul
Karachi   Kuala Lumpur   Madrid   Melbourne   Mexico City   Mumbai
Nairobi   Paris   São Paulo   Singapore   Taipei   Tokyo   Toronto   Warsaw

and associated companies in
Berlin   Ibadan

Published by Oxford University Press, Inc.,
198 Madison Avenue, New York, New York, 10016
http://www.oup-usa.org

Library of Congress Cataloging-in-Publication Data
Anthropology in public health : bridging differences in culture and society /
edited by Robert A. Hahn, with the assistance of Kate W. Harris.
p. cm. Includes bibliographical references and index.
ISBN 978-0-19-512902-1 (cloth).—ISBN 978-0-19-511955-8 (paper)
1. Public health—Anthropological aspects.
I. Hahn, Robert A., 1945- . II. Harris, Kate W.
[DNLM: 1. Public Health Practice. 2. Anthropology, Cultural.
3. Community Health Planning. 4. Developing Countries. 5. Health Services. Indigenous.
WA 30A6347 1999] RA427.A58 1999 306.4'61—dc21 DNLM/DLC for Library of Congress 98-34571

15 14 13 12 11

Printed in the United States of America
on acid-free paper

Contents

Contributors, ix

Introduction, xv

1. Anthropology and the Enhancement of Public Health Practice, 3
   Robert A. Hahn

I   Infectious Disease

2. Folk Flu and Viral Syndrome: An Anthropological Perspective, 27
   Susan C. McCombie

3. The Role of Anthropological Methods in a Community-Based Mosquito
   Net Intervention in Bagamoyo District, Tanzania, 44
   Peter J. Winch

4. Engaging Indigenous African Healers in the Prevention
   of AIDS and STDs, 63
   Edward C. Green

5. Anthropological Perspectives on Childhood Pneumonia in Pakistan, 84
   Dorothy S. Mull

II Cancer

6. Ethnography and Breast Cancer Control among Latinas
   and Anglo Women in Southern California, 117
   Leo R. Chavez, F. Allan Hubbell, and Shiraz I. Mishra

7. A Policy Approach to Reducing Cancer Risk
   in Northwest Indian Tribes, 142
   Roberta L. Hall, Kerri Lopez, and Edward Lichtenstein

III Pharmacy and Nutrition

8. The Rational Basis of "Irrational" Drug Use: Pharmaceuticals
   in the Context of Development, 165
   Nina L. Etkin, Paul J. Ross, and Ibrahim Muazzamu

9. Cultural Tailoring in Indonesia's National Nutrition
   Improvement Program, 182
   Marcia Griffiths and Michael Favin

IV Injury and Occupational Health

10. Road Warriors: Driving Behaviors on a Polynesian Island, 211
    Judith C. Barker

11. Balancing Risks and Resources: Applying Pesticides without
    Using Protective Equipment in Southern Mexico, 235
    *Linda M. Hunt, Rolando Tinoco Ojanguren, Norah Schwartz,
    and David Halperin*

V Community Health

12. Prospects for Family Planning in Côte d'Ivoire: Ethnographic
    Contributions to the Development of Culturally Appropriate
    Population Policy, 257
    Ruth P. Wilson, Carolyn F. Sargent, Shegou Darret, and Kale Kouamé

13. Integrating Mental Health Care and Traditional Healing in Puerto Rico:
    Lessons from an Early Experiment, 279
    Joan D. Koss-Chioino

14. Project Community Diagnosis: Participatory Research as a First Step toward Community Involvement in Primary Health Care, 300
Mark Nichter

VI Health Institutions

15. Neglect of Cultural Knowledge in Health Planning: Nepal's Assistant Nurse-Midwife Program, 327
Judith Justice

16. Bureaucratic Aspects of International Health Programs, 345
George M. Foster

Appendix: Resources in Anthropology, 365

Glossary, 367

Index, 371

Contributors

JUDITH C. BARKER, PH.D.; Medical Anthropology Program, University of California, San Francisco—Chapter 10. Barker is a medical anthropologist whose current research primarily investigates the day-to-day experience of chronic illness, especially among the frail elderly. Along with a focus on gender and ethnic differences in the assessment and management of health and disease, Barker looks at social organization of health care.

LEO R. CHAVEZ, PH.D.; Professor, Department of Anthropology, and Center for Health Policy and Research, University of California, Irvine—Chapter 6. Chavez received his doctorate in anthropology from Stanford University in 1982. His research focuses on issues of access to health care for Latino immigrants and the role of culture in the control of cancer.

SHEGOU DARRET, M.D.—Chapter 12. Darret is the Assistant Coordinator of Family Planning Activities, Ministry of Health and Social Protection, Abidjan, Côte d'Ivoire.

NINA L. ETKIN, PH.D.; Professor of Anthropology, University of Hawaii—Chapter 8. Etkin's research in Nigeria, Hawaii, and Indonesia combines inquiry in ethnomedicine, diet, pharmaceuticals, and the pharmacology of foods and medicinal plants. She is president of the International Society for Ethno-pharmacology and editor-in-chief of the journal *Reviews in Anthropology*.

MICHAEL FAVIN, M.A., M.P.H.—Chapter 9. Michael Favin is an international health specialist with experience in more than 20 countries. For more than a decade, at the Manoff Group, he has worked in social marketing and health communication, focusing on qualitative research methods and community participation in program design, implementation, and evaluation.

GEORGE M. FOSTER, PH.D.; Professor Emeritus of Anthropology, University of California, Berkeley—Chapter 16. Foster's research interests include peasant society, applied anthropology, international health, ethnomedicine, and culture change. In addition to long-term research in Mexico and Spain, he has served as consultant with USAID, WHO, and other organizations in Asia, Africa, and Latin America.

EDWARD C. GREEN, Ph.D.—Chapter 4. Green is an applied medical anthropologist who consults for international development organizations, mostly in Africa. His newest book on African ethnomedicine is *African Theories of Contagious Disease* (Sage Publications, in press).

MARCIA GRIFFITHS, M.Sc.—Chapter 9. Griffiths, president of the Manoff Group, is a nutritional anthropologist who has worked for more than two decades to bring the voice of participants to program planning and operations. She has worked in health and nutrition programs in Asia, Africa, and Latin America that have specialized in social marketing approaches and community work.

ROBERT A. HAHN, PH.D., M.P.H.; Epidemiologist, US Centers for Disease Control and Prevention, Atlanta, Georgia—Editor and Chapter 1. Hahn received his PhD in anthropology (1976) and an MPH in epidemiology (1986). He has conducted anthropological and public health research in Brazil, the United States, Niger, and the Cameroon, and published on chronic diseases, syphilis and AIDS, obstetrics and internal medicine, ethics, racial/ethnic classification, poverty and death, and the nocebo phenomenon. He is the author of *Sickness and Healing: An Anthropological Perspective* (Yale University Press, 1995).

ROBERTA L. HALL, PH.D.; Professor of Anthropology, Oregon State University, Corvallis—Chapter 7. Hall earned her PhD in 1970 at the University of Oregon. She taught at the University of Victoria from 1970 to 1974 and held a postdoctoral fellowship at the University of Connecticut Alcohol Research Center from 1981 to 1983. Her main interests are human biological variation and health.

DAVID HALPERIN, M.D., M.P.H.; Director of the Comitan Center for Health Research, Comitan Chiapas; Coordinator of the Division of Population and Health of the Colegio de la Frontera Sur (ECOSUR), San Cristóbal de Las Casas, Chiapas, México—Chapter 11. Halperin received his MD from the University of Chicago and his MPH from the Harvard School of Public Health. He has conducted health research in Chiapas for 13 years.

F. ALLAN HUBBELL, M.D., M.S.P.H.; Chief of the Division of General Internal Medicine and Primary Care, Director of the Center for Health Policy and Research, and Professor of Medicine and Social Ecology at the University of California, Irvine—Chapter 6. Hubbell received his MD from Baylor College of Medicine in 1974, completed an internal medicine residency at the University of California, Irvine, in 1978, and received an MSPH from UCLA in 1983. His research focuses on access to medical care and cancer control needs of special populations.

LINDA M. HUNT, PH.D.; Assistant Professor of Nursing Research, University of Texas Health Science Center, San Antonio—Chapter 11. Hunt received her PhD in anthropology from Harvard University. Her research interests include illness concepts and treatment practices in Mexico and south Texas, focusing on chronic illness and reproductive health.

JUDITH JUSTICE, PH.D., M.P.H.; Medical Anthropology Program and Institute for Health Policy Studies, University of California at San Francisco—Chapter 15. Justice's research interests include international and national health policy, foreign assistance and health development, cultural context of emerging and re-emerging infectious diseases, and reproductive and child health. Current research includes two multisited comparative studies on child immunization and another on tuberculosis. She has worked in South and Southeast Asia, Africa, and the United States conducting research and consulting with foundations, international organizations, and non–governmental organizations.

JOAN D. KOSS-CHIOINO, PH.D.; Department of Anthropology, Arizona State University—Chapter 13. Koss-Chioino's main research activities are interdisciplinary, focusing on cross-cultural approaches to psychological and psychiatric clinical concerns regarding traditional healing, psychotherapy, and psychiatric nosology, particularly among Hispanic peoples.

KALE KOUAME—Chapter 12. Kouamé is on the faculty of the National Institute of Public Health in Abidjan, Côte d'Ivoire. He has consulted for numerous internationally and nationally sponsored public health projects in Côte d'Ivoire, and has co-authored this and other articles addressing public health issues.

EDWARD LICHTENSTEIN, PH.D.; Research Scientist, Oregon Research Institute, and Professor Emeritus of Psychology, University of Oregon—Chapter 7. Lichtenstein received his doctorate in psychology from the University of Michigan (1961). His interests are in health psychology, especially the development and evaluation of smoking cessation programs.

KERRI LOPEZ, B.A.; Health Resources Coordinator, Northwest Portland Area Indian Health Board—Chapter 7. Lopez served as the interventionist in the Tribal Tobacco Policy Project and as director of the Western Tobacco Prevention Project at the Northwest Portland Area Indian Health Board. She is an enrolled member of the Smith River Tolowa Tribe of Northern California.

SUSAN C. McCOMBIE, PH.D.; Independent Consultant—Chapter 2. McCombie received her PhD in anthropology from the University of Arizona in 1986. Her research centers on the relationship between culture and infectious disease and has included studies of AIDS, diarrhea, measles, and malaria. She has designed and implemented evaluations of public health communication programs in several countries in Africa.

SHIRAZ I. MISHRA, M.D., PH.D.; Assistant Professor of Medicine and Social Ecology, and faculty associate at the Center for Health Policy and Research, University of California, Irvine—Chapter 6. Mishra received his MD from Bombay University, Bombay, India, in 1982 and his PhD in social ecology from the University of California, Irvine, in 1992. His research centers on cultural and behavioral determinants of cancer and HIV/AIDS prevention and control among ethnic minorities.

IBRAHIM MUAZZAMU; Research Fellow, Department of Medicinal Plants of the National Institute for Pharmaceutical Research and Development in Abuja, Nigeria—Chapter 8. Muazzamu's work centers on medical ethnobotany among Nigeria's diverse populations.

DOROTHY S. MULL, PH.D.; Center for Health Policy and Research at the University of California, Irvine, and Department of Family Medicine at the University of Southern California—Chapter 5. Mull is a medical anthropologist who has written extensively on maternal and child health issues in Mexico and Pakistan.

MARK NICHTER, PH.D., M.P.H.; Department of Anthropology, University of Arizona—Chapter 14. Nichter is a professor of anthropology and coordinator of the graduate program in Medical Anthropology at the University of Arizona. An active participant in the fields of health and development, he continues to work in South and Southeast Asia.

ROLANDO TINOCO OJANGUREN, MSc; Colegio de la Frontera Sur (ECOSUR), San Cristóbal de Las Casas, Chiapas, México; Head of Operations for the Comitan Center for Health Research, Comitan Chiapas—Chapter 11. Tinoco is an agronomist and researcher. He is involved in a variety of health-related research projects, including the health effects of pesticides in southern Mexico.

PAUL J. ROSS, R.N., O.C.N., M.S.N.(c); Adjunct Instructor, Department of Anthropology, University of Hawaii—Chapter 8. Ross is a member of the Oncology Staff at The Queen's Medical Center, Honolulu. His present inquiries focus on applications in transcultural nursing.

CAROLYN F. SARGENT, PH.D.; Professor of Anthropology and Director of Women's Studies at Southern Methodist University—Chapter 12. Sargent received her doctorate from Michigan State University. Her interests include women's reproductive health, child survival, and bioethics. She has done fieldwork in Africa and the Caribbean. She is the author of *The Cultural Context of Therapeutic Choice* and *Maternity, Medicine and Power*, and she is co-editor of *Medical Anthropology: A Handbook of Theory and Method*; *Gender in Cross-Cultural Perspective*; and *Gender and Health: An International Perspective*.

NORAH SCHWARTZ, M.P.A.; Visiting Researcher at the Colegio de la Frontera Norte, Tijuana, México—Chapter 11. Schwartz is a doctoral candidate in The Joint Medical Anthropology Program, University of California at San Francisco and Berkeley. She is currently studying respiratory illness in a border city of northern Mexico.

RUTH P. WILSON, PH.D.; Associate Professor of Anthropology, Southern Methodist University—Chapter 12. Wilson earned a doctorate in Social Anthropology from Stanford University. She has provided technical expertise to USAID-sponsored child survival programs in sub-Saharan Africa. Her publications address the social and cultural dimensions of public health issues including family planning, pediatric acute respiratory illnesses, diarrheal disease control, and HIV/AIDS. Her latest research focuses on HIV/AIDS caregivers in Dallas.

PETER J. WINCH, M.D., M.P.H.; Assistant Professor, Department of International Health, Johns Hopkins University, School of Hygiene and Public Health—Chapter 3. Winch's areas of research are community participation in disease control and use of qualitative research methods to improve the design of control programs. He has been involved in research on prevention of dengue hemorrhagic fever in Puerto Rico, Mexico, Honduras, and Brazil; malaria control in Tanzania; and schistosomiasis control in Egypt.

Introduction

In 1955, Benjamin Paul introduced his seminal anthology, *Health, Culture, and Community*, by noting that "application of our available health knowledge is the weakest link in our chain of health protection" (Paul, 1955:iii). The case studies in Paul's anthology illustrate the many ways in which culture and social organization affect the health of communities and can foster or hinder the effectiveness of health care programs. Although the roles of culture and community in health have been increasingly recognized since the publication of Paul's book, systematic use of this knowledge to translate public health techniques into effective practice is far from commonplace. In the practice of public health today, more than 40 years after Paul's work, relevant anthropological knowledge and methods have grown substantially, but application remains a weak link.

Anthropology in Public Health is written for a public health audience, including practitioners and policymakers; its 15 recent case studies illustrate the potential for understanding and improving public health by using anthropological approaches. All but one of the lead authors are anthropologists, one is a physician with anthropological expertise, and several have collaborators from other disciplines. Authors describe their anthropological theories, methods, and findings, and they provide resource references for further exploration. The chapters in this book are by no means typical of the academic writing of anthropologists. Theoretical discussions are focused on the public health problem addressed.

In the rare instances in which anthropological jargon is particularly useful, it is explained to the reader, and a glossary of the anthropological terminology used is included. The chapters were edited to facilitate communication with readers who are not anthropologists.

The studies included in this volume were conducted in North and South America, Africa, Europe, Asia, and Oceania (see the map on the title page). Topics range from beliefs and practices regarding infectious agents to the culture of international health agencies. Each chapter illustrates one way in which anthropological methods have been applied to public health. All the chapters describe methods, present results, and make recommendations; several also describe interventions developed and assessed on the basis of anthropological results. Each chapter indicates the utility of, if not the need for, translating knowledge of public health practices for use in specific social and cultural settings.

The chapters were selected to demonstrate the role of anthropology in addressing a wide range of public health problems. The case studies use a variety of anthropological methods and cover diverse geographic and sociocultural settings. This breadth is intended to provide public health practitioners specializing in particular topics and particular places with examples of how anthropology may help in their own work, and to indicate as well the uses of anthropology elsewhere and on other matters of public health. The topics addressed in the book are by no means an exhaustive list of public health issues where anthropology is relevant; indeed, it is difficult to imagine community health programs in which anthropology could not make contributions. For example, even in the study of pathogenesis in some settings, it may be important to consider how local social and cultural patterns have made the physical environment more hostile or more hospitable to pathogens, their vectors, or physical agents of disease (Hahn, 1995; Inhorn and Brown, 1997).

An assumption of many chapters in this volume is that public health is inevitably a cross-cultural enterprise carried out in interpersonal relationships across social and, often, national boundaries. Minimally, cross-cultural and cross-societal interactions in public health include two parties, the "donor" agency and the "recipient" population. More commonly, public health interactions also include collaborating sponsors, consultants, academic institutions, national and local governments, and social groups within recipient communities. Because such interactions are likely to involve substantial differences among participants in beliefs, values, and rules of action, "translation" is required for effective communication and program design. Failure to recognize and take into account these differences is likely to result in misunderstanding and inappropriate action, if not failure of the program.

In essence, this book is about (1) how to take into account the social organization, cultural beliefs, and practices of the communities involved in public health programs and (2) the potential benefits of doing so, such as gaining an understanding of local settings and designing socially effective programs. However, as several authors note, "taking into account" is not only, or even primarily, a matter of using knowledge of the local setting to achieve public health objectives as perceived by the public health practitioner; rather, it is a matter of understanding, addressing, and responding to local perspectives, concerns, and values. It is a matter of basic respect for the perspectives and goals of others. In applied fields of anthropology, such as anthropology in public health, "taking into account" may also mean responding.

The examination of three contexts of anthropology in public health is critical: the context of politics, the context of public health bureaucracy, and the context of anthropology itself. Rapid and substantial political change, including revolution and civil and other wars, commonly has disastrous health effects. But the civil political process also affects the distribution of disease and injury in the population through its effect on the work, residence, and recreation of individuals and groups, and through consequent exposure to pathogenic agents and activities; the civil political process also affects the allocation of health care resources. While several chapters in this volume focus on the global, administrative, and political aspects of public health, others show that changes in the political environment led to failure to adopt or extend a public health project. The political process can make or break, and, between these extremes, facilitate or hinder a well-designed project.

Public health projects are often conceived and born in public health agencies and/or academic settings. The last two chapters of this book, in particular, indicate the powerful effects of the culture and organization of public health agencies themselves in the shaping of public health projects and broader agendas. It is clearly critical for public health practitioners to examine the values of their own institutions and those offering to solve or support solutions for public health problems. Applying anthropology in public health may contribute to the reform of these institutions, making them more effective and responsive to their public health objectives.

Finally, the anthropological research community itself plays an obvious role in applying anthropology to public health. Perhaps the greatest challenge for anthropologists in public health is the recognition of social and cultural differences between their own and other communities, and the need for translation of concepts, principles, and language to facilitate communication of their messages. Successful use of anthropological knowledge in the translation of public health knowledge into effective action may depend on translation of anthropological knowledge into the language of public health personnel and policymakers.

The chapters that follow indicate how anthropology in public health embraces not only a complex array of social institutions, but also many disciplines, theories, methods, and findings beyond those of anthropology itself. Individual chapters use theoretical and substantive findings from biomedicine (principally on

infectious diseases), from epidemiology and public health, and from pharmacology, communications, sociology, and social psychology. The authors also
employ methods from epidemiology (principally the case-control design), statistics (principally sampling methods and tests of association), and the findings
and methodologies of "natural" sciences such as botany and experimental design.

Anthropological approaches and skills facilitate interaction and communication with populations often regarded as "hard to reach," for example, groups
engaged in illegal activities and individuals with secret knowledge. Difficulties
of access to hard-to-reach populations may be associated with ignorance about
them, with their exposure to socially unwanted and possibly harmful environments, and with their lack of basic health care resources; they may thus be at
greater risk of sickness and have fewer resources. Two chapters, one involving
illegal immigrants, the other traditional healers with secret knowledge, illustrate
anthropological approaches to engagement. Recognizing the importance of social and cultural differences, anthropologists are cautious not to be offensive and
not to establish alliances before understanding a community's organization. They
are careful to build rapport, itself an anthropological undertaking, both as part
of and prerequisite to research.

Engagement of recipient communities in diverse aspects of public health
programs accords well with the premises of the discipline. Minimally, anthropology in public health involves community participation in the sense that
projects are designed to respond to the local culture and society. But anthropologists may also invite more active community participation, including participation in project selection, design, management, implementation, and evaluation. Many projects described in this book involve researchers from the nations
where the projects are conducted; some employ researchers and interviewers
from the community studied; some receive guidance from community advisers;
one includes community review of reports submitted for publication; one involves "participatory research," in which the training of community-based researchers provides a major source of program information. Public health is traditionally a practice directed at the health *of* the public and at programs *for* public
health. Anthropology in public health indicates an additional role of the public
in public health, that is, public health *by* the public.

The book is divided, somewhat arbitrarily, into an introduction and six parts,
each focused on a different kind of public health problem or issue. Chapter 1
introduces readers to the roles that anthropology can play in contemporary public
health. It describes underlying principles and premises of anthropology and notes
ethical mandates as well. It gives an overview of the stages and techniques of
anthropological methodology. And it suggests directions for the future development of anthropology in public health.

Part I includes four chapters and focuses on a traditional topic of public health:
diseases induced by infectious agents. Chapter 2, "Folk Flu and Viral Syndrome:

An Anthropological Perspective," examines how the word "flu" has different meanings for the general population, for physicians and other clinical personnel, and for epidemiologists in a county health department in the southwestern United States. The author, Susan McCombie, both conducted field research in a health department for her dissertation and worked as a disease control staff member. In this dual role, she used anthropological methods to examine the meanings of terms such as "flu" (a popular concept) and "viral syndrome" (a diagnostic label used by clinicians) and the behavior associated with these terms. She demonstrates how differences in terminology lead to miscommunication and, consequently, to the avoidable spread of disease. Effective disease control requires understanding the concepts, vocabularies, and related behaviors of those involved with the disease—patients, clinicians, and public health personnel.

Chapter 3, "The Role of Anthropological Methods in a Community-Based Mosquito Net Intervention in Bagamoyo District, Tanzania," shows how anthropological approaches can explain and enhance the use of bednets for prevention of malaria, a major cause of death. The author, Peter Winch, collaborated with five Tanzanians, including two with degrees in sociology. Winch demonstrates how failure to use bednets corresponds to local concepts of malaria. Educational programs developed in this project, regrettably, were not as successful as expected because of local factional politics and lack of national commitment.

Chapter 4, "Engaging Indigenous African Healers in the Prevention of AIDS and STDs," describes a program to enhance prevention of the spread of AIDS and sexually transmitted disease (STD) in Mozambique by collaborating with traditional healers who see many patients with these conditions. At the request of the Mozambique Ministry of Health, the chapter author, Edward Green, designed a program to communicate with traditional healers, who could then influence their patients regarding AIDS and STD prevention. Green indicates that programs similar to that developed in Mozambique are now in place in several settings in Africa and have effectively modified the practices of traditional healers.

Chapter 5, "Anthropological Perspectives on Childhood Pneumonia in Pakistan," examines how Pakistanis in diverse settings—village and hospital, rural and urban, northern and southern—recognize and respond to pneumonia in their children. The author, Dorothy Mull, summarizes four studies conducted with Pakistani researchers, using anthropological and other methods. She discovers Pakistani ideas about anatomy and physiology that correspond to their treatment of respiratory problems; several practices impede diagnosis and exacerbate the disease. But public health personnel can use Pakistani concepts to teach effective diagnosis and appropriate response.

Part II has two chapters on the use of anthropological methods to understand and develop interventions that can control the morbidity and mortality associated with different cancers. Chapter 6, "Ethnography and Breast Cancer Control among Latinas and Anglo Women in Southern California," assesses beliefs about breast cancer, its causes, and its prevention. Leo Chavez and colleagues use in-depth ethnographic interviews, supported by surveys, to compare the beliefs, attitudes, and practices of Latina immigrants to the United States, US-born women of Latin origin, non-Latina white women, and physicians from several ethnic groups. Chavez is bilingual (in English and Spanish) and a Chicano whose family has lived for many generations in the southwestern United States. On the basis of findings from the first part of the study, Chavez and colleagues designed an intervention for Latinas to increase awareness of breast cancer risk factors and the benefits of mammography.

Chapter 7, "A Policy Approach to Reducing Cancer Risk in Northwest Indian Tribes," reports an experimental trial—rare in anthropology—in which Roberta Hall and colleagues randomly assigned 39 Indian tribes in the Pacific Northwest to receive either an early or late intervention; the intervention consisted of an information program on health issues related to tobacco and its control through policies on smoking in public places. The project emphasized community participation in several phases of the research, including review of the chapter for this book. A particular challenge in establishing tobacco use guidelines is the culturally appropriate ceremonial use of tobacco, which has to be distinguished from recreational use.

Part III has two chapters, one on adoption of pharmaceuticals in a non-Western setting, the second on a program to enhance nutrition in early childhood. In Chapter 8, "The Rational Basis of 'Irrational' Drug Use: Pharmaceuticals in the Context of Development," Nina Etkin and colleagues use anthropological approaches, including ethnobotany, to understand the use of Western medicines in a Hausa community in northern Nigeria. One co-author is a Nigerian specialist on medicinal plants and has maintained regular contact with the study community over the more than 20-year course of the project. Etkin and colleagues demonstrate that beneficial introduction of pharmaceuticals requires an understanding of the logic of local medical and nutritional theory and practice.

In Chapter 9, "Cultural Tailoring in Indonesia's National Nutrition Improvement Program," Marcia Griffiths and Michael Favin describe a program intended to decrease severe and moderate malnutrition among young children in Indonesia. The program involves the participation of Indonesians from the Ministry of Health, national organizations, and community organizations. Dietary practices in households are assessed and modifications tested for program development. With input from social marketing, the program is then implemented in two regions by community volunteers, and is shown to be successful in changing knowledge, practice, and nutrition.

The chapters on injury and occupational health in Part IV indicate how local environment and culture affect the use of technology. In Chapter 10, "Road

Warriors: Driving Behaviors on a Polynesian Island," Judith Barker investigates high rates of vehicle crashes, injuries, and death in the island nation of Niue. To explore this phenomenon, she uses participant observation, supplemented by review of hospital records. She notes environmental causes of high rates of injury but concludes that social organization, beliefs, and values are more powerful determinants. Barker recommends that local social organization and cultural values be examined in the design of vehicle safety programs and that alternative outlets for harmful traditional values be developed when current outlets exact too heavy a personal and social toll.

In Chapter 11, "Balancing Risks and Resources: Applying Pesticides without Using Protective Equipment in Southern Mexico," Linda Hunt and colleagues use in-depth ethnographic interviews and ethnographically based surveys to understand why peasant farmers in southern Mexico do not use protective equipment when applying pesticides. She shows that failure to use protective equipment is not due to lack of knowledge. Hunt argues that effective and widespread promotion of protective equipment and procedures will require attention to local ideas about symptoms and health, and design of equipment and procedures that are inexpensive, available, and acceptable.

The three chapters in Part V discuss diverse facets of community health. In Chapter 12, "Prospects for Family Planning in Côte d'Ivoire: Ethnographic Contributions to the Development of Culturally Appropriate Population Policy," Ruth Wilson and colleagues report on a research project, designed at the request of the Ministry of Health in Côte d'Ivoire, to assess Ivoirian attitudes about the value of the family and family planning, and about the responsibility of individuals, households, and the government for family planning. Two of the co-authors are Ivoirians, and additional Ivoirians were trained to conduct some of the study interviews. The study indicated a need for a national family planning policy that considered traditional values regarding the family as well as the challenges of the economy.

In Chapter 13, "Integrating Mental Health Care and Traditional Healing in Puerto Rico: Lessons from an Early Experiment," Joan Koss-Chioino describes a three-year project to integrate Spiritist healing, a century-old tradition in Puerto Rico, with approaches to mental health from biomedicine and Western psychology. The project was not institutionalized following its development, in part because of political change and also because of the career changes of project personnel. Despite many social hurdles, participants from both approaches learned from each other, and there appeared to be an increase in the referral of patients from one practice to the other.

Chapter 14, "Project Community Diagnosis: Participatory Research as a First Step toward Community Involvement in Primary Health Care," describes a research project designed to understand local health concerns and attitudes about a pending program of community health committees and community health workers in a state in southern India. The author, Mark Nichter, trained researchers at the community level to engage members of their communities in discussions about health and the upcoming program. Findings from the study were not used because of changes in state leadership. A community health program was hastily implemented and short-lived, apparently because of poor administration and lack of responsiveness to local concerns.

Public health institutions themselves are the subject of the final part. In Chapter 15, "Neglect of Cultural Knowledge in Health Planning: Nepal's Assistant Nurse-Midwife Program," Judith Justice analyzes how decisions were made in developing an assistant nurse-midwife program in Nepal designed to provide maternal and child health services. She examines policy at the World Health Organization (WHO) and Nepali institutions, as well as the actual working of the program in Nepal. Justice describes agency and bureaucratic obstacles to the use of available knowledge.

The anthology concludes with Chapter 16, "Bureaucratic Aspects of International Health Programs," an analysis by George Foster of the bureaucratic culture and structure of international health agencies, including WHO. Foster's analysis is based on 40 years of participant observation in international health programs, discussions with development personnel, and examination of documents and published literature. He poses a number of challenges that international health bureaucracies should address if they are to overcome internal, bureaucratic obstacles and more effectively address the health needs of those they purport to serve.

References

Hahn RA (1995) Sickness and Healing: An Anthropological Perspective. New Haven: Yale University Press.

Inhorn MC, Brown PJ (1997) The Anthropology of Infectious Disease. International Health Perspectives. Amsterdam: Gordon and Breach.

Paul BD (1955) Health, Culture, and Community. New York: Russell Sage Foundation.

Anthropology in Public Health

1

Anthropology and the Enhancement of Public Health Practice

ROBERT A. HAHN

Advances in world health in the twentieth century have occurred at a rate unprecedented in human history. In both the developed and the developing world longevity has increased markedly, owing largely to basic research and application of discoveries and inventions in biomedicine and public health.[1] Causative agents of major infectious disease have been discovered and methods for investigation have revealed findings unimagined in 1900. Principal causes of major chronic diseases, such as lung cancer and heart disease, have been identified; injuries (both intentional and unintentional) are now seen as matters of public health, and their prominent modifiable risk factors are recognized.

Medical and public health sciences have also produced powerful technologies and interventions. The use of screening, for example, can prevent some congenital defects and reduce the consequences of various cancers. Immunization can now prevent infection, morbidity, and death from many diseases that were previously mass killers. Indeed, the global eradication of smallpox by campaigns of vaccination based on public health surveillance may be counted as one of the major world achievements of the century. Polio has been eliminated in the Americas and elimination is well under way on other continents. Therapies for diarrhea provide seemingly simple means of reducing extensive developing-world morbidity and mortality. Although demonstrated capacity to control chronic diseases and injuries has been less dramatic, public education and modification of the physical and social environment have been shown to reduce exposure to prominent risk factors for many of these conditions. Overall, the armaments of medicine and public health are formidable and have made major contributions to human health.

Yet wide gaps separate public health capacities to advance global health and the fulfillment of these capacities. Available knowledge and resources potentially allow far more control of human suffering than has been achieved. An index of this gulf is the difference in longevity between Japan, with the highest life expectancy, and Sierra Leone, with the lowest; the Japanese can expect to live more than twice as long as the Sierra Leonese (males—76.3 years and 37.5 years, respectively; females—82.5 and 40.5, respectively) (United Nations, 1996). Such large divergences in health status are probably attributable not to biological differences between populations, but to differences in social and political environment (Polednak, 1989). The almost 80-fold difference between health care expenditures in established market economies and the nations of sub-Saharan Africa (World Bank, 1993) undoubtedly contributes to the wide range in longevity—by affecting efforts both to prevent and to treat disease and injury. Expenditure is inversely proportional to need.

Progress and Problems in World Health at the End of the Twentieth Century

It can be argued that there are four major obstacles to the implementation of available techniques to reduce morbidity and mortality, as well as gaps in morbidity and mortality, worldwide. First is the ongoing *deliberate production of illness, suffering, and death* by human acts such as warfare, homicide, and persecution (Desjarlais et al., 1995). In 1990, warfare was the 16th leading cause of disability-adjusted life years (DALYs)[2] in the world; by the year 2020, warfare is projected to be the eighth leading cause (Murray and Lopez, 1996). In 1993, there were approximately 20 million refugees worldwide, and approximately the same number of persons displaced within their own countries (UNHCR, 1993); refugees and other displaced persons together accounted for almost 1 in every 100 people in the world. The dominant causes of such conflict and disruption are nationalism and ethnocentrism—belief that one's own culture and society are the only true and worthy ones.

A second obstacle to solving public health problems is *poor allocation of resources, including misallocation and inefficient allocation*, both within and among nations of the world. Discrimination and unequal access to resources based on gender, race/ethnicity, age, religion, socioeconomic status, and region are well recognized; lack of access to resources can have substantial detrimental effects on health (see, for example, Doyal, 1995). Moreover, allocation of health resources on the basis of suffering, efficacy, and cost-effectiveness is far from the standard procedure (Murray et al., 1994). Again, ethnocentrism and nationalism, in addition to racism, sexism, ageism, and other forms of prejudice, have been, and continue to be, underlying factors in the unequal distribution of resources.

A third and related obstacle is *lack of commitment of needed resources* on the part of those who control the resources and technology and/or on the part of those who control access to suffering populations. Public health rests on a moral assumption that response to the perceived suffering of others is a worthy action, deserving commitment of resources and effort. Implementation requires the agreement, if not the active participation, of the host country. Some of the interventions described in the chapters of this anthology failed because of lack of national and/or international commitment to projects designed to address the perspectives and concerns of the populations in need.

A fourth obstacle is the *inadequate translation of public health knowledge into effective action* across the social and cultural boundaries that separate those who have specific preventive and curative capacities and resources from those who may need them. Social and cultural separation occurs not only across, but also within, national borders. The failure of some public health agencies to reflect on their own strengths and weaknesses may result in programs based on misleading concepts and erroneous theories and information. The failure of some public health programs to study and take into account the culture and society of the community toward which the program is directed has sometimes led to only partial program success or even to program demise.

Together, these obstacles signify the lack of full moral, economic, and scientific commitment to the solution of critical public health problems.

Anthropology in Public Health

This anthology addresses the fourth of these obstacles, in particular, the lack of routine and systematic use of anthropological theory and methods to make health knowledge and techniques available to other cultures and societies. This may be attributed partly to anthropologists who, with unfortunate irony, have often failed to apply a basic anthropological premise to themselves: they have not consistently acknowledged their own cultural position and thus the need to make their perspectives understandable for the cultures of others, for example, the public health community. The chapters in this anthology illustrate the use of anthropological knowledge and methods for the public health community through 15 case studies on diverse public health topics in different places around the world.

The remainder of this introduction briefly:

- describes underlying principles of anthropology, indicating their application to public health;
- gives an overview of anthropological methods, noting sources of more detailed information; and
- proposes directions for the future of anthropology in public health.

A list of basic literature on anthropology and its methods, as well as major anthropological organizations, is found in the appendix of this book.

Principles of Anthropology

Anthropology is a discipline that examines diverse aspects of human social life, its processes and causes, the interrelations of its elements, and its relations with phenomena studied by other disciplines, for example, human biology, ecology, economics, politics, and religion. The annual meetings of the American Anthropological Association, undoubtedly the largest regular gatherings of anthropologists in the world, indicate the field's rich variety as its practitioners examine facets of social life taken for granted by most.

Anthropology is roughly divided into four major subfields: *archaeology* examines the physical remains of societies—most often societies of the past—to reconstruct as much of their social and cultural life as possible; *physical anthropology* focuses on human biology and its relation to society, culture, and history; *linguistics* examines various facets of human language and its relationship to social and cultural life; and *social and cultural anthropology* examine the organization of societies and their cultural systems, that is, their beliefs, values, and norms and patterns of behavior. Although the division into four subfields reflects differences in interests, theories, and methods, these also may be shared among the subfields. Medical anthropology, which focuses on the interrelationships of society, culture, and biology, on the one hand, and sickness and healing, on the other, is the anthropological field most central to anthropology in public health. Medical anthropology draws most heavily from social and cultural anthropology, and, in the remainder of this introduction, this subfield is referred to simply as "anthropology."

Like scholars in other disciplines, anthropologists have diverse views and approaches to their discipline. Nevertheless, there are perspectives shared by most anthropologists. The following discussion summarizes four basic anthropological premises and their corollaries as well as indicating their application in public health. The chapters in this volume illustrate these assumptions.

Premise One: Cultural Relativity

Undoubtedly, the most basic premise of anthropology is *cultural relativism*, the assumption that "cultures" (the systems of beliefs, values, and norms of behavior found in all societies) are more or less coherent, systematic, and rational within their own context. Beliefs about health and sickness, and their causes and treatment, commonly referred to as "ethnomedicines," are elements of these cultural systems. Politics, the economy, and religion are also cultural elements; in many technologically less developed societies, there is considerable overlap of ethnomedicines and other cultural elements. Cultural relativity is essentially the opposite of ethnocentrism, cited earlier as a source of failure to address major global health problems. While there are limits to the anthropological acceptance of cultural relativity (few if any anthropologists would find slavery or the culture of Nazi Germany in the 1930s and 1940s legitimate), most anthropologists subscribe to some version of cultural relativity and value the integrity and worthiness of all human societies.

A question of relativity critical to the role of anthropology in public health is whether the predominant medical system of Western civilization, that is, biomedicine, is superior—entirely, in general, or in specific aspects—to the ethnomedical systems of non-Western societies (Hahn, 1995). An operating principle of public health is that biomedicine and public health have at least some superior knowledge or technique which justifies addressing the health problems of others.

Several corollaries follow from the premise of cultural relativity.

First, *societies and cultures are best understood as whole systems, that is, "holistically."* If the elements of a cultural system do not "make sense" on their own, then the way in which cultural elements fit together is critical for understanding the individual elements. Anthropology traditionally addressed this corollary of relativism by means of holistic studies of communities, referred to as "ethnographies." These are studies that examine not simply a focal topic, but the interrelationships of physical environment, principal activities, economics, and social organization, including kinship and marriage, politics, science, and religion. In contemporary anthropology, holistic studies are exceptional, perhaps in response to the limitations of funding. Yet even focused, topical studies, which are now the rule, frequently provide some contextual information.

Second, *Western civilization is also a culture, or rather a combination of many cultures.* Similarly, the discipline of *anthropology, largely an intellectual product of the Western world, is itself a culture with many subcultures.* A consequence of this corollary is that anthropologists have their own distinct worldviews; they have theories of the way the world is, along with their own, possibly distinctive, values and behavioral norms.

For public health, an implication of the culture of anthropology is that, to communicate with practitioners of other disciplines, even within their own society, anthropologists need to translate their concepts and methodologies into the concepts and languages of other disciplines and practices, for example, public health and policy-making. While this corollary—the need to translate across cultural boundaries—seems basic to the discipline of anthropology, many anthropologists appear to ignore it in dealing with the nonanthropological world. Many anthropologists direct their discourse to other practitioners. Some anthropologists may resist translation because they regard the application of anthropology to the solution of real world problems as tainting the discipline with politics and values—as if their own practices were apolitical and value-free. Anthropologists who do not acknowledge their own culture or who disdain application of their knowledge may fail to communicate adequately their perspective, its methods, and usefulness.

Third, *local populations, not the outsiders, are the experts on their own sociocultural environment.* If appropriately enlisted, community members can become the teachers of local perspectives, values, and social life. Anthropologists are schooled to be the students of others. They often acknowledge that, in many instances, they do not even know what knowledge is relevant in new cultural settings. When they do develop questionnaires, they do so based on their understanding of the local culture and society. The humble assumption that expertise resides in others is common in anthropology, but rare in other academic disciplines.

Fourth, a corollary especially important to programs of technical assistance, such as public health, is that *those who seriously interact with foreign cultures have a moral obligation to take those cultures seriously, including their social organizations and values.* Anthropologists have noted that technical assistance in the past was often based on the assumption that the communities for which programs were planned were "empty vessels," lacking the relevant knowledge of how to improve some facet of their lives; it was assumed that the problem would be solved by adding the developer's knowledge and techniques. Anthropologists reject this assumption.

Taking seriously the culture and society of others involves two related steps. First is coming to know the social organization and values of the other culture. The methods outlined below and exemplified in the chapters of this book indicate how such knowledge is achieved. This knowledge may make public health and other interventions more effective and efficient. But there is a second step, which some regard as essential, in taking the local social setting seriously and in using knowledge of this setting to develop local interventions. This is a *moral* step of respecting, attending to, and addressing local perceptions, interests, and ways of life. At the least, it requires listening and sympathetic understanding; at the most, it requires helping to serve local interests.

The challenge of taking others seriously may be couched as a question: "Are we providing a benefit that the recipient does not recognize or value as a 'benefit'?" Members of the recipient society may reject our offering because they do not understand it—at least in the same way that we do—or because they understand it, but give this potential benefit a relatively low priority. We might then be motivated to act paternalistically—a morally hazardous course, particularly when dealing with communities that include adults. In the design or implementation of many public health programs, local concerns are not a critical consideration. The anthropological approach provides moral grounds for routinely making local concerns a primary criterion in public health decision making.

The 1998 Code of Ethics of the American Anthropological Association[3] recognizes the many individuals and communities involved in research, including the anthropologist, his or her students and institution, the broader society, informants and their communities, and funding agencies. The code emphasizes obligations to the population studied:

> A. Responsibility to people and animals with whom anthropological researchers work and whose lives and cultures they study.
>   1. Anthropological researchers have primary ethical obligations to the people, species, and materials they study and to the people with whom they work. These obligations can supersede the goal of seeking new knowledge, and can lead to decisions not to undertake or to discontinue a research project when the primary obligation conflicts with other responsibilities, such as those owed to sponsors or clients. These ethical obligations include:
>   • To avoid harm or wrong, understanding that the development of knowledge can lead to change which may be positive or negative for the people or animals worked with or studied
>   • To respect the well-being of humans and nonhuman primates . . .
>   • To consult actively with the affected individuals or group(s), with the goal of establishing a working relationship that can be beneficial to all parties involved. (American Anthropological Association, 1998:2)

Premise Two: Theoretical Foundations of Knowledge and Practice

A second anthropological premise is that *knowledge and practice are founded in theory*, that is, one's beliefs and actions are based on underlying beliefs about how the world works. The theory may be explicitly recognized by the believer/actor, or it may be unconscious and implicit. Some anthropologists, though, believe themselves to be "theory-free"; they then assume that their conclusions follow logically from their theory-free observations. Most anthropologists, however, would regard this assumption as anthropologically naive. This is not to say that revision of theory on the basis of observations does not occur; it does. The testing of hypotheses may be regarded as an assessment of a theory's implications; results may indicate the need for revision of the theory. Most anthropologists hold a "constructivist" position, recognizing that what one observes and concludes are profoundly shaped, or "constructed," by one's underlying assumptions about the way things are. Constructivist principles of knowledge and practice apply to different disciplines as well, including public health.

In an insightful review of the development of anthropological theory from the 1960s to the 1980s, Ortner wrote: "We are no longer sure of how the sides are to be drawn up, and of where we would place ourselves if we could identify the sides" (Ortner, 1994: 372). Recent and contemporary theory in anthropology indicate rich and productive ferment (Dirks et al., 1994). In particular, anthropologists have recognized that cultures are not always single, unified systems, but are often fragmented within societies, and that such fragmentation is associated with history and with the social distribution of power.

> Culture as emergent from relations of power and domination, culture as a form of power and domination, culture as a medium in which power is both constituted and resisted; it is around this set of issues that certain anthropologists and certain historians . . . are beginning to work out an exciting body of thought. (Dirks et al., 1994:6)

These developments suggest a need to attend to the historical context of health programs as well as to the political environment in which they are embedded.

Anthropologists have proposed a wide range of theories to account for the forms of human illness found in different social and cultural settings. The range of theoretical positions is suggested by the following rough categorization (Hahn, 1995):

Ecological/evolutionary theory claims that the physical environment and human adaptations to it are the principal determinants of sickness and healing.

Cultural theory posits that cultural systems of beliefs, values, and customs are the basic determinants.

Political/economic theory proposes that economic organization and contending relationships of power are the principal forces controlling human sickness and health.

These theories have substantially different consequences for public health. They are not exclusive of one another and may be combined.

It is important that public health practitioners recognize that knowledge and practice are founded in theory and that they be aware of their own theories. Awareness of the underlying theory allows deliberate assessment of the extent to which its elements are reasonable and compatible with observations; unreasonable and noncorresponding elements need further assessment and may need revision. Where there is a literature on the theory of the public health issue in question, available theories may confirm one's own theory or suggest revision.

Anthropological theory may be useful in public health in at least two ways. First, theories may help explain particular circumstances, for example, the health conditions and problems of a particular community for which a program is being planned. Second, theories of behavior and community change may also suggest effective (as well as ineffective) project design.

Premise Three: Research as Sociocultural Process

A third basic premise of anthropology is that *research and intervention are sociocultural processes*. Research about (and by) human beings involves social relationships. In anthropology, and in many other disciplines as well, this relationship is frequently "cross-cultural." Within one's own sociocultural setting, it may be reasonable to assume that people share some of one's values, concepts, and behavioral norms; this assumption cannot reasonably be made when crossing sociocultural boundaries. For example, one cannot assume that information about a different setting will be provided just for the asking or absorbed when given. There are societal rules for interaction, including the proper way to ask questions, which may be different for political and religious leaders, men and women, and children and elders, and that must be recognized to gather information effectively. Moreover, to interpret responses, it is important to know how one is regarded by the community being studied. For example, in communities where investigators are believed to represent "the government," information may be withheld or distorted so as to maximize the benefits (or minimize the losses) of a potential governmental response.

Similarly, *intervention, including public health action, is fundamentally a process of social and cultural exchange*. Again, there are at least two sociocultural systems involved, those of "donor" and "recipient." As in cross-cultural research, there are rules for behavior that must be recognized to effectively implement an intervention. Here too, it is important to know how one is regarded by the community examined in order to know how to interpret community members' responses to an intervention.

Another corollary more recently given credence by many anthropologists is the *national and global context of local society and culture*. Anthropologists recognize that, while individual cultures are more or less internally coherent systems, they are also part of nations which are, in turn, connected with other nations of the world. Thus local cultures are not autonomous, independent systems; they are influenced by international circumstances and events. Researchers must take the global context into account. Societies may once have lived in relative isolation, little affected by the activities of other societies, but in the late twentieth century such isolation is rare, if it still exists. An implication for public health is that agents of change must take into account not only the society for which the intervention is intended, but also its social, economic, and political environment. Local programs are often subject to control at higher levels of authority; they may succeed or fail, depending on their attention to this environment.

Premise Four: Human "Nature" Is also Cultural and Social

A fourth premise shared by some, but not all, anthropologists is that *human "nature" is not only natural (i.e., a matter of the "basic" sciences of physics, chemistry, and biology), but it is also cultural and social.* Interdisciplinary connectedness has two basic facets, one substantive, the other methodological.

The subject matters of anthropology and other disciplines, including psychology, political science, and history, as well as biology and the physical sciences, are fundamentally connected. Many anthropologists assume, for example, that human culture and social organization are substantially affected by human biology and the physical environment, as in the contrast between arctic and desert cultures. Similarly, human biology is affected by human culture and social life, as suggested by studies of migrants whose health status often tends to change when they leave their country of origin to live in a new country. The integrated sociocultural and biological aspect of human nature is critical for public health, insofar as populations for which programs are designed cannot be assumed to be biologically identical to the populations of the program designers. The understanding of sociocultural and biological effects on public health problems may be essential in addressing those problems. Thus, in addition to social and cultural anthropology, physical anthropology may also be important in public health. Population differences can lead to the success of a program in one setting and to failure in another.

A second connection is methodological: If the subject matters of different disciplines are interconnected, then *the methodologies of those disciplines are also mutually relevant.* Anthropologists, for example, may need to be aware of the methodologies of fields closely linked with their particular study foci. In addition, different disciplines have developed methodologies that may be useful to the practices of other disciplines, independent of disciplinary subject matter; anthropologists sometimes use at least rudimentary statistics and medical anthropologists often use techniques from epidemiology (Hahn, 1995; Inhorn, 1995; Trostle and Sommerfeld, 1996).

Anthropological Methods in Public Health

Foundations

Given its basic objectives and premises, anthropology's methodological challenge is to develop a cultural and disciplinary framework through which the differing cultural frameworks and details of other, varied societies can be understood. At least initially, the anthropologist has no choice but to use his or her own framework to know the culture of others. To this end, anthropological methods are designed to be flexible and to allow comprehension of other ways of seeing and organizing reality.

Many aspects of human social life, such as beliefs and values, are subjective and resist quantitative measurement. Such subjective phenomena may, nevertheless, be determinants of behavior and are thus critical to assess. Subjectivity of research topic does not imply subjectivity of the research method used to assess the topic. Subjective characteristics may be measured by the qualitative approaches developed by anthropologists and others (Bernard, 1994); once measured, individuals and communities may be systematically compared.

Within anthropology, there are two distinct views regarding quantification in anthropological research. This "qualitative–quantitative" division is associated with underlying differences in views of the discipline, its methods, and its results. Some anthropologists regard qualitative information, which examines the concepts, values, and meaning of sociocultural life, as the essence and foundation of anthropological knowledge. From this perspective, causation among social and cultural elements may not be an appropriate goal of anthropological inquiry; other forms of explanation, such as creating a coherent description or "making sense" of information, are the primary goal. Other anthropologists view quantitative information and statistical analysis as the basic sources of anthropological knowledge. From this perspective, causal or other quantified analysis is a central task, although "making sense" of information may also be a goal of quantified analysis.

Many anthropologists take the middle ground in this qualitative–quantitative division, using both approaches in complementary fashion, each indicating support (or lack of support) for the other. Anthropologists, including contributors to this volume, often adopt a mixture of methods. It has been argued that, while there are differences in practice between quantitatively and qualitatively oriented disciplines—for example, between epidemiology and anthropology—there is no radical difference in underlying principles; indeed, both approaches implicitly use each other and may be enhanced by explicit use and collaboration (Hahn, 1995; Inhorn, 1995).

As in many disciplines, anthropological research usually has several phases. The anthropologist generally begins by posing a research question; reviewing prior approaches, theories, and results; and specifying research design. Next, a study is conducted and the findings analyzed; and finally a book, series of articles, or other report is prepared. The anthropological research process gives primary importance to the societies being studied and their cultural perspectives. And, depending on the setting, anthropologists may encourage participation of the study population in the research process, in phases ranging from formulation of the initial research question through review of the results and final report.

Formulating a Research Question

Anthropological research commonly has many sources, including the personal interests of the researcher and colleagues, the "magnitude" of potential study problems, the state of theory, method, and findings in the discipline, sources of support, and research opportunities. The anthropologist must select a focus, however general, and develop a coherent proposal balancing these realities. In particular, anthropology in public health commonly addresses practical solutions for specific public health problems.

Because the culture an anthropologist studies generally differs greatly from the anthropologist's own culture, it may be difficult to specify in advance the exact information sought in research. Respondents may think of the research topic in a fashion entirely different from that of the researcher, a difference critical to the anthropologist's process of understanding. Thus the phases of research do not always follow the same course. Newly discovered topics may be critical to the researcher's original interests, and alternative methods of information collection or analysis may be indicated. Nevertheless, it is incumbent on the researcher to specify clearly at the start what he or she intends to do, why and to what end, and how. It is also an intellectual prerequisite that the researcher demonstrate how the proposed study responds to the theory, methods, and prior findings on the chosen topic.

Anthropology in public health may also differ in several ways from the approaches of other anthropological subdisciplines. Because it is directed toward solution of a problem, the questions it seeks to answer generally have practical import, such as why some intervention did not work, or how new knowledge can provide a solution. Also, because it is directed to solution of a problem, the research may examine not simply a question of current health conditions, but also a means of improving those conditions. The anthropological researcher may observe or even participate in an intervention and evaluate its outcome. Finally, rather than, or in addition to, producing books and articles, anthropology in public health may result in action-oriented reports of findings (and theory and methods) that may include recommendations to policymakers, public health practitioners, or the communities studied.

Anthropological research, like all other research, needs to be funded. Traditionally, support was needed for prolonged field research in remote locales. Today, support may be required more for equipment and research teams. It is critical that researchers attend to funding sources, while also being aware of and nurturing institutional connections, particularly with host countries and study communities. The American Anthropological Association's Code of Ethics regards informed consent of the study community and its members (though not necessarily written or signed) as a prerequisite for anthropological research.

Ethical issues of research and action should always be paramount in research design. In an important sense, they are part of what the project is about.

Fieldwork: Collecting and Analyzing Anthropological Information

The research setting of much anthropology is referred to as "the field." "Doing fieldwork" or "ethnography" is a rite of passage in anthropological training and an ongoing activity in the careers of many anthropologists. Basically, fieldwork means living or working for an extended period (and for purposes of research) at the site of one's research—an obvious precondition of participant observation, described below. Anthropologists refer to community members who provide them with information as "informants." For anthropologists, the term does not carry the connotation of espionage associated with "informer"; moreover, it avoids the connotation of domination associated with anthropology's own history of research in colonial settings and with a term of other behavioral disciplines, that is, "subject."

Because fieldwork often fully and sometimes abruptly engages the anthropologist in a setting very different from his or her own home setting, it is commonly an intense and personal experience. It is often wonderful, but it sometimes results in "culture shock," that is, a personal disturbance fostered by abrupt immersion in a new cultural setting where one may not understand the language, expectations, and one's standing, and where one's own sense of cultural and social order is not shared. While many anthropologists experience such strains, most gradually transform their uncertainty into understanding.

Anthropologists recognize the need to establish rapport with the community in which they conduct their study, and particularly with the community informants. Rapport is a relationship of mutual trust. Building rapport is a critical step in research, because information given by informants may be substantially affected by their relationship with the researcher and by their understanding of what the researcher is doing. From an anthropological perspective, it involves the interaction of two social and cultural systems. Once rapport is established, the likelihood that informants will behave abnormally—out of character—in front of the newcomer diminishes. But rapport is not simply of methodological interest, as a tool for gathering information; it is of ethical importance as well in affirming the observer's obligations to the people studied.

A renowned principle of anthropological research is *participant observation*. Participant observation is not so much a specific method as an approach to the collection of information by means of the presence and participation of the researcher in the social life of the study setting. The participant observer makes anthropological observations while participating; participation is a means of observation. Anthropologists rarely attempt to "go native," fully adopting local customs and beliefs; most retain some distance while participating. The observer's participation may diminish the effects his or her presence might otherwise have on "normal" events.

Anthropologists traditionally assess basic background information about the research setting, some of which may be based on unobtrusive measures (Scrimshaw and Hurtado, 1987). They make maps of the community, collect information on its physical environment, including the "man-made" environment, and approximate population size and demographic characteristics. Much of this information can be collected by use of unobtrusive measures, which do not involve the observer's presence in, and thus potential alteration of, the local setting. Such information not only gives a sense of what the place is like, but is often critical to the substance of the project.

Beyond background information, basic anthropological information collected in the field may be roughly categorized into two types: *cognitive*, that is, mental or ideational (including local concepts, beliefs, attitudes, and values); and *behavioral*, that is, describing what people actually do and how they interact. Anthropologists have developed substantial expertise for eliciting local concepts of how things (e.g., types of diseases) are classified and defined (Bernard, 1994). They regard the understanding of concepts as a guide to local views of the world. Anthropologists have also developed techniques for assessing how concepts are woven into belief systems (e.g., about the etiology and treatment of diseases). And they have methods (Bernard, 1994) for the assessment of attitudes and values, that is, ideas about what is good and bad, right and wrong, beautiful and ugly. Values are important because they are associated with local priorities, for example, whether treatment of one person or one condition is regarded as more or less important than treatment of another person or another condition.

Interviews are the principal source of cognitive information collected by anthropologists in the field; they also make sense of observed behavior, as described below. Anthropological interviews, like interviews in other disciplines, are commonly described in terms of their relative "structure," that is, the degree to which they are intended to control interviewer–informant dialogue (Agar, 1980; Bernard, 1994; Fetterman, 1998; Spradley, 1979). Informal interviews are barely interviews at all; the researcher participates in normal conversation and records comments of interest to the research topic. Informal interviews are a side benefit of participant observation.

In formal interviews—classified as unstructured, semistructured, or structured—interviewee and interviewer both know there is a specific goal: the interviewer's collection of certain information. Degrees of structure are the extent to which the interviewer is supposed to follow a fixed sequence of questions and the interviewee is supposed to choose from a fixed set of response options. In unstructured interviews, while the interviewer may have a chosen topic, he or she learns both by attempting to move the discussion to flesh out the topic and by allowing informants to explain their points of view on topics of interest and to lead in directions yet unknown to the anthropologist. Except for specific purposes, anthropologists carefully avoid leading questions, because rather than eliciting a response that reflects the respondents' own beliefs about the question, these might yield an answer that is thought to be expected by the questioner.

Bernard (1994) provides a list of "probes" useful in unstructured interviews to elicit different kinds of responses by informants. For example, the *echo probe* responds to an informant's statement with a brief summary of the statement; the *silent probe* waits silently for the informant to continue speaking; and the *leading*, or *baiting, probe* (Agar, 1980) suggests to the informant knowledge on the part of the interviewer, to encourage the informant to reveal information that might otherwise be secret. Since the rules vary by setting, the usefulness of probes depends on the cultural circumstances. For example, cultures differ in the time allowed between turns of speech, so that what the interviewer regards as a silent probe may be a normal wait in some settings, and thus not a probe at all.

A particularly useful probe for anthropology in public health is the question, "What happens when someone has such-and-such disease?" The question may be about a current episode of the disease or a past one. Case histories elicited by such questions allow assessment of local theories of disease origins, perceived importance and implications, consultation and diagnosis, home and healer treatment, and follow-up; they may be complemented by observation of disease-related actions.

In structured interviews, the interviewer has a fixed set of questions or a questionnaire. Several structured interview techniques have been developed by anthropologists for assessing local concepts, beliefs, and values (Bernard, 1994). They include *free listing*, in which the informant is asked to list all items in a given category, such as skin diseases; *ranking*, in which the informant is asked to rank items by specified criteria, such as most severe or most common; *triad tests*, in which the informant is asked to indicate which two of three items are most similar and which most different; and *pile sorts*, in which the informant is asked to put like items together in piles. These techniques allow analysis of how informants divide up their universe and what dimensions connect and distinguish the elements.

Anthropologists also use questionnaires, generally built on established knowledge of local concepts and beliefs. Although widely used in other behavioral disciplines, questionnaires raise special issues in anthropology, largely because of differences in culture and society between questioner and respondent. Not only literacy, but also, for example, rules of speech, privacy, and secrecy may affect the design, administration, and usefulness of questionnaires. Questionnaires presume that the researcher knows what to ask and how.

There are also semistructured interviews, in which the interviewer may have an interview guide containing a list of questions he or she wants addressed, but the specific questions asked and the response options are not determined in advance. Semistructured interviews are particularly useful when there are time constraints on the interview, when there may not be subsequent opportunities for interviews, and when teams of interviewers must collect comparable information (Bernard, 1994).

Each form of interviewing has its particular use: unstructured interviews are an excellent means of exploring new topics, exploring topics in greater depth, and in designing more structured interviews; semistructured interviews allow more directed exploration and facilitate systematic coverage of a topic; and structured interviews are best for examining the distribution of specific beliefs in populations (Bernard, 1994).

In recent years, anthropologists have also used *focus groups* as an interview technique (Krueger, 1994). In focus groups, individuals from a community are selected by chosen criteria and interviewed together by a trained interviewer. The interviewer guides discussion with a semistructured list of questions and analyzes the results to assess group attitudes and/or practices on a given topic. While focus group methodology suffers the anthropological handicap of occurring out of normal social context, it is useful for rapidly assessing a community's ideas about a topic.

Because language is a principal instrument of their research, particularly in interviews, anthropologists give great importance to the local language in conducting field research. Ideally, the researcher uses the local language. In practice, though, even if language instruction is available, it is often difficult, if not impossible, to learn the local language in advance, and it may require years to learn a language in the field. Anthropologists, therefore, use interpreters, when available. The use of interpreters, however, hinders a basic anthropological task—the recognition and comprehension of conceptual differences in culture, commonly represented in language. For this reason, anthropologists are careful about translation; for example, when they translate questionnaires or educational materials into a local language, they may "back translate," that is, check the accuracy of the translation by translating the material back to the researcher's language.

In addition to asking questions about the cognitive world of the local population, anthropologists also gather information through systematic observation of local behaviors and social interactions. The behaviors observed are not simply physical movements, but also actions that are intentional and meaningful to the actor, including "verbal behaviors" (speech).

Behavioral observations form part of the background description of an anthropological report, allowing characterization of the basic activities of the population, such as work, rituals, and recreation. Systematic observation of behavior requires selection of settings and persons to be observed, as well as definition and classification of behaviors of interest. For purposes of public health, background information may indicate sources of exposure to various pathogenic agents, substances, or events.

Beyond background characteristics, anthropologists may also observe health-related behavior, such as how people respond to the health conditions they recognize, diagnose themselves and others, consult and make decisions with family members and others regarding home treatment, and resort to healers of different sorts. By assessing behaviors in households, anthropologists can estimate the distribution of these behaviors in the population. On the basis of information collected in a systematic way, the researcher should be able to describe community response to health conditions of interest. Applying anthropological methods in public health, assessments of behavior in settings such as clinics, hospitals, and health bureaucracies allow analysis of treatments, healer–patient interactions, and the control of health resources.

The analysis of "social organization" is a common anthropological practice that involves both cognitive and behavioral information. Social organization is the framework in which the society operates; its components include institutions and other organizational structures as well as behavioral roles. Social organization is a broad notion that interrelates societal groups and membership, societal and community factions, and leadership and decision making, as well as marriage and postmarital residence, kinship, and inheritance. Law and its sanctions, as well as politics and economics, may be regarded as elements of social organization. Cognitive information indicates the rules and rationale of social organization, while behavioral information indicates what people actually do (including violation of organizational rules and consequent sanctions). Social organization may be important in public health for many reasons, including societal allocation of work and other activities (some of which may, in turn, be associated with harmful exposures), allocation of treatment resources and control of access, certification of healers and healing institutions, and provision of public education, health-related information, and programs.

The systematic recording of observations in the field is a critical step in anthropological research. This may be especially true with an open-ended research agenda, in which observations that do not make sense to the observer initially may become comprehensible later. Bernard (1994) provides a useful classification of types of information recorded in the field, including logs of intended and actual daily activities, a personal diary, and methodological and descriptive field notes of observations and analyses. Computer software developed for anthropology allows for the analysis of such notes (Bernard, 1994).

Traditionally, anthropological research required at least a year and sometimes more than two years of field study, followed by a thorough analysis and written account. Anthropology is often criticized by action-oriented professions as too time- and resource-consuming in producing results. Partly in response to such concerns, anthropologists have formulated a variety of quicker and more focused approaches to the collection of information. *Rapid Assessment Procedures* (RAPs) have been developed (Scrimshaw and Hurtado, 1987) to survey the research setting and address particular health issues in one or two months, using a systematic set of questions and methods. First developed to understand issues of nutrition and primary care, RAPs are applicable and have been used in the assessment of a far broader array of issues (Scrimshaw and Gleason, 1992). Scrimshaw and Hurtado (1987) provide guides for the rapid and systematic elicitation of health-related information at the community, household, and biomedical resource (i.e., clinicians and pharmacy) levels. These guides can be tailored to particular studies and particular settings; they are not rigid protocols. Both RAP and a similar approach, the *Focused Ethnographic Study* (FES), directed toward the understanding of specific disease conditions and programs, have been used by applied medical anthropologists in the 1990s (Pelto and Pelto, 1997). Although more time generally allows for the gathering of more and better information, the results of rapid, pointed approaches are more likely to meet the needs of public health programs and personnel.

The computer age offers enormous benefits to qualitative as well as quantitative analysis in anthropology. Computers allow the filing, analysis, and transmission of vast amounts of information (Bernard, 1994; Weitzman and Miles, 1995). Without the assistance of computers, some analyses would (and formerly did) require enormous amounts of time and resources. But there are also hazards in the use of computers in anthropological (and other) research. Perhaps the greatest hazard is the distance between the researcher and the information that computers readily allow, easily producing so-called results that do not accord with what the researcher has observed. Researchers may simply enter the information they have collected, decide on a coding strategy to sort the information, and establish an analytic approach to assess relationships in the sorted information. With a few computer keystrokes, an "analysis" is produced. What is missing is the intense scrutiny, pondering, review, and revision that are traditional in anthropology and that give the anthropologist a familiarity with what he or she has observed. Experts in the use of computers for analysis in anthropological research recognize the need for analysts to remain close to their information in the course of computer analysis.

Ethnographic and Other Reports

The format of anthropological reports often differs from that of other disciplines, but usually includes descriptions of research objectives, methods used, results or findings obtained, and their implications. A critical feature of anthropological studies in public health is that they often include recommendations for action or policy; they may recommend specific actions or policies, or they may even recommend not intervening. For purposes of anthropology in public health, the contents, language, and accessibility of reports are critical determinants of their use and application. Minimally, anthropological reports that are readily available but full of jargon and esoteric language, abstract theoretical or methodological discussions, and factual details not clearly relevant to application will not be read—an obvious obstacle to their effective use. While these characteristics may be efficient, if not necessary, for communication within the discipline of anthropology, they are most often inappropriate and ineffective in communication with nonanthropologists.

Integrating Anthropology in Public Health

The objectives of this anthology are to provide examples for public health and kindred audiences of how anthropology is useful, if not necessary, in public health and to describe the discipline and indicate resources for its further exploration and application. I propose three courses of action to increase the integration of anthropology in public health: (1) enhancement of the translation of anthropology into public health; (2) further development of medical anthropology as a basic subdiscipline in schools of public health; and (3) enhancement and establishment of links among anthropological organizations and public health institutions and agencies.

1. Translating Anthropology into Public Health

Anthropologists are accustomed to communication within their own community. As in many other disciplines, much of what they produce is not comprehensible to those in other fields, and it is sometimes not clear to anthropologists from other schools or subfields. A major effort in the preparation of this book was the translation of anthropological studies into a language accessible to public health audiences. What would be useful, particularly for anthropologists who apply their scholarship to the solution of social problems, is the development and use of curricula to teach anthropologists how to communicate beyond the discipline. Such a curriculum should emphasize:

- Common language and concepts and the avoidance of jargon.
- Clear description of methods.
- Theoretical exposition focused on solution of the problem at hand.
- Ethnographic detail focused on the problem.
- Reports organized to clearly indicate the utility of the information provided, theories and methods used, findings, and implications.

- Practical conclusions that address solution of the problem, even when the conclusion is that the problem should not be addressed or that the proposed project will be ineffective and should be revised or abandoned.

2. Integrating Medical Anthropology into Schools of Public Health

Medical anthropology is a fundamental public health discipline and should be routinely taught in schools of public health. This book might serve as an introduction to anthropology in public health for students, practitioners, administrators, and policymakers. It is by no means intended as a comprehensive or freestanding guide to anthropological theory and method. The field of anthropology and its medical subfield offer rich resources for further study. (Additional resources are indicated in the appendix.)

3. Establishing Links among Anthropological and Public Health Organizations

Hand in hand with better communication of anthropology to other communities, and the subsequent increased awareness within the public health community of the roles of anthropology in public health, establishing connections among institutions would facilitate collaboration of anthropologists in public health. Anthropologists have been consulted and employed by public health agencies for decades; at the US Centers for Disease Control and Prevention (CDC), there are currently 15 PhD anthropologists at work on diverse public health matters. Closer working relations of, for example, the American Anthropological Association and its Society for Medical Anthropology, with WHO, CDC, and the public health agencies of other nations, would facilitate the exchange of relevant perspectives, information, and personnel, and the improvement of programs.

Anthropology is commonly regarded as a discipline that studies the communities of others: "them." While this view may be historically valid, much of current anthropology has a far broader reach that includes not only other communities, but the global physical and social environment and the political, economic, and administrative contexts of those communities, as well as the community of anthropological investigators themselves. Through its methods for understanding communities and populations, contemporary anthropology lessens the distinction between "us" and "them." It recognizes expertise, rationality, and authority in others. Rather than ethnocentrically assuming that only we are right and just, anthropology begins with the humanizing assumption that others, like ourselves, live in more or less orderly conditions. While the Western world has much to offer, its donors will be more respectful and effective when they respond to local realities, values, and social life.

Notes

1. Biomedicine is distinguished from public health in its focus on pathology in individual patients and its orientation toward laboratory science and clinical practice (Hahn, 1995). Public health focuses on the pathology and health of populations; it builds on biomedicine but examines a broader array of causes.

2. The DALY is a measure of disease burden that takes into account not only death from specific causes, but also the youthfulness of the decedent and the sickness, disability, and suffering associated with these causes.

3. The Code of Ethics is available on the Internet at www.ameranthassn.org.

Acknowledgments

I am especially grateful for the constructive comments of my colleagues Marcia Inhorn (Department of Anthropology, Emory University) and G. David Williamson (Division of Prevention Research and Analytic Methods, Epidemiology Program Office, CDC).

References

Agar MH (1980) The Professional Stranger. An Informal Introduction to Ethnography. New York: Academic Press.

American Anthropological Association (1998) Code of Ethics of the American Anthropological Association.

Bernard HR (1994) Research Methods in Anthropology. Qualitative and Quantitative Approaches. Thousand Oaks, Calif: Sage Publications.

Desjarlais R, Eisenberg L, Good B, Kleinman A (1995) World Mental Health. New York: Oxford University Press.

Dirks NB, Eley G, Ortner SB, eds. (1994) Culture/Power/History. A Reader in Contemporary Social Theory. Princeton, NJ: Princeton University Press.

Doyal L (1995) What Makes Women Sick. New Brunswick, NJ: Rutgers University Press.

Fetterman DM (1998) Ethnography. Step by Step, 2nd ed. Thousand Oaks, Calif: Sage Publications.

Hahn RA (1995) Sickness and Healing. An Anthropological Perspective. New Haven: Yale University Press.

Inhorn MC (1995) Medical anthropology and epidemiology: divergences or convergences? *Social Science and Medicine* 40:285–290.

Krueger RA (1994) Focus Groups. A Practical Guide for Applied Research. Newbury Park, Calif: Sage Publications.

Murray CJL, Kreuser J, Whang W (1994) Cost-effectiveness analysis and policy choices: investing in health systems. *Bulletin of the World Health Organization* 72:181–192.

Murray CJL, Lopez AD (1996) The Global Burden of Disease. Cambridge, Mass: Harvard University Press.

Ortner SB (1994) "Theory in anthropology since the sixties." In Culture/Power/History. A Reader in Contemporary Social Theory. NB Dirks, G Eley, SB Ortner, eds. Princeton, NJ: Princeton University Press, pp. 372–411. [Reprinted from *Comparative Studies in Society and History* 1984; 26:126–166.

Pelto PJ, Pelto GH (1997) Studying knowledge, culture, and behavior in applied medical anthropology. *Medical Anthropology Quarterly* 11:147–163.

Polednak AP (1989) Racial and Ethnic Differences in Disease. New York: Oxford University Press.

Scrimshaw NS, Gleason GR, eds. (1992) RAP. Rapid Assessment Procedures. Qualitative Methodologies for Planning and Evaluation of Health Related Programmes. Boston: International Nutrition Foundation for Developing Countries.

Scrimshaw SCM, Hurtado E (1987) Rapid Assessment Procedures for Nutrition and Primary Health Care. Anthropological Approaches to Improving Programme Effectiveness. Los Angeles: University of California, Latin American Center Publications.

Spradley JP (1979) The Ethnographic Interview. New York: Holt, Rinehart and Winston.

Trostle JA, Sommerfeld J (1996) Medical anthropology and epidemiology. *Annual Review of Anthropology* 25:253–274.

UNHCR (United Nations High Commission on Refugees) (1993) The State of the World's Refugees 1993. The Challenge of Protection. New York: Penguin.

United Nations (1996) Demographic Yearbook 1994. New York: United Nations.

Weitzman EA, Miles MB (1995) Computer Programs for Qualititive Data Analysis. Thousand Oaks, Calif: Sage Publications.

World Bank (1993) World Development Report 1993. Investing in Health. New York: Oxford University Press.

I

INFECTIOUS DISEASE

2

Folk Flu and Viral Syndrome:
An Anthropological Perspective

SUSAN C. McCOMBIE

In the United States, a majority of the research on lay perceptions of illness has focused on ethnic minorities and recent immigrants. With the development of clinically applied anthropology in the 1970s and 1980s, a growing number of anthropologists turned their attention to health culture in mainstream America. They reasoned that understanding popular views of health and illness had the potential to enhance physician–patient communication, facilitate health education, and increase patient compliance.

The need for an understanding of American illness perceptions has been recognized by the medical profession. Interest was triggered partly by the growth of medical malpractice litigation. There has been increasing recognition that middle-class Americans may see illness differently from the physicians' biomedical model, and that patient dissatisfaction with biomedicine may be related to this incongruity. In 1985, an article in the *New England Journal of Medicine* recommended that physicians attempt to elicit their patients' disease beliefs (Gillick, 1985).

While some analysts have emphasized understanding patients' perceptions of illness, others have suggested that since clinicians do not always employ a single coherent explanatory model, their models and medical decision making also need to be studied. Eisenberg described the distinction between medical models of disease and popular models of illness and noted that physicians combined both in their actual practice (Eisenberg, 1977). Kleinman distinguished "scientific explanatory models" from the "clinical explanatory models" evident in practice and stated that the latter may diverge greatly from the former (Kleinman, 1980).

These distinctions are apparent when studying the treatment of common illness in general medical practice. Between 1973 and 1977, while working as a general practitioner, physician-anthropologist C. G. Helman investigated folk beliefs about "colds" and "fevers" in a London suburb. He characterized the folk belief system as a fluid one that easily incorporated biomedical treatment and concepts. Helman noted that the "operational model" used by general practitioners in Britain was in some respects closer to the folk model than to the biomedical model; moreover, the diagnoses given to patients reinforced the folk model (Helman, 1978). In a subsequent study, Helman described the experiences of a patient with presumed angina to illustrate that the biomedical model is actually a cluster of many explanatory models, the use of which is moderated by a number of factors, including audience, type of condition, and characteristics of the physician (Helman, 1985).

There are also important differences between biomedical practice and public health practice (O'Reilly, 1985). In medical practice the focus is on the treatment of illness in individual patients. In contrast, public health practice involves the application of preventive medicine to populations. The major focus is on prevention of diseases, rather than cure. Prevention requires an understanding of the factors that spread disease, which is the province of epidemiology.

The discipline of epidemiology is concerned with the distribution and determinants of disease in human populations. Application of epidemiological methods provides the data to design and evaluate public health measures. Epidemiologists search for associations between disease patterns and other phenomena. They seek to minimize bias and avoid misclassification that might hide true relationships or create false ones (Hahn, 1995).

Epidemiologists working in communicable disease control attempt to stop the spread of infection by identifying its source. They construct "case definitions," which are sets of criteria for counting cases of a disease. These criteria do not always match physician diagnoses, and one of the first rules of epidemiology is to *confirm the diagnosis*. Epidemiologists tend to approach a disease outbreak with skepticism, and they find some satisfaction when they can demonstrate that a presumed outbreak is due to an unanticipated factor. If an outbreak is "real," the highest achievement is being able to apply control measures to stop further transmission. This accomplishment is sometimes described in metaphorical terms. An example of this is "removing the pump handle," a phrase which summarizes the achievement of John Snow during a cholera epidemic in nineteenth-century London, where a pump handle provided access to cholera-infected water. This chapter illustrates how inattention to the cultural understandings of lay and medical participants in disease outbreaks may hinder the search for the "pump handle."

Methods

Ethnographic and epidemiological data were collected between 1983 and 1988 in a county in the southwestern United States. The county has both rural and urban areas, with the majority of its 600,000 residents clustered in one major city. According to the county's office of vital statistics, the county population was 83.0% white, 2.9% black, 2.8% Native American, 0.9% Asian and Pacific Islander, and 10.4% "other" races. Twenty-one percent of the population is of Spanish origin, any race (1981 estimates). Tourism, mining, agriculture, and industry form the basis of the economy. According to 1980 census data, in 1979 the median family income in the county was $15,796. Nine percent of households had incomes below the federal poverty level ($8,414 for a family of four in 1980).

The Communicable Disease Division of the County Health Department consisted of four units. The Venereal Disease Section (with a staff of seven), Tuberculosis Control Section (staff of eight), and Immunization Section (staff of two) were supported by federal block grants and funds from the state health department in addition to county funds. The Epidemiology Section initially consisted of one county-funded epidemiologist who was responsible for surveillance and investigation of all other diseases. In October 1983, I offered my services to the epidemiologist as a volunteer. I was interested in studying the relationship between popular beliefs and the transmission of infectious disease. I was a graduate student in anthropology, in search of data for a dissertation. Ultimately I became a paid employee, finished my dissertation, and remained on staff in the role of epidemiologist until 1988.

During the course of this study, my role evolved from that of observer to active participant. I became a public health worker and carried out official duties as a disease investigator. Interaction with physicians, nurses, administrators, and the public occurred daily. In the process of investigating outbreaks and reports of communicable diseases, I interviewed patients and physicians and reviewed patients' charts. I attended meetings such as the local infection control association and pediatric society as well as grand rounds presentations at the university hospital.

After my initial training in the health department, I spent a considerable amount of time providing public education in schools, in medical settings, and on the telephone. Telephone inquiries were frequent, and much time was spent responding to inquiries from the public and medical practitioners. This gave me firsthand experience in various situations involving infectious disease control.

For the first 18 months of fieldwork, I kept a daily log, recording the events of the day. Initially I attempted to record everything that transpired, with a focus on situations that related to disease beliefs and behaviors. When possible, I made notes during the day, for example, when responding to telephone inquiries or conducting investigations by telephone. Both nonelicited statements from individuals and responses to informal interviews were noted. Later I reviewed my notes, collating items that dealt with specific diseases or concepts, such as "flu."

I also interviewed colleagues at the health department about various issues, using a tape recorder both for these interviews and for discussions in the latter stages of fieldwork. However, with respect to the public and the private medical community, I asked only those questions that were related to fulfilling my official role and simply listened to the responses. I learned more from the questions people asked of me than I did from questioning them.

After a period of several months, I decided to focus on all forms of viral hepatitis as a dissertation topic and began systematically to record information on situations that involved hepatitis. Later I received funding to conduct a special research project on shigellosis, which ultimately involved the use of a standardized questionnaire with some open-ended questions. "Flu" and "viral syndrome" were not central research topics. However, they emerged repeatedly in situations I recorded involving hepatitis, shigellosis, and many other reportable communicable diseases and outbreaks, that is, those diseases that must, by law, be reported for purposes of public health.

With respect to the analysis presented here, I acted as a participant observer, using neither a standardized questionnaire nor other data collection instruments. The method of participant observation involves making observations while engaging in the same daily activities as the people under study (Fetterman, 1989; Spradley, 1980). The approach had pros and cons. Because I was a participant, I was not an intruder. Like Helman, who did research while working as a physician, I had an official role to carry out and was much more than an observer. I benefited from an insider's view that would not have been possible had I begun with a specific research question and proceeded to conduct focused interviews. I discovered that hypothetical questions and attempts to elicit abstract disease beliefs revealed little of interest. Yet a single outbreak or situation in which an infection was involved yielded a wealth of information about people's beliefs and attitudes about specific diseases and the nature of their fears of contagion. While this approach had the limitations of being an informal, rather than a formal, study, it was invaluable in gaining insight into many of the social factors affecting the spread of disease.

"Influenza": The Epidemiologist's Perspective

To an epidemiologist, "flu" or "influenza" refers to an infection of the respiratory tract caused by several closely related viruses of the orthomyxoviridae family (Douglas and Betts, 1985). The characteristic symptoms are fever, headache, sore throat, runny nose, and muscle aches (Benenson, 1985). Influenza is defined by an epidemiologist as infection with a single-stranded RNA virus. Influenza has a marked seasonal pattern. In temperate climates, influenza activity is restricted to late fall and early winter months. Surveillance during this time is important to evaluate the efficacy of influenza vaccine and to monitor antigenic changes in virus strains so that appropriate vaccines can be developed. Waldman states:

> The term influenza should be reserved for that illness caused by influenza virus. This is unfortunately not the case with respect to most of the lay public and many in the health industry. Such terms as "intestinal flu" are particularly misleading and inaccurate because one of the characteristics of influenza epidemics is the very small percentage of patients who have intestinal symptoms. (Waldman, 1984:485)

"Folk Flu": The Layperson's Perspective

"Flu" emerged as a common American illness category in the initial stages of fieldwork. It quickly became apparent that "flu" does not mean the same thing to the epidemiologist that it does to the public, who include illnesses with a number of clinical presentations. Lay diagnoses of flu are often made during outbreaks of gastrointestinal disease. For some informants, nausea, vomiting, and diarrhea are the defining features of the flu, whereas an illness whose symptoms are compatible with influenza is classified as a bad cold. Others lump illnesses with gastrointestinal and respiratory symptoms together under flu, and sometimes make distinctions by using terms such as "stomach flu." Confusion surrounding the definition of flu is increased by articles in the popular press and medical literature that describe the symptoms of diseases such as malaria, encephalitis, and AIDS as "flu-like."

Individuals frequently contacted the health department seeking advice about an episode of illness. Usually their questions were directed at finding out "what's going around" and whether or not they should see a doctor. One of the first calls I took after my initial orientation proved to be a typical example:

CALLER (a young male): I just wanted to ask a question. Is there anything going around right now that I should know about?

HEALTH DEPT: We receive reports of several different types of diseases every week. Are you ill right now, or is someone you know feeling sick?

CALLER: Well, I think I might have it.

HD: What do you think you have?

CALLER: I guess it's the flu.

HD: What kind of symptoms do you have?

CALLER: You know, just regular flu symptoms.

HD: What kind of symptoms exactly?

CALLER: I've been sick to my stomach a lot.

HD: Do you have a fever? Or diarrhea?

CALLER: I don't know, I haven't taken it. I don't really have the diarrhea yet. Maybe it's just too much partying. Should I go to the doctor? Do they give you a shot for this flu?

This type of interaction occurs frequently, as individuals seek a diagnosis for their illness over the telephone, perhaps to avoid unnecessary visits to the doctor. The symptoms that are reported as characteristic of flu in this context vary, but gastrointestinal complaints are common. Between October 1983 and February 1985, the symptoms of 26 callers who attributed their illness to "flu" were recorded. Twenty-three percent reported symptoms of diarrhea alone, while 19% reported vomiting alone. Overall 81% reported vomiting or diarrhea, along with other symptoms, while only 15% reported any respiratory symptoms that would characterize influenza.

Effect of Differences in Perspective on Outbreak Investigation

The discrepancy between the lay and epidemiological definitions of flu is more than a matter of semantics. Or, rather, semantics is an epidemiological issue. For the epidemiologist whose task is to investigate and control outbreaks of communicable disease, this discrepancy in categorization and the associated health behaviors is a major obstacle and may become a source of frustration. The words of an epidemiologist who worked for the County Health Department for nine years illustrate this:

> For years, I would talk to people on the phone, ask them what they had, or go out to try to do an investigation of diarrheal disease in a day care center, knowing that there were cases of *Giardia* in the center, and they would say no, nobody's sick, we just have the flu. And I would ask them what have you had, and they all had diarrhea. And it got to be so damn repetitive that I just got so angry every time somebody said flu. I'd give a lecture, and try and talk about disease, and the first question would be ah, it's the flu, stomach flu. It drove me crazy.

I encountered the same problem at a day care center, when the director attributed diarrhea to "the flu," not as a symptom of giardiasis. "Folk flu" therefore becomes a problem for epidemiologists because people say they have the flu when they have something else. In addition to giardiasis, viral hepatitis and bacterial infections caused by *Shigella, Salmonella,* and *Campylobacter* are often attributed to flu. These infections are not uncommon in the United States.

Also complicating epidemiological investigation is the failure of the lay population to recognize identical symptoms in different people. Folk diagnoses of "teething" and "milk allergy" are common in the presence of infectious diarrhea in infants and young children and often accompany "flu" diagnoses in the folk explanation of outbreaks. In the summer of 1984, an outbreak of shigellosis (bacterial dysentery) occurred in a day care center in the county. Investigation revealed explanations for the illness which tended to be individualized for each child. The staff had failed to recognize that an outbreak was occurring in spite of the fact that more than half the children had diarrhea in a three-week period.

In this outbreak, several distinct explanations were given for cases of diarrhea. Those without individual explanations were attributed to flu. One female staff member who also had an infant in the center attributed her own diarrhea to flu and that of her infant to teething. Another woman consulted a physician when her infant experienced an episode of bloody diarrhea. She was told that the diarrhea was probably due to breastfeeding and was advised to discontinue nursing. Because gastrointestinal illness is so often attributed to "flu" or to noninfectious processes, outbreaks of bacterial and parasitic diarrheal diseases can go undetected for weeks.

Folk flu not only obstructs epidemiologic control of diarrheal outbreaks, but it is also an obstacle to surveillance for influenza virus itself. Epidemiologists often spend considerable time following false leads. Between October 1983 and October 1984, medical staff from three nursing homes reported outbreaks of flu. Two of the outbreaks turned out to be gastroenteritis (vomiting and diarrhea), while only one was influenza. The health department typically received more calls about flu outbreaks when influenza was absent from the community than when it was present.

In addition, the public health importance of influenza is not recognized. During one outbreak of influenza A, the health department was called to investigate a claim of disease caused by pigeon droppings in the ventilation system of a public school. On arriving to begin the investigation, I was told that the fears were based on the fact that a large number of students were absent with complaints of respiratory disease. When I suggested that the influenza outbreak might be responsible for this, the teacher became somewhat annoyed. She replied, "We have a lot more than just flu here!"

The investigation of foodborne outbreaks is also hampered by folk beliefs about "flu." In one instance, 17 of the 50 members (34%) of a minor league baseball team became ill after a common meal in a restaurant. The health department was contacted after 13 of the players visited an emergency room. Cooperation from the restaurant owner in identifying the probable source was limited. Quick to defend the quality of his food, he maintained that the players were simply "suffering from the flu."

Such explanations are often used even when lay diagnosticians have no vested interest in denying the possibility of foodborne illness. In September 1984, I attempted to investigate an outbreak of campylobacter gastroenteritis[1] in a fraternity house. Three laboratory-confirmed cases were reported to the health department by a physician in the Student Health Service, who reported that there were others with diarrhea at the house. The students found my presence amusing, since it was obvious to them that the outbreak was "just the flu" or "just something contagious." One of the fraternity members pointed out that it couldn't be "food poisoning" since they all had fevers. The students shared a popular misconception: that food poisoning comes on quickly after a meal and can be distinguished from flu by the absence of a fever. Because of these beliefs, very few of the residents responded to the food history questionnaire, and the investigation could not be completed.

In the epidemiological investigation of an outbreak of an infectious disease, the first step is to locate individuals who may be ill and obtain symptom histories. This "case finding" activity allows the epidemiologist to characterize the outbreak and construct hypotheses about the source of the infection. If case finding is incomplete, the epidemiologist's ability to determine the source of infection is weakened. In many cases, attempts to identify additional persons who are ill fail because the illness has already been classified by lay diagnosticians as flu.

An example of obstacles to case finding involved a small outbreak of hepatitis A that occurred among the members of a college athletic team. Three cases with onset in a one-week period were reported. Initial interviews with the first patients and their teammates did not uncover any more infected team members. However, on further questioning, it was discovered that another teammate had been ill, but it was stated that "she really just had the flu." As it turned out, her illness was characterized by vomiting and fever, symptoms that are compatible with hepatitis A infection.

The frequency with which flu diagnoses are made by laypersons indicates that the category has important functions in American society. It acts as a ready label that can be applied to many kinds of illness. The anxiety of an ill person is reduced when a diagnosis is made, and the diagnosis of flu carries several important messages. Since everyone is susceptible to the disease, individuals do not feel responsible for contracting the disease as they might, for example, for contracting a sexually transmitted disease. As Helman observed regarding "colds" and "fevers":

The patients were relieved to find that there is a "Bug going round" and that they are blameless and not socially deviant in their behavior; they also no longer feel uneasy or unsure of their condition, particularly as their illness is now a disease within the biomedical world—and by definition capable of being cured, or at least palliated. (Helman, 1978:126)

The diagnosis of flu is also reassuring because it is believed that the condition is temporary and full recovery will be prompt. This is evident in the frequent use of the term "just" to describe flu. It is "just the flu"—not something worse. While the illness may be severe, it is not considered serious.

"Flu" allows people to explain illness in a reassuring and socially acceptable manner. When an individual feels the need to exclude himself from professional or social responsibilities, a complaint of flu can legitimize absence without generating embarrassment or undue concern. Perhaps because of its greater social acceptability, "flu" often replaces excuses that involve admissions of diarrhea, menses, hangovers, or more serious symptoms. However, from the perspective of epidemiologists who are responsible for the investigation and control of communicable diseases, this popular illness category hinders communication and creates obstacles to appropriate intervention.

"Viral Syndrome": The Perspective of Practicing Physicians

The category "viral syndrome" as used by physicians and medical personnel also engenders problems for epidemiological investigation and disease control. Like folk flu, it does not correspond to any single disease recognized by epidemiologists. During routine investigation, viral syndrome was the initial diagnosis by medical personnel in a number of bacterial infections, notably typhoid fever, shigellosis, campylobacter enteritis, and neurosyphilis.

"Viral syndrome" is to the practitioner what "flu" is to the layperson. Like the folk diagnosis of flu, the medical diagnosis of viral syndrome labels many types of illness. Usually when a physician diagnoses a virus, the message is "it's just a virus, you'll get over it." Although ignorant of the exact cause of the illness, the physician expects recovery without intervention.

Viral syndrome first came to my attention in October 1983. Active surveillance was initiated following extensive flooding that carried the potential for fecal contamination of the water supply. To determine if any increase in gastrointestinal disease had occurred, surveillance systems were set up in nine locations: four emergency rooms, one hospital clinic specializing in digestive disorders, one pediatric clinic in a community hospital, one rural primary health care clinic, and two laboratories. In reviewing medical records in these facilities for an 11-week period, I discovered that the diagnosis of viral syndrome was a frequent one in physician office visits and emergency rooms, and it was often made in the absence of any laboratory testing to rule out bacterial disease or identify specific viruses.

Viruses are the causal agents of a large number of diseases which have widely varied clinical manifestations. The diagnosis of viral syndrome is not linked to any particular set of symptoms; it is made on the basis of many different patient complaints including fever, headache, dizziness, abdominal pain, sore throat, shortness of breath, vomiting, and diarrhea. This diagnosis does not correspond to a specific viral disease or to any particular syndrome and cannot be used as an epidemiological datum. The only diagnoses that could be counted in our surveillance were gastroenteritis, viral gastroenteritis, and viral enteritis, with the assumption that all three of these would correspond to complaints of vomiting and/or diarrhea. Although the results of the flood surveillance did not indicate any increase in gastrointestinal illness subsequent to the flooding, it is impossible to know how many cases of gastrointestinal illness were diagnosed as viral syndrome.

Daily summaries of physician diagnoses in a community hospital's outpatient pediatric clinic illustrate the potential magnitude of this effect (Table 2.1). Viral syndrome was the most common communicable disease diagnosis, accounting for more than a third of diagnoses. Prior to the flooding, 94 cases of gastroenteritis (14.6% of total communicable disease diagnoses) were recorded in one month. The month after the flooding, 58 cases of gastroenteritis (9.3%) were recorded. This suggests a decrease in gastrointestinal illness after the flooding. However,

Table 2.1 Number of Communicable Disease Diagnoses in a Pediatric Clinic

| | SEPTEMBER 1983 | | OCTOBER 1983 | |
DIAGNOSIS	N	%	N	%
Viral syndrome	220	34.2	250	40.1
Otitis media	208	32.3	196	31.5
Gastroenteritis	94	14.6	58	9.3
Upper respiratory infection	45	7.0	37	5.9
Conjunctivitis	31	4.8	13	2.1
Beta Streptococcus	17	2.6	28	4.5
Croup	12	1.9	17	2.7
Flu-like illness	5	0.8	0	—
Bronchiolitis	4	0.6	8	1.3
Pneumonia	3	0.5	11	1.8
Scarlet fever	2	0.3	1	0.2
Viral meningitis	1	0.2	2	0.3
Campylobacter	1	0.2	0	—
Giardiasis	0	—	1	0.2
Total	643	100.0	622	100.0

Source: Flood surveillance data, County Health Department.

the number of cases of viral syndrome increased over the same time period, from 220 (34.2%) to 250 (40.1%). If the label "viral syndrome" was applied to gastrointestinal illness seen in children in the clinic, the apparent decrease in gastroenteritis and increase in viral syndrome might represent differences in reporting rather than changes in disease patterns. I questioned two nurses at the clinic about the diagnosis of viral syndrome. One stated that "sometimes it means runny nose and a sore throat." The other nurse found the question amusing and said, "That's what they [the doctors] put when they aren't sure!"

In addition to interfering with epidemiological investigation and disease control, a diagnosis of viral syndrome may endanger a patient's health when a serious bacterial infection is the true cause of the illness. In one case that occurred in the county, a handicapped child with fever and diarrhea was diagnosed by her physician as having "viral syndrome." After the symptoms persisted for several days, the child was again brought for medical care. After being transferred to a second hospital, the child died. An autopsy established a diagnosis of shigellosis (bacterial dysentery). Leopold (1986) describes a similar case in which a 14-month-old child was brought to a pediatric clinic with a fever of 104°F. The initial diagnosis was viral syndrome, with a recommendation of treatment with acetaminophen. Three days later, the child died, and the postmortem exam established a diagnosis of septicemic plague (*Yersinia pestis*). In both these cases, appropriate antibiotic therapy might have prevented death, but the specimen cultures that would have established the diagnosis and indicated the need for specific antibiotic therapy were not performed, possibly because a diagnosis of viral syndrome had obscured the problem.

Because much illness is self-limited, extensive laboratory testing to establish an exact etiology is often of little value to the patient, since recovery often occurs before laboratory reports are received. Only when patients return with continued symptoms are diagnostic procedures implemented. A 13-year-old girl was brought to the emergency room three times. On the first visit, the mother was told that her child had "intestinal flu." On the second, pancreatitis was the diagnosis. Only on the third visit was a stool culture performed, which established the diagnosis of typhoid fever, after which appropriate antibiotic treatment was initiated. Even when they are the cause of an infection, viruses may be difficult to isolate and are expensive to test. This explains why laboratory tests are not often ordered.

There is considerable semantic overlap in the diagnoses of folk flu and viral syndrome. This is apparent when a doctor tells a patient he has the flu but writes viral syndrome or viral infection in the medical record.

Thus far I have described "flu" as part of a lay model and "viral syndrome" as part of a medical model. However, this dichotomy is an oversimplification. Laypersons frequently talk about viruses and often diagnose themselves as having a virus. Some individuals appear to make a distinction between flu and viruses, evident in statements such as, "I don't know whether I have the flu or just a virus." Others appear to use an explanatory model that is closer to the medical model, in which flu is a subset of a larger category of viruses. In this model all types of flu ("stomach flu" included) are seen as being caused by viruses, but viruses are also recognized to be the cause of illnesses that would not be called flu, such as warts and cold sores.

The details of laypersons' and practitioners' definitions of flu and virus vary considerably. There has been no systematic study to investigate patterns of these beliefs. Colleagues have suggested that there are geographic differences in the extent to which flu is associated with diarrhea. It is also likely that there are differences in the frequency of diagnosis of viral syndrome by medical specialty. These are important and virtually untouched research questions.

Effects of Differences in Perspective on Spread of Infection

From the standpoint of an epidemiologist, the effects of lay and practitioner beliefs on disease investigation and control are generally equivalent, regardless of the specific features of the explanatory models. For example, it doesn't matter whether an individual who is suffering from fever and diarrhea classifies his illness as the "flu," a "virus," or, possibly, a "flu virus." If the patient doesn't seek medical care, the specific type of infection will not be identified. Even if a medical evaluation is sought, the information important to an epidemiologist may not be obtained.

There is also a great deal of variability in the extent to which diagnoses of folk flu and viral syndrome affect the spread of communicable disease. Transmission may be limited or facilitated, depending on the mode of transmission of a particular disease and subsequent individual behaviors of the physician, the patient, and his or her contacts.

Consider antibiotic therapy in the case of bacterial infections that spread by the fecal-oral route. In the absence of treatment, a person with *Shigella* or *Campylobacter* infection who is diagnosed as having viral syndrome can continue to transmit the disease. This does not always happen, however, as physicians sometimes prescribe antibiotics even when diagnosing viral disease. In this case two wrongs may make a right, and the physician prescribes an effective treatment despite misdiagnosis and treatment inappropriate for that diagnosis.

There is sometimes no direct relationship between diagnosis and treatment, as illustrated by information obtained during the investigation of a large outbreak of shigellosis that occurred in the county in August 1986. The outbreak occurred among individuals who had eaten at a local restaurant. Fifty individuals who ate the contaminated food and had symptoms of diarrhea and fever were interviewed. Of the 28 who sought medical care, 8 (29%) were diagnosed as having shigellosis, but 2 of these did not receive appropriate antibiotic therapy; 7 (25%) of the patients were diagnosed with the "flu" or a "virus" ("virus"—4, "flu"—2, "summer flu"—1). Of these, 2 received no treatment, 2 received antibiotics, 1 received Lomotil and 1 received Imodium (both contraindicated in the treatment of *Shigella*), and 1 received an unknown type of suppository.[2] Of the remaining 13 individuals, 11 were not informed of any diagnosis. One was told simply that he had "diarrhea," and one was told he had "gastroenteritis," which is simply a term that describes the symptoms of diarrhea and/or vomiting. Two of these 13 received antibiotics, 2 received Compazine, and 2 received Imodium. The rest were not treated. Overall, only 36% of patients seen by a physician received appropriate antibiotic therapy, while 21% received antidiarrheals, which can be harmful in cases of bacterial dysentery.

Treatment with antibiotics in the absence of a specific diagnosis is extremely common (Hamm et al., 1996; Mainous et al., 1996; Nicole et al., 1996). The medical rationale for such treatment is that even if it is a virus, antibiotics won't do any harm. Prescribing antibiotics also reduces the anxiety experienced by physicians when uncertain about a diagnosis (McCombie, 1989). In an article about how physicians talk about patients, Hardison gives an example of this:

> I think the patient has the flu, but I am going to give him broad spectrum antibiotics until his blood cultures come back negative. It is better to be safe, and after all, it won't hurt to give him antibiotics, and besides I won't have to worry about gram-negative septicemia. (Hardison, 1986)

However, in the case of bacterial gastroenteritis, the choice of antibiotic is important and tied specifically to the etiologic agent. In addition, antibiotic therapy may not be necessary, or may even be contraindicated. For instance, treatment with antibiotics usually prolongs the carrier state for infections caused by *Salmonella* and is related to relapses (Hook, 1985).

When individuals with the bacterial infections mentioned above are interviewed as part of a health department investigation, lack of knowledge regarding the disease they suffer from is a common finding. Many do not know the name of the disease they have and state that the doctor told them that they had "a bug," "an infection," "the flu," or "a virus." Those individuals who have been told the scientific name of their infection are often anxious to find out more about it. During the course of these investigations, it is rare to find patients who understand that they have an infection which is transmitted by the fecal-oral route, although some have a vague idea that they have something contagious.

In the initial stages of the shigellosis research project, in which detailed patient interviews were conducted by health department staff, we asked 53 patients whose infections had been reported by physicians what instructions the physician had given them. Only six (11.3%) reported that they were told to be sure to wash their hands after going to the bathroom. Some of the more common responses were, "He told me to take Tylenol," "He told me to give the baby clear fluids," "He told me to take the medicine," and, "He didn't tell me anything."

Another common infection in which patient and practitioner behaviors are important determinants of disease spread is viral hepatitis A. Physicians frequently diagnose "flu" as well as "viruses" in the presence of hepatitis symptoms. In reviewing the medical records of hepatitis patients, assessments such as "Intestinal flu" and "Probably influenza—Rule out hepatitis" were observed. The early symptoms of viral hepatitis are characterized by fever, anorexia, nausea, vomiting, and abdominal pain. These symptoms are also typical of flu. Visible jaundice occurs in only a small proportion of cases, and only late in the course of illness. When there are delays in seeking medical care and in diagnosis, it is often too late to prevent illness in household members and other close contacts by giving immune serum globulin injections. If delay occurs in diagnosing a food preparer who has hepatitis A, transmission to the public can be considerable.

Individuals diagnosed as having hepatitis often report that they initially thought they had a bad case of flu. When physicians are consulted they often concur with this diagnosis. In one case, a male cook employed at a local restaurant contacted me at the health department requesting prophylactic injections because a close friend had been diagnosed as having hepatitis A. The individual stated that he had the "flu" now, and didn't want "to get hepatitis on top of that!" He reported symptoms of vomiting, fever, and headache. He was advised to see a physician for evaluation of this condition. When he visited an emergency room, he was told he had "stomach flu" and no diagnostic tests were performed. Subsequent testing by the health department revealed that he had hepatitis A.

In addition to problems caused by failure to diagnose hepatitis, problems were also common when physicians actually did diagnose hepatitis and then made recommendations. Often these recommendations reflected the view that all forms of hepatitis were as contagious as the "flu." Frequently, persons who were not capable of transmitting hepatitis were excluded from schools and workplaces. Health department staff spent a considerable amount of time responding to crisis situations that arose from misconceptions about viral hepatitis and misdiagnoses of the diseases, despite the availability of diagnostic tests for several forms of hepatitis. Time spent in these investigations meant that other investigations were neglected. In many cases, members of the public acted on the basis of information received from physicians, which was considered incorrect by the county health department disease control staff. People frequently became hostile, insisting, "But my doctor said. . . . " Responding to these situations was difficult because of the unwritten rule that prohibits questioning a physician's diagnosis or telling a patient "your doctor is wrong." These situations were a constant source of frustration for the health department staff.

Discussion

The need for an understanding of popular health culture is as real for modern industrial societies as it is for developing countries. Infectious disease control in public health is dependent on successful epidemiological investigation, which is ethnographic in nature. What individuals report is filtered through their own perception of what is relevant. When people believe that they have the flu, an epidemiologist finds that it is even more difficult to obtain the information needed to determine the cause of outbreaks. Complete and accurate case reporting, which is crucial for disease control, is never reached, even under the best conditions. Many cases of food poisoning and reportable infectious diseases never come to the attention of disease control specialists because laypersons categorize the symptoms as "flu" and/or "virus."

There is increasing awareness among public health practitioners of the need to design culturally appropriate health care interventions and understand cultural conceptions of illness. However, the major focus is on "different" cultures that might be found among immigrants and minorities. Mainstream and middle-class Americans are sometimes viewed as "culture-less," or as homogeneous carriers of the biomedical model. The apparent congruity between the disease models of middle-class Americans and the biomedical model, however, is a fiction created by the use of an apparently similar vocabulary. Terms like "flu," "virus," and "infectious" have different meanings for laypersons, epidemiologists, and physicians.

Differences in the language and behavior of laypersons and those of clinical practitioners are often noted. Less recognized is the difference between clinical practitioners and epidemiologists. In clinical practice, physicians use explanatory models that differ from scientific explanatory models and are closely related to popular models of illness. In addition, there is a wide range of variability in theory and practice among biomedical practitioners in the United States. This variability often acts as an obstacle to epidemiological investigation and disease control. The nature of the clinical models used by physicians in actual practice and the extent to which these diverge from scientific explanatory models are important areas for future medical anthropological research.

In spite of the fact that the clinical explanatory model of disease in the United States is closely related to the epidemiological model, some important discrepancies regarding specific disease entities may contribute to the spread of infectious diseases. Although vague diagnoses and failure to order laboratory tests are sources of annoyance for epidemiologists, physicians may simply be practicing culturally appropriate health care when they tell patients they have the "flu." Their working models of disease are based on healing individuals, and their daily activities have goals and objectives that differ from those of epidemiologists concerned with preventing the spread of disease in populations. Recognition of the different goals of public health and medical practice can place these behavior patterns in perspective.

Anthropological research can do more for public health than simply elucidating patterns of beliefs and behaviors among laypersons. Medical practitioners are another important target population for public health officials. In many instances, they are considered "difficult to reach." Attempts to elicit their cooperation and change their behavior also need to be based on an understanding of their belief systems and rationales. Anthropologists can contribute to improving public health by studying the relationship among illness categories, beliefs, and health behavior and by elucidating the variety of common disease terms used by laypersons and professionals.

Notes

1. Like *Salmonella* infections, *Campylobacter* infections are often traced to foods such as chicken.

2. The antidiarrheal agents Lomotil and Imodium are contraindicated in the treatment of diarrhea caused by toxigenic bacteria such as *Shigella*.

Acknowledgment

An earlier version of this paper, "Folk Flu and Viral Syndrome: An Epidemiological Perspective," was published in *Social Science and Medicine* (1987) 25, no. 9: 987–993.

References

Benenson AS (1985) Control of Communicable Diseases in Man. Washington, DC: American Public Health Association.

Douglas RG, Betts RF (1985) "Influenza Virus." In: Principles and Practice of Infectious Diseases. GL Mandell, RG Douglas Jr, JE Bennett, eds. New York: Wiley, pp. 846–866.

Eisenberg L (1977) Disease and illness: distinctions between professional and popular ideas of sickness. *Culture Medicine and Psychiatry* 1:9–23.

Fetterman DM (1998) Ethnography: Step by Step, 2nd ed.. Newbury Park, Calif: Sage Publications.

Gillick MR (1985) Common sense models of health and disease. *New England Journal of Medicine* 313:700–703.

Hahn RA (1995) Sickness and Healing. An Anthropological Perspective. New Haven: Yale University Press.

Hamm RM, Hicks RJ, Bemben DA (1996) Antibiotics and respiratory infections: are patients more satisfied when expectations are met? *Journal of Family Practice* 43:56–62.

Hardison JE (1986) Benefit of the doubt. *Cutis* 37:150–151.

Helman CG (1978) "Feed a cold, starve a fever": folk models of infection in an English suburban community, and their relation to medical treatment. *Culture Medicine and Psychiatry* 2:107–137.

Helman CG (1985) "Disease and Pseudo-Disease: A Case History of Pseudo Angina." In: Physicians of Western Medicine. RA Hahn, AD Gaines, eds. Dordrecht: Reidel, pp. 293–331.

Hook EW (1985) "Salmonella Species Including Typhoid Fever." In: Principles and Practice of Infectious Diseases. GL Mandell, RG Douglas Jr, JE Bennett, eds. New York: Wiley, pp. 1256–1265.

Kleinman A (1980) Patients and Healers in the Context of Culture. Berkeley: University of California Press.

Leopold JC (1986) Septicemic plague in a 14 month old child. *Pediatric Infectious Disease* 5:108–110.

Mainous AG, Huestion WJ, Clark JR (1996) Antibiotics and upper respiratory infection: do some folks think there is a cure for the common cold? *Journal of Family Practice* 42:357–361.

McCombie SC (1989) The politics of immunization in public health. *Social Science and Medicine* 28:843–849.

Nicole LE, Bentley D, Garibaldi R, Neuhaus E, Smith P (1996) Antibiotic use in long-term-care facilities. *Infection Control and Hospital Epidemiology* 17:119–128.

O'Reilly KR (1985) "Applied Anthropology and Public Health." In: Training Manual in Medical Anthropology. CE Hill, ed. Washington, DC: American Anthropological Association, pp. 8–20.

Spradley JP (1980) Participant Observation. Fort Worth, Tex: Harcourt Brace Jovanovich.

Waldman RH (1984) "Influenza Virus." In: Infectious Diseases. RH Waldman, RM Kluge, eds. New Hyde Park, NY: Medical Examination Publishing Company, pp. 485–500.

3

The Role of Anthropological Methods in a Community-Based Mosquito Net Intervention in Bagamoyo District, Tanzania

PETER J. WINCH

In 1898, the simultaneous discovery of the role of anopheline mosquitoes in malaria transmission (by Ronald Ross in India and Giovanni Battista Grassi and colleagues in Italy) made possible modern malaria control. One hundred years after this discovery, malaria is a greater threat to public health than ever, causing an estimated 300 million to 500 million clinical cases and between 1.5 million and 2.7 million deaths per year (WHO, 1996). The majority of the deaths occur in young children living in endemic areas of Africa. Mosquito nets (bednets), treated every 6 to 12 months with pyrethroid insecticides, are a simple, low-cost malaria prevention measure ideally suited to conditions in rural Africa. Regular treatment with insecticide significantly increases the impact of the nets on malaria transmission. A recent study in The Gambia provided evidence that untreated mosquito nets confer some individual protection against malaria, but not as much as insecticide-treated mosquito nets (D'Alessandro et al., 1995b). Pyrethroid insecticides such as permethrin, used in this project, break down quickly and do not accumulate in the tissues (Lines, 1996a). Insecticides on nets pose minimal health risks.

There are now calls for operational research into how best to promote the use of insecticide-treated nets on a large scale (Lengeler et al., 1996). This operational research must address a wide range of questions, including how to achieve high rates of use and regular retreatment with insecticides, and how to make programs promoting the use of insecticide-treated nets sustainable (Carnevale and Coosemans, 1995; Fielden, 1996; Lines, 1996b; Zimicki, 1996). As part of this effort, applied anthropologists have been asked to investigate local practices related to febrile illnesses and biting insects, and to develop behavior change strategies that are both acceptable and result in increased use of treated nets by people living in malarious areas.

The Bagamoyo Bed Net Project

This chapter provides examples of the role that anthropology played in the Bagamoyo Bed Net Project (BBNP) from 1991 to 1995 (Makemba et al., 1995, 1996; Mfaume et al., 1997; Winch et al., 1994, 1996, 1997). BBNP was a community-based malaria control research project that aimed to develop a sustainable system for distributing and promoting the use and regular insecticide treatment of mosquito nets. Its purpose also was to evaluate the impact of the nets on mosquito densities; on rates of infection in mosquitoes (sporozoite rates); and on clinical malaria, anemia, and mortality in young children, the group most affected by the disease (Makemba et al., 1995; Premji et al., 1995b).

The study area was divided into four geographic zones, each with three to four villages (Makemba et al., 1995; Premji et al., 1995b). The project villages are located in Bagamoyo District on the coastal plain of Tanzania, 50 km north of the capital, Dar es Salaam, with a total population of approximately 22,000. Most of the people are either fishermen or subsistence farmers, the principal crops being rice and cassava. The predominant ethnic groups are the Zaramo, Kwere (Beidelman, 1967) and Swahili (Middleton, 1992). A number of people have migrated into the area in recent years from southern Tanzania.

The intervention was implemented one group at a time, at intervals of six months. In each village five representatives were nominated for the village mosquito net committee and confirmed in a village-wide meeting. Village mosquito net committees were responsible for sales, distribution, and treatment of the nets. Nets were sold to villagers for between three and five US dollars, depending on the size. Retreatment of nets with insecticide was initially free and later cost 40 cents per net.

This chapter discusses three research questions in which anthropological methods played a key role:

- Why did many villagers not view malaria control as a high priority, even though malaria is one of the leading causes of childhood mortality in the study area?
- How could year-round net use be promoted?
- How could the project create a demand for regular retreatment with the insecticide?

Malaria in the Project Area

The project villages are located in an area of endemic or "stable" malaria trans-mission, meaning that malaria is transmitted every month of the year. Although endemic and epidemic malaria are caused by the same *Plasmodium* parasites, they produce distinct impacts on health. In a region of epidemic transmission, malaria is present only a few months of the year, and the population has little or no immunity to the disease. When transmission occurs, the entire population is subject to acute attacks of malaria. The occurrence of symptoms in close prox-imity, temporally and spatially, to increases in mosquito populations both facili-tates the recognition of malaria and makes the role of mosquitoes in disease trans-mission easier to recognize.

In endemic areas, continuous (stable) transmission results in high levels of immunity in the human population. Instead of affecting all age groups rela-tively equally (as does epidemic malaria), most morbidity and mortality asso-ciated with endemic malaria occur in young children and pregnant women, and for this reason the Bagamoyo Bed Net Project focused on the health of children. As a result of their immunity, adults suffer acute attacks much less frequently, so much so that they may not view the control of fevers as a prior-ity. Endemic malaria produces a wide range of health impacts beyond acute attacks of fever. Some, such as cerebral malaria and severe malarial anemia in young children, are accompanied by fever. Others, including increased inci-dence of stillbirth, low birthweight, and premature delivery related to malaria in pregnancy, kidney failure, Burkitt's lymphoma, ruptured spleen, and poor performance at school or work secondary to anemia, may all develop in the absence of fever (Greenwood, 1987).

Monitoring of children aged 6–36 months in Bagamoyo District found at enrollment in the project that 86% were infected with malaria parasites, pri-marily *Plasmodium falciparum* (Premji et al., 1995b). Chloroquine resistance was present in 57% of malaria infections (Premji et al., 1994). The infant mortality rate was 131 per 1,000 live births. Verbal autopsies conducted for deaths in children less than four years of age found that 56% of deaths were due to malaria (Premji et al., 1997). The majority of young children were iron deficient, and malaria was the major cause (Premji et al., 1995a). People liv-ing in the study area received an average of 234 infective mosquito bites per year.

In Bagamoyo District, Tanzania, there are two rainy seasons, the long rains from March to June and the short rains from October to January (see Table 3.1). Mosquito populations show two annual peaks, one in May toward the end of the long rains and a much smaller one in December toward the end of the short rains. The months of May through July see the highest levels of infection in the

Table 3.1 Locally Defined Seasons and Their Perceived Characteristics Contrasted with Results of Mortality Surveillance and Collections of Mosquitoes with Light Traps

	JAN	FEB	MARCH	APRIL	MAY	JUNE	JULY	AUG	SEPT	OCT	NOV	DEC
Local term for the season												
English	Hot season of the new year		Long rains			Cold season and rice harvest			Hot season of the short rains		Short rains	
Swahili	Kiangazi cha mwaka		Masika			Kipupwe			Kiangazi cha vuli		Vuli	
Perceived health problems	Hernia "Fever of problems"		Mild febrile illnesses such as homa ya malaria			Severe febrile illnesses (e.g., degedege) and death, especially due to supernatural causes, weakness, "low blood"			Few problems, blood is strong		Mild febrile illnesses such as homa ya malaria	
Mean number of child deaths per month in study area, 1992–94	4.0	4.5	3.5	5.5	8.0	9.0	15.0	14.0	10.0	6.0	5.0	6.5
Mean number of Anopheles gambiae mosquitoes caught per trap per night	0.57	0.48	0.95	3.66	59.48	29.60	3.14	0.76	0.52	0.47	1.05	3.71
Percentage of mosquitoes infected	18%	7%	4%	5%	5%	7%	25%	9%	9%	6%	2%	5%

anopheline mosquitoes that transmit malaria. A peak of childhood mortality, to which malaria is one of the main contributors, occurs in July and August, although there are far fewer mosquitoes than in April and May.

Why Was Malaria Not a Community Priority?

The Problem

People who use nets perceive a wide range of benefits, including protection from mosquitoes and bedbugs, malaria prevention, privacy, decoration, and protection from roof debris dropping on the bed (Aikins et al., 1994; MacCormack and Snow, 1986). Projects promoting use of treated nets sometimes stress protection from biting insects, reasoning that this is a visible and immediate benefit, while protection from malaria is less tangible and less immediate. The BBNP chose to emphasize treated nets as a way of specifically preventing malaria because (1) in some villages, mosquito densities are low even during the long rains, and protection from mosquitoes would not motivate people to use nets; and (2) we wanted to promote the idea that using insecticide-treated nets is a community-wide activity that would have a greater impact on malaria transmission if everyone participated.

In an initial series of meetings with leaders of each of the villages, it was found that malaria control generally was not a high priority. It was felt that this situation might be due to problems of terminology. As noted by Helitzer et al. (1993), planners of malaria control programs commonly assume that one single local word or phrase can be found which corresponds to "malaria," and that it can serve multiple uses within the program. We therefore decided to investigate the vocabulary people use for the various health outcomes associated with clinical malaria, and specifically to look at which terms are thought to be serious.

Methods

A step-by-step approach for investigating local terminology and classification systems is described by Spradley (1979). Initially data on social and cultural characteristics of the 13 study villages were collected through group meetings in each village to which local government officials, religious leaders, teachers, and health workers were invited. "Free listing" is a method in which an individual or group is asked "what are all the types of X?" and prompted until an exhaustive list is obtained (Bernard, 1994; Weller and Romney, 1988). From free listing of illnesses conducted in these meetings, a list of 41 illness terms was compiled. "Pile sorting" was then performed with eight respondents (Bernard, 1994; Weller and Romney, 1988). Each illness term was written on a card, and respondents were then asked to put the cards into piles of similar illnesses and justify the groupings they had made, a process that took about two hours per respondent. Respondents who were unable to perform pile sorting because they were illiterate, were asked to talk about the different illnesses one by one. Pile sort data were analyzed using the computer program ANTHROPAC (Borgatti, 1996).

In a subsequent series of 40 unstructured interviews and focus groups, a comprehensive description of each illness, including perceived cause, symptoms, method of diagnosis, and treatment was elicited, as described by Scrimshaw and Hurtado (1987), with modifications specifically for malaria described by Agyepong et al. (1995). Finally, a survey was administered to a systematic random sample of 567 respondents from all 13 villages, which included items on symptoms and sources of treatment for locally defined illnesses compatible with clinical malaria.

Results and Use of the Findings

Based on pile sorting and unstructured interviews, seven groupings of illness terms were defined: routine fevers, fevers due to spirits, childhood illnesses, illnesses due to witchcraft and sorcery, swellings, illnesses of the genital organs, and skin conditions. The grouping of routine or mild fevers includes five terms: malaria fever (*homa ya malaria*), fevers due to personal problems, periodic fevers, ordinary fever, and fever from boils. The fact that *homa ya malaria* is placed in this group along with other non-serious fevers is evidence that people do not view it as a severe illness.

The term most commonly used to translate the word malaria was *homa ya malaria* or malaria fever, and for residents of the study area it is an illness closely associated in people's minds with formal health services (Winch et al., 1996). Survey respondents presented with a list of sources of treatment and asked which febrile illnesses could be treated at each one reported *homa ya malaria* as the illness least likely to be treated in the home (6.7%) or by a traditional healer (5.5%), and most likely to be treated by a village health worker (24.5%) or at the dispensary or hospital (96.5%). *Homa ya malaria* was said to be readily treatable with chloroquine. Among survey respondents, 92.9% agreed that the defining characteristic of *homa ya malaria* is that it is caused by mosquitoes.

The symptoms of *homa ya malaria* are those of acute malaria: episodic fever, chills, and headache. People diagnose *homa ya malaria* if they develop fever during the long or short rains when mosquitoes are numerous. *Homa ya malaria* was said to be mild, and several respondents stated outright that malaria is not an important problem.

Illnesses having symptoms compatible with severe malaria were seen as distinct from *homa ya malaria* and were placed either with severe fevers or with illnesses due to witchcraft and sorcery. Such conditions were referred to as "out-of-the-ordinary fevers" or "fevers which do not respond to hospital treatment." A serious attack by a spirit leads to very high fever (*homa kali*), along with signs that the brain is affected, such as "speaking other languages" and convulsions. Such attacks are regarded as best treated by traditional practitioners.

Among the terms for childhood illnesses, *degedege* was extremely important. It is used to refer to an illness with symptoms compatible with severe malaria (including cerebral malaria), yet most informants did not link it with *homa ya malaria*. Health workers use *degedege* to refer to convulsions in children. Although informants understood the meaning given to the word by health workers, their own use of the word denotes an illness with its own specific cause, symptoms, and treatments.

Degedege is recognized by the sudden onset of severe fever, trembling and/or stiffness of the limbs, frothing at the mouth, babbling incomprehensibly (which is sometimes interpreted as speaking foreign languages), and a high mortality rate. This illness is greatly feared, especially because of its sudden onset. *Degedege* is so feared that people hesitate to mention the illness by name, as its very mention might invite its occurrence in the household. This condition and others similar to it are thought by many to be unrelated to malaria; this leads people to underestimate the importance of malaria as a cause of death in children. A few people stated that *degedege* is caused by *homa ya malaria* going to the brain. Most others explained that it resulted from a spirit attacking the child. This spirit assumes the form of a bird and flies over houses, producing illness in the children sleeping inside.

There was little awareness of the relationship between malaria and anemia. In unstructured interviews, weakness and "low blood" were related to seasonal variations in temperature, work, and food availability, but not to *homa ya malaria*. The blood is said to be very low (dilute) from April to July due to lack of food, hard work in the fields, and the cold at night. If one is cut, the blood that comes out is almost like water. During November and December, the blood is said to be strong (concentrated) or "happy"—features associated with the availability of fruit such as mangoes and the hot weather. If one is cut, the blood that comes out is dark red.

In unstructured interviews with midwives and mothers of young children, malaria was not recognized as a problem in pregnancy. Special problems in the first pregnancy in young women are said to be seizures, headache, pains in the loins and stomach, hookworm, swollen calves of the legs, low blood, spontaneous abortions, and high mortality among newborns. When asked why some women tend to have more febrile illnesses during their first and second pregnancies, people stated this happened because they were young. Fever is perceived to be a normal sign of pregnancy instead of a symptom of *homa ya malaria*.

To summarize, there were numerous local terms for different illnesses that had symptoms compatible with clinical malaria. Given this situation, *homa ya malaria* (and the mosquitoes that bring it) was seen as just one of a large number of febrile illnesses found in the area, and not of any particular importance. Most people did not associate *homa ya malaria* with anemia, malaria in pregnancy, or cerebral malaria. People appeared to have little difficulty in accepting that mosquito nets are an effective way to prevent *homa ya malaria*, as it is, by definition, that type of *homa* illness caused by mosquitoes.

The research made it clear that there were major differences in perceptions of "malaria" and terminology used to describe conditions compatible with clinical malaria. A number of measures were taken to facilitate communication between project staff and villagers. Early in the project, personnel were briefed on the findings: they were told that local people have perceptions of malaria quite different from those of health workers, and implications for how this would affect interactions with the residents of the study area were discussed. Since *homa ya malaria* was seen as a mild illness with few consequences, efforts were made to make people aware of the other consequences of malaria infection. Whenever *homa ya malaria* was mentioned in plays, booklets, or clinics, consequences of infections—such as anemia, *degedege*, missing school, tiredness, and adverse pregnancy outcomes—were also mentioned. This was done without being judgmental about local medical knowledge. It was not stated that local illnesses, such as those caused by spirits, do not exist, or that they are the same thing as *homa ya malaria*. Instead it was stated that *homa ya malaria* can cause *degedege* and other serious illnesses.

Another key finding was that control of *homa ya malaria* was not a high priority for many people because it was only one of many different types of fever and also because people had a number of competing priorities such as transport, water, and food. Again, several approaches were adopted to address this issue. Meetings were held in every village to discuss the results of epidemiological studies. Many people saw the symptoms and the long-term consequences of *homa ya malaria* as synonymous, so project personnel attempted to draw a distinction between the symptoms (*dalili*) of malaria, such as fever, and the negative effects (*madhara*) of the disease, such as anemia. Communicating this proved to be extremely difficult. When asked about the negative effects of malaria, most people still spontaneously mentioned the symptoms of acute disease, such as fever and chills, although some then went on to mention anemia and malaria in pregnancy.

Traditional healers were found to treat many of the cases of severe malaria (Makemba et al., 1996). Efforts were made to involve traditional healers in promoting the nets, while at the same time neither denigrating their practices nor denying the existence of conditions that they treat, such as spirit possession. Some traditional healers served as members of village mosquito net committees, and one even purchased mosquito nets for all the beds in his inpatient ward. The messages and approaches discussed here were incorporated into posters, village meetings, and plays written and performed during net distribution and before clinics.

Perceptions of Seasonal Variation in Risk of Malaria

The Problem

There have been several reports of seasonal variation in use of mosquito nets (e.g., Cattani et al., 1986). People will sleep under nets during the peak of the mosquito season, but when mosquito densities drop and the rains stop, nets may be put into storage until they are thought to be needed again. Thus a problem the project faced was convincing people to sleep under nets in months when mosquitoes were few, especially July and August, when the level of infection in mosquitoes is high and a peak in childhood mortality occurs (Table 3.1).

Methods

Three steps were involved in examining perceptions of seasonality. In the first step, a list of terms used for seasons and/or seasonal events was obtained primarily through discussing the yearly cycle of agricultural activities with farmers and fisherman in several different villages. Informants were asked for a detailed description of what happened in each season: weather, agriculture, fishing, ceremonies, and illnesses.

The purpose of the second step was to obtain a visual impression of the changes occurring over the year. A chart with 7 columns and 12 rows was drawn on the inside of a file folder, the central column representing the calendar months. Columns on either side of the central column represented items of interest to the study: rainfall, the direction the wind blows from, the numbers of mosquitoes, the frequency of fevers (homa), whether people have "high" or "low" blood, and the foods commonly eaten. A set of cards was made up for each column. For example, for the mosquito column, cards had many mosquitoes drawn on one side, but only one mosquito drawn on the other. For the rain column, one side showed clouds and rain, and the other side showed sun. For each column, informants went down the months and indicated which side of the card should be facing up. For example, for the rain column, the respondent was asked whether each season or month was rainy or sunny and then to indicate that by placing the card either "sunny side up" or "rainy side up" in the row corresponding to that month. For the few informants who did not understand calendar months, names of local seasons were used instead, although this was problematic because local seasons overlap considerably. In the final step, questions concerning perceptions of seasonality were placed on the survey to confirm the results of the qualitative research in a broader, systematic sample of the population.

Results and Use of Findings

Villagers' descriptions of seasons and of seasonal variation in mosquito populations differed little from the findings of project staff. Differences between residents of the study area and project personnel lay in perceptions of seasonal variation for various illnesses, as noted earlier.

Informants stated that the long rains (*masika*) typically start in March, are very heavy in April and May, and taper off in June (Table 3.1). This was said to be the worst time of the year for mosquitoes, with heavy biting from dusk until dawn, and an increase in all types of fevers due to hard work, getting caught in the rain while working in the fields, and mosquitoes.

The cold season (*kipupwe*) occurs in the months of June, July, and August (Table 3.1). The cold is thought to make the body very weak and susceptible to illness, as well as making the blood flow sluggish. The blood, in addition, is said to be very dilute during the *kipupwe*, as a result of both the cold and the poorer quality of foods available in the preceding months.

One of the most prominent features of the *kipupwe* is said to be a steep drop in the number of mosquitoes. Mosquitoes are said to be weakened by the cold, just as humans are. Typical comments were "the mosquitoes have no strength" and "they lose their voice," the latter referring to the decrease in the number of mosquitoes buzzing in people's ears at night.

Other events at this time are the rice harvest and circumcision rites for adolescent males. This time of the year is closely associated with sickness and death from febrile illnesses, severe fevers due primarily to spirits, witchcraft, and sorcery (Table 3.1). Some respondents stated that spirits attack people during the rice harvest because food is plentiful and people can eat until they are full, a version of the idea that bad luck befalls those who are doing well. Rites known as *madogoli*, which last one to two days, are performed during the rice harvest (see Swantz, 1970). The function of these rites can be either to placate spirits, such as *kinyamkera*, that attack people at this time of year, or to treat people made ill by these spirits.

To summarize, the months of June, July, and August are associated with cold weather, a decrease in the number of mosquitoes, weak blood, the south wind, the rice harvest, circumcision and initiation rites, severe fevers caused by spirits and witchcraft and the rites to placate these spirits. *Homa ya malaria* is not thought to be common at this time, because mosquitoes are weak and few in number. The lower mosquito densities and cooler temperatures at night lead people to conclude that mosquitoes are not a major cause of illness at this time and to explain the occurrence of fevers through causes not related to malaria, such as the malevolent influence of spirits.

As the main peak in malaria-related mortality and rates of infection in mosquitoes occurs in July and August, well after the peak in mosquito densities in May and June, many of the cases of severe and fatal malaria are attributed not to *homa ya malaria*, but rather to other causes. This had two unwanted effects, from the perspective of the project: (1) It reinforced the idea that *homa ya malaria* was not a serious condition, making it more difficult to build community interest in malaria control; and (2) People failed to see the need to use mosquito nets during the months of June, July, and August.

"Malaria is a big threat every month of the year" became one of the central messages in educational activities, including plays and public meetings. A local artist was commissioned to create a panel with a drawing for each season, each drawing depicting typical activities for that season. The panel, with five locally defined seasons and recommendations to sleep under nets throughout the year, was used to spread the message. It was reproduced on the center pages of a booklet about how to use a net and given to people when they purchased their nets; the panel also formed the top half of a 1993 wall calendar which was distributed free throughout the project area.

A series of interviews with 40 respondents conducted after the calendars were distributed showed that people understood the message the calendars were communicating. Several respondents thought the sole purpose of the calendar was to remind people about when the nets needed to be retreated with insecticide, and two individuals mentioned that the calendar showed that nets are needed only during the rainy season. Illiterate people were less likely to understand the message. Future calendars might show someone sleeping under a net during each of the seasons to make the point more explicit.

The January 1993 Net Usage Survey

In January 1993, a net usage survey was conducted in the second group of villages to receive the nets. This is the hottest and driest period of the year, and a time when mosquito densities are low, so we would expect net use to be at a minimum. One purpose of the survey was to see whether messages about the importance of using nets even during the hot months were having any effect.

In a systematic sample of the three villages surveyed, 666 households were visited, in which a total of 2,713 people were living. The survey located 641 nets, or an average of 0.96 net per household, and 477 (74%) of the nets had been used on the previous night. Few households yet had enough nets to cover all members in the household. An average of almost 2 nets per household would be necessary to allow all adults and children to sleep under nets.

During the regular monthly meetings held with village mosquito net committees and during interviews described in the next section to investigate reasons for low rates of retreatment of nets, reasons for the low coverage and inadequate usage in some parts of these villages were explored. Some of the factors included greater access to nets for males in the household, seasonal migration, the inconvenience and/or discomfort associated with using nets during the hottest season of the year, and the continued perception that there is no reason to sleep under nets when there are few mosquitoes.

Some households had more than enough nets for every bed, but one or more nets were set aside for guests. In many households, nets were bought one at a time over the duration of the project. The first to have access to the nets were adult men, then women, then children. Most spouses were found to sleep separately, largely because of the heat, so that the wife did not automatically gain access to a net along with her husband. Very young children sleep with their mothers and are therefore more likely than older children to sleep under a net. Most children over two years of age do not sleep with their mothers; they are in the group least likely to sleep under nets. The problem of children not sleeping under nets was addressed specifically in a new version of the plays that emphasized the importance of purchasing nets for children.

Seasonal variation in patterns of work affected net usage in two ways. First, some people migrate to the city during the dry season. They may take a net with them for protection from urban mosquitoes, although many of these are *Culex* species and do not transmit malaria. This deprives one or more of the household members remaining in the village of use of the net. Second, seasonal patterns of work result in seasonal access to cash, thus restricting the ability to purchase nets and retreat them. Owners of small plots of land said they had the most cash income from November to February, when cashew nuts and mangoes are harvested, and very little income from March to June, before the rice harvest. People working as day laborers in agriculture have no work when it is hot and dry, while those who work in the salt mines (harvesting salt from seawater) on the Indian Ocean have the opposite pattern: when it rains they have no work.

Some people found net use to be inconvenient, for reasons such as the following: interference with getting in and out of bed; the need to wash and retreat the net with insecticide; and, when people sleep outside to guard the crops just before the harvest season, the difficulty of watching for animals from under a net.

Creating a Demand for Retreatment of the Nets

The Problem

Although the initial phase of sales and distribution of treated nets enjoyed considerable success in the 13 project villages (Makemba et al., 1995), during the first cycle of retreatment in three coastal villages in November and December 1992 rates of retreatment (59%–77%) fell far short of the desired minimum level of 80%, and they fell further (20%–55%) when cost recovery was instituted in May–June 1993.

Methods

First Phase. A series of 60 semistructured open-ended interviews was conducted in September and December 1993 in the three coastal villages where retreatment had first taken place. Interviewers asked 20 respondents to list all the different types of *dawa* they knew (a local term that refers to both insecticide and pharmaceuticals), and to discuss benefits of treating nets with the insecticide, side effects of the insecticide, and barriers to bringing nets in for retreatment. Members of village mosquito net committees and of village governments were also interviewed. As a result of these interviews, a series of neighborhood (hamlet) meetings was held in all study villages to discuss people's concerns about the insecticide and ways to increase rates of retreatment. Changes were made in the procedure for retreatment to make it more convenient, but subsequent rates of retreatment (43%–65%) were still lower than expected and showed marked variation within as well as between villages.

Second Phase. In February 1994, four members of the research team spent one week in a village where variation in retreatment rates was present, to try to understand the causes. During this time they carried out participant observation of sleeping patterns, 20 unstructured key informant interviews about factors that might affect rates of retreatment, and informal discussions with villagers during the evenings. Notes from semistructured and unstructured interviews, hamlet meetings, and participant observation were expanded, entered into word processing files, and coded for different reasons for not retreating nets.

Results of the First Phase of Investigation

Whenever villagers referred to the insecticide, the Swahili word invariably used was *dawa*. The meaning of *dawa* that emerged from the interviews is very broad and encompasses almost any substance that produces noticeable effects, including drugs obtained at the pharmacy, treatments prescribed by traditional practitioners, and poisons for controlling rodents (Winch et al., 1997).

Twenty respondents were asked to list all the types of *dawa* they knew. Types of *dawa* mentioned three or more times were the chemical fungicide used to treat the cashew trees (18 mentions); chloroquine, or "bitter medicine" (9); aspirin (8); and three proprietary pain medications, Aspro (3), Panadol (3), and Cafenol (3).

All 60 respondents in the initial set of interviews felt that the insecticide "works," or has beneficial effects. Respondents also stated that overall mosquito densities, as well as fevers, had diminished since the introduction of the nets. When describing the impact of the insecticide on insects, respondents used words such as poison (*sumu*), danger (*hatari*), harsh/strong (*kali*), and kill/death, as in statements such as "It's strong *dawa*, it even kills cockroaches." The permethrin insecticide used in this project was either referred to as *dawa* with no qualification, or as *dawa ya chandalua* (*dawa* for the net).

In 60 semistructured interviews and meetings with members of village mosquito net committees and local leaders in the three coastal villages, four principal reasons were cited for the low rates of retreatment of nets: (1) the fee; (2) the inconvenience of bringing a net to a central point for retreatment; (3) lack of net use; and (4) concerns about toxicity of the insecticide. Of the four reasons, the first three were common to all villages, while concern about toxicity was a focal problem strongly influenced by local leaders.

The main reason people stated that they could not pay the fee was that they had not had sufficient advance notice. Information about payment of the fee was disseminated only in the month before the retreatment exercise. Villagers asserted that they needed three or more months advance notice to put aside money for the fee. Others objected to the change in policy: retreatment had been free during the first round (November–December 1992), then a fee equivalent to 40 cents (US) per net retreated was instituted (May–June 1993). People who disapproved of the fee sometimes cited the fact that other types of modern *dawa*, such as agricultural chemicals and medicines, are given away free by the government. Although many could afford to pay for retreatment, they objected to the principle of paying for modern *dawa*. Finally, some people objected to paying for the *dawa* while the foreigners (*wazungu*) were still around: why couldn't they pay for it?

Efficacy and toxicity of the *dawa* were felt to go hand-in-hand: the greater the demonstrable effects of any given *dawa*, the greater the potential for toxicity. Some respondents considered any *dawa* to be potentially poisonous. Certain aspects of the way the nets were treated with insecticide amplified concerns about toxicity. Villagers who were treating the nets had to wear gloves, and people were told not to touch the insecticide and to burn or bury the plastic bag that they used to carry the nets home, all of which heightened concerns about toxicity, especially where children were concerned. Some people felt that if the *dawa* was so toxic for insects and other small animals, it would also be toxic for children. Another reason that children were said to be particularly vulnerable to the toxic effects of the insecticide was that they might chew or suck on the netting while asleep.

In response to concerns about access to retreatment, more retreatment stations were organized, and they operated for three days instead of one. Demand for retreatment was stimulated through meetings at the neighborhood or hamlet level (*kitongoji*) and in mosques (Mfaume et al., 1997) to stress the importance of retreatment and to answer any questions people might have. Previously only village-wide meetings had been held, and these were found primarily to reach men living at the center of the village, as they were the ones who attended and sat near the front of the audience.

Results of the Second Phase of Investigation

As a result of these changes in the procedure for retreatment of nets, it was expected that rates of retreatment would be much higher in the second group of three villages than in the first group of three coastal villages. Rates of retreatment in this second group of villages in December 1993 were 43.4%, 43.3%, and 44.3%, a disappointing result. These low overall rates masked the fact that some sectors (hamlets) of the villages had high rates, while others had low rates. In each of the villages, the sectors with the lowest rates tended to be older, long-settled, central parts of the village whose residents were mostly from local (coastal) ethnic groups (Zaramo and Kwere). The sectors with the highest rates tended to be newer, recently settled, peripheral parts of the village whose residents were mostly immigrants from southern and central Tanzania.

To investigate this situation further, four members of the research team each spent one week in a different sector of Mapinga village. They found that most of the variation in rates of retreatment was attributable to economic and political factors. Mapinga village is divided into two major groups, a pattern also observed in neighboring villages. One group, dominated by the Zaramo, consists of people that live at the center of the village and speak local languages. The other group is referred to as the "guests" (*wageni*) by the first group. They have migrated to the coast from the interior of Tanzania, and they are predominantly Christian. They live on the periphery of the village where land is more plentiful, cultivate larger plots of land, grow a greater variety of crops including maize, and are insistent that their children attend public school.

Many, but far from all, in the first group stated either directly or indirectly that their power and way of life are being eroded by the influx of government employees, migrants, and externally funded projects into Bagamoyo District. Those in the second group, the guests, had a different point of view. They considered treatment of diseases with modern medicines and treatment of nets with modern *dawa* to be a positive step, and one of a number of modern behaviors and technologies in which they are eager to invest. They have moved into the area to improve their lives and those of their children.

It was also found that the *balozi*, local leaders who each represent 10 households and attend village meetings, are highly aware of the rates of retreatment achieved in their neighborhood. High rates of retreatment are interpreted as a sign of support for the *balozi*, as well as for the village mosquito net committees and the village government. Factionalism in the center of villages apparently results in some people not bringing in their nets for retreatment. Conversely, the social cohesion and strong leadership found in peripheral areas of the villages favor higher rates of retreatment. Leaders in the three peripheral hamlets reiterated their support of the project in interviews and sent strong messages to their fellow villagers to buy nets and bring them in for retreatment. The research team also noted that there is more trust between neighbors in the peripheral areas, which allows people to borrow money to have their nets retreated and pay it back later.

The interviews demonstrate that although logistical problems were the common explanation for failure to bring nets for retreatment, political or social divisions within the community needed to be taken into account to explain variation in rates of retreatment within villages. In subsequent rounds of retreatment, efforts were made to address these political factors. Attempts were made to have all different groups in the village represented on the village mosquito net committee. To promote net sales and retreatment, the source of information or channel of communication was changed according to the group being addressed; for example, if one group had low rates of retreatment, another person from the same group was sent to speak to them. More politically neutral channels of communication were used, for example, elementary schools instead of the village government.

Even with these changes, rates of retreatment did not increase to an acceptable level in all villages. Timing the retreatment opportunity to the seasonal cash flow of local residents is much more complex than at first glance, as each occupational group has its own best time for cash availability, and each neighborhood may contain a variety of occupational groups. One solution to this problem is to have sachets containing sufficient insecticide to treat one net on sale in local shops, so that people can retreat their own nets whenever they see the need. This approach has three disadvantages: (1) great effort is needed to develop unambiguous instructions suitable for illiterate people, so the correct dosage of insecticide is applied to the nets; (2) people will use whatever container is available in the household to treat their net, which may be a cooking pot or container for storing food; and (3) higher rates of retreatment may be achieved when the entire community is mobilized to bring in their nets on the same day.

Discussion

The investigations described in this chapter indicate the utility of anthropological approaches in efforts to promote insecticide-treated mosquito nets in Africa. The flexible nature of these methods allowed them to address a wide range of problems. The findings changed the attitudes of project personnel toward local knowledge and enabled them to communicate more effectively with villagers. Rather than viewing local ways of naming, diagnosing, and treating illnesses as "wrong," project personnel could see that local knowledge was internally consistent and had its own logic. This recognition led them to negotiate with villagers about how to implement the project, rather than imposing predefined plans and procedures.

In retrospect, the greatest problem in sustaining the intervention has been political and administrative in nature, including lack of either a public or private system to make nets and insecticide available at the village level and difficulties in implementing cost recovery. When cost recovery was implemented, rates of retreatment fell, as has also been found in The Gambia (D'Alessandro et al., 1995a). While village mosquito net committees (Makemba et al., 1995) are still functioning and the demand for nets is still high, there has been considerable difficulty in obtaining the political commitment at all levels (national, regional, district) needed to make the intervention sustainable. This raises the question of whether it would have been profitable to employ anthropological methods to investigate perceptions of the intervention among decision makers, as Justice (1986) and others have suggested, rather than focus exclusively on the villagers.

References

Agyepong IA, Aryee B, Dzikunu H, Manderson L (1995) The Malaria Manual. Geneva: World Health Organization. TDR/SER/MSR/95.1

Aikins MK, Pickering H, Greenwood BM (1994) Attitudes to malaria, traditional practices and bednets (mosquito nets) as vector control measures: a comparative study in five west African countries. *Journal of Tropical Medicine and Hygiene* 97:81–88.

Beidelman TO (1967) The Matrilineal Peoples of Eastern Tanzania. London: International Africa Institute.

Bernard HR (1994) Research Methods in Anthropology. Thousand Oaks, Calif: Sage Publications.

Borgatti S (1996) ANTHROPAC 4.92. Columbia, SC: Analytic Technologies Ltd.

Carnevale P, Coosemans M (1995) Some operational aspects of the use of personal protection methods against malaria at individual and community levels. *Annales de la Société Belge de Médecine Tropicale* 75:81–103.

Cattani JA, Tulloch JL, Vrbova H, Jolley D, Gibson FD, Moir JS, Heywood PF, Alpers MP, Stevenson A, Clancy R (1986) The epidemiology of malaria in a population surrounding Madang, Papua New Guinea. *American Journal of Tropical Medicine and Hygiene* 35:3–15.

D'Alessandro U, Olaleye BO, McGuire W, Langerock P, Bennett S, Aikins MK, Thomson MC, Cham MK, Cham BA, Greenwood BM (1995a) Mortality and morbidity from malaria in Gambian children after introduction of an impregnated bednet programme. *Lancet* 345:479–483.

D'Alessandro U, Olaleye BO, McGuire W, Thomson MC, Langerock P, Bennett S, Greenwood BM (1995b) A comparison of the efficacy of insecticide-treated and untreated bed nets in preventing malaria in Gambian children. *Transactions of the Royal Society of Tropical Medicine and Hygiene* 89:596–598.

Feilden R (1996) "Experiences of Implementation." In: Net Gain. Operational Aspects of a New Health Intervention for Preventing Malaria Death. C Lengeler, J Cattani, D de Savigny, eds. Geneva: World Health Organization/TDR and Ottawa: International Development Research Center, pp. 55–110.

Greenwood BM (1987) Asymptomatic malaria infections: do they matter? *Parasitology Today* 3:206–214.

Helitzer DL, Kendall C, Wirima JJ (1993) The role of ethnographic research in malaria control: an example from Malawi. *Research in the Sociology of Health Care* 10:269–286.

Justice J (1986) Policies, Plans, and People: Culture and Health Development in Nepal. Berkeley: University of California Press.

Lengeler C, Lines JD, Cattani J, Feilden R, Zimicki S, de Savigny D (1996) Promoting operational research on insecticide-treated netting: a joint TDR/IDRC initiative and call for research proposals. *Tropical Medicine and International Health* 1:273–276.

Lines J (1996a) "The Technical Issues." In: Net Gain. Operational Aspects of a New Health Intervention for Preventing Malaria Death. C Lengeler, J Cattani, D de Savigny, eds. Geneva: World Health Organization/TDR and Ottawa: International Development Research Center, pp. 17–53.

Lines JD (1996b) Mosquito nets and insecticides for net treatment: a discussion of existing and potential distribution systems in Africa. *Tropical Medicine and International Health* 1:616–632.

MacCormack CP, Snow RW (1986) Gambian cultural preferences in the use of insecticide-impregnated bed nets. *Journal of Tropical Medicine and Hygiene* 89:295–302.

Makemba AM, Winch PJ, Kamazima SR, Makame V, Sengo F, Lubega PB, Minjas JN, Shiff CJ (1995) Implementation of a community-based system for the sale, distribution and insecticide impregnation of mosquito nets in Bagamoyo District, Tanzania. *Health Policy and Planning* 10:50–59.

Makemba AM, Winch PJ, Makame VM, Premji Z, Minjas JN, Shiff CJ (1996) Treatment practices for *degedege*, a locally recognized febrile illness, and implications for strategies to decrease mortality from severe malaria in Bagamoyo District, Tanzania. *Tropical Medicine and International Health* 1:305–313.

Mfaume MS, Winch PJ, Makemba AM, Premji Z (1997) Mosques against malaria. *World Health Forum* 18:35–38.

Middleton J (1992) The World of the Swahili. An African Mercantile Civilization. New Haven: Yale University Press.

Premji Z, Hamisi Y, Shiff C, Minjas J, Lubega P, Makwaya C (1995a) Anaemia and *Plasmodium falciparum* infections among young children in an holoendemic area, Bagamoyo, Tanzania. *Acta Tropica* 59:55–64.

Premji Z, Lubega P, Hamisi Y, Mchopa E, Minjas J, Checkley W, Shiff C (1995b) Changes in malaria associated morbidity in children using insecticide treated mosquito nets in the Bagamoyo District of Tanzania. *Tropical Medicine and Parasitology* 46:147–153.

Premji Z, Minjas JN, Shiff CJ (1994) Chloroquine resistant *Plasmodium falciparum* in coastal Tanzania. A challenge to the continued strategy of village based chemotherapy for malaria control. *Tropical Medicine and Parasitology* 45:47–48.

Premji Z, Ndayanga P, Shiff C, Minjas J, Lubega P, MacLeod J (1997) Community based studies on childhood mortality in a malaria holoendemic area on the Tanzanian coast. *Acta Tropica* 63:101–109.

Scrimshaw SCM, Hurtado E (1987) Rapid Assessment Procedures for Nutrition and Primary Health Care. Anthropological Approaches to Improving Programme Effectiveness. Los Angeles: University of California, Latin American Center Publications.

Spradley JP (1979) The Ethnographic Interview. New York: Harcourt Brace Jovanovich.

Swantz M-L (1970) Ritual and Symbol in Transitional Zaramo Society: With Special Reference to Women. Studia Missionalia Uppsaliensia 16. Uppsala: Gleerup-Lund.

Weller SC, Romney AK (1988) Systematic Data Collection. Thousand Oaks, Calif: Sage Publications.

WHO (1996) Division of Control of Tropical Diseases, Progress Report 1996. Geneva: World Health Organization.

Winch PJ, Makemba AM, Kamazima SR, Lurie M, Lwihula GK, Premji Z, Minjas JN, Shiff CJ (1996) Local terminology for febrile illnesses in Bagamoyo District, Tanzania and its impact on the design of a community-based malaria control programme. *Social Science and Medicine* 42:1057–1067.

Winch PJ, Makemba AM, Kamazima SR, Lwihula GK, Lubega P, Minjas JN, Shiff CJ (1994) Seasonal variation in the perceived risk of malaria: implications for the promotion of insecticide-impregnated bed nets. *Social Science and Medicine* 39:63–75.

Winch PJ, Makemba AM, Makame VR, Mfaume MS, Lynch MC, Premji Z, Minjas JN, Shiff CJ (1997) Social and cultural factors affecting rates of regular reimpregnation of mosquito nets with insecticide in Bagamoyo District, Tanzania. *Tropical Medicine and International Health* 2:760–770.

Zimicki S (1996) "Promotion in Sub-Saharan Africa." In: Net Gain. Operational Aspects of a New Health Intervention for Preventing Malaria Death. C Lengeler, J Cattani, D de Savigny, eds. Geneva: World Health Organization/TDR and Ottawa: International Development Research Center, pp. 111–147.

based on the premise that it is critical to discover the indigenous or ethnomedical system of beliefs relating to a domain of health in which there is to be an attempt at behavior change—in fact, this is far more useful than KAP surveys which simply demonstrate lack of biomedical knowledge.

The program involving traditional healers aimed to reduce the spread of HIV not only through the promotion of responsible sexual behavior and condom use but also by means of treatment and prevention of other sexually transmitted diseases (STDs),[1] which themselves increase the likelihood of HIV infection. Specifically, a proposed program objective was to reduce STD incidence and thereby HIV seropositivity by first modifying the behavior of traditional healers (in their referral if not their treatment practices) and then, through them, modifying the behavior of their clients. Another objective was to promote reduction in numbers of sexual partners by reinforcing indigenous beliefs about the dangers of sex with strangers.

A basic hypothesis was that AIDS prevention efforts could take advantage of the prestige, credibility, authority, and widespread availability of traditional healers to promote behavior change and the adoption of new technology (such as condoms) among their clients. Research suggests that traditional healers see and attempt to treat many or most STD cases in southern Africa, if not in all of Africa (Good, 1987; Green, 1994; Nzima, 1995). Healers also provide vaccinations and participate in ritual scarification, using razor blades, thus facilitating transmission of AIDS. It is generally accepted that about 80% of the people of sub-Saharan Africa rely on traditional healers for treatment of all conditions, even if many also visit hospitals (Bannerman et al., 1983). In Mozambique, the proportion relying on traditional healers may be even higher because of poverty, inaccessibility of biomedical health services, and years of attacks against the government's rural health personnel and infrastructure during Mozambique's civil war (1976–1992). Preliminary census studies by the Department of Traditional Medicine (Gabinete de Estudos de Medicina Tradicional, or GEMT) of the Mozambique Ministry of Health suggest a ratio of roughly 1 traditional healer for every 200 people. This estimate is comparable to estimates made elsewhere in sub-Saharan Africa (specified in Green, 1994:19). Given a national population of about 17 million, Mozambique can be estimated to have approximately 85,000 healers. The physician to population ratio in Mozambique is about 1:50,000, with some 52% of doctors concentrated in the capital city.

My GEMT colleagues and I proposed a three-year program to establish a foundation for public health collaboration between traditional healers and the National Health Service (Green et al., 1991). In 1991, I designed and directed preliminary ethnomedical research in Manica province in a pilot program focusing on child diarrheal disease and sexually transmitted disease, including AIDS. These foci were chosen because (1) both diseases were and are priority areas of preventive and promotive health care for the Ministry of Health; (2)

the GEMT lacked the resources to work directly in more than two health topics, at least initially; (3) there was prior experience collaborating with traditional healers in diarrheal disease control elsewhere in Africa, and (4) there was already interest on the part of Mozambique's National AIDS program in such collaboration. The first phase of the pilot program consisted of what has come to be called rapid ethnographic research (Yoder, 1997). This was followed by development of a research-based communications strategy, a "training" workshop, and, finally, impact evaluation.

The current program of indigenous–biomedical collaboration was funded for at least three years by the Swiss Development Cooperation (beginning 1994). I served as program adviser for the first year. Following the pilot program in Manica, there have been additional GEMT collaborative programs based on the pilot model, in Gaza, Maputo, Inhambane, and Nampula provinces.

Healers in our study came from Shona ethnolinguistic groups: Ute, Ndau, Manica, and Sena. There are roughly 10 million Shona living today in Zimbabwe and another roughly 1.8 million in west-central Mozambique. The Shona occupy a geographical position between the Central Bantu to the north and west and the Nguni to the south. They are primarily agricultural, raising maize as well as millet, rice, beans, manioc, groundnuts, pumpkins, and sweet potatoes. Animal husbandry is practiced by the Shona but it is not as important as among some neighboring groups. They live in dispersed hamlets or homesteads (kraals). Group membership is primarily patrilineal, unlike their matrilineal Central Bantu neighbors. Historically, the Shona were organized in relatively complex states: a king lived with advisers in a royal court in a capital village or town and received tribute from outlying chieftaincies (Murdock, 1959). The Shona have undergone great social changes in the last two or three generations, due to major conflicts related to independence, wage labor, urbanization, and government policies intended to rapidly modernize people in both Zimbabwe and Mozambique.

Development of Cultural Sensitivity in Mozambique Since Independence

Before 1989, the concept "culturally appropriate" would have made little sense in the context of government programs, including health programs. A brief sketch of Mozambique's history since independence is needed to explain this. The Frelimo party fought Portuguese colonial rule, eventually winning independence for Mozambique in 1975. Mozambique's health system in the late 1970s and 1980s was in some ways a model for Africa, "in the forefront internationally" of primary health care (Hanlon, 1984:55). For the majority indigenous population this represented a great improvement over the health system under colonial rule: whereas the old system had emphasized curative services for whites, the new system emphasized rural outreach and prevention and established a widespread system of health centers, health posts, and village health workers.

On the other hand, the new system was centralized and top-down in the extreme. It was unresponsive to existing local health beliefs, values, felt needs, priorities, and social organization. There was no attempt to understand indigenous health systems, which were equated with witchcraft practices and spirit beliefs, both of which had no place in Frelimo's program of "scientific socialism." The government felt its mission was to enlighten "the masses," to show them the error of their superstitious ways. Accordingly it attempted to suppress indigenous medicine and its practitioners, along with other backward-seeming features of local cultures, such as polygyny, bride payments, initiation rites, and the system of chiefs and their councils. In response, the indigenous health system (along with the political system, initiation rites, etc.) simply went underground and continued much as before despite the official ideology.

By the Fifth Frelimo Party Congress in 1989, the government formally recognized the mistakes it had made in its zeal to create a new, equitable, unified, national society. In late 1990, because of my background in applied anthropology in Africa (ethnographic and survey research in Swaziland [1981–1990], Nigeria [1985–1988], and Liberia [1988]), I was asked to assist the Ministry of Health in defining a role for traditional healers. The pilot and the current program are direct outcomes of this consultancy. The Frelimo party, elected in Mozambique's first multiparty election in 1994, is today a party that has been humbled by recognition of the power of culture (Green, 1995).

Pilot Program: STI-Related Beliefs and Practices of Traditional Healers

Research Methods

Prior to the GEMT program, little was known about indigenous Mozambican theories and healing practices related to STIs. Our pilot research was exploratory in nature and related to complex beliefs and behaviors which Africans, including Mozambicans, tend to keep secret from those (such as government interviewers) who may hold unsympathetic or even derisive views. Systematic in-depth interviews and focus group discussions were conducted with a representative sample of traditional healers, as described below. Interviewers approached healers with respect and sincere interest, and this helped to overcome their suspicion; however, a few healers would not be interviewed or participate in the program.

Our research does not qualify as ethnographic in the traditional sense; it was of the "rapid research" or "focused ethnographic study" type (Bentley et al., 1988; Yoder, 1997). I did not live in the region prior to the study; in fact, I spent only a few weeks in the study area. However, I trained and collaborated with four Mozambican health workers, three of whom were from the local groups under investigation. Such applied, rapid research methods have become the norm in applied or operations research in international health. There is not enough time to conduct the long-term, ethnographic research distinctive of anthropology. Fortunately, anthropological studies of African societies—or neighboring societies—where health programs are to be carried out are usually available and can provide applied researchers with a general sociocultural context, if not more specific ethnomedical information. In the present case, there was abundant ethnographic material on the Shona from across the border in Zimbabwe.

Why interview traditional healers rather than those who consult them? First, since they are the immediate group with whom we wished to collaborate directly, we needed to understand how they perceive illness. Second, healers presumably represent the beliefs of clients who consult them and they are often better able than their clients to articulate such beliefs, both because of their specialized knowledge and because their status in the community makes them less likely to be intimidated by an interviewer (Bishaw, 1989; de Sousa, 1991; Green and Nzima, 1995; Nzima, 1995; Reis, 1994). On the other hand, healing knowledge is considered sacred and secret in much of Africa. Some healers feel constrained by their empowering spirits not to reveal secret information to interviewers. Again, approaching them with sincerity and respect helped overcome resistance, as did taking the time to fully explain the purpose and objectives of the GEMT program.

Random sampling was not attempted since we lacked an adequate sampling frame. To select healers to be interviewed, we collaborated with the Manica branch of AMETRAMO, the national healers association, which helped to provide balance by gender, age, and district. As with the membership of AMETRAMO itself, there may have been a selection bias in favor of more urbanized, Portuguese-speaking healers. Considerations of war and security for interviewers biased the sample in the same direction. This choice had a useful side effect in that urbanized, Portuguese-speaking healers were more willing to attend workshops than their rural counterparts.

Between February and October 1991, in-depth interviews were conducted with 51 traditional healers reporting a specialty in sexually transmitted illnesses. A semistructured interview schedule was used, with some 90% of interviews conducted in the Shona language, and 10% in Portuguese. Interviews took place in the homes of healers in the five districts of Manica province accessible by road. Key informants were sometimes interviewed again to clarify points that arose in earlier interviews. Interview schedules had to be flexible as information gained in interviews might generate new questions. For example, before the initial interviews, we had no idea about the complex concept of *nyoka* (see below), which required exploration through a new series of questions.

We also used focus group discussion (FGD), a type of research that has been used increasingly in public health and behavioral science in recent years. As a qualitative method, it has more in common with in-depth interviews than with survey research using a fixed questionnaire. A moderator guides discussion to focus on specific topics of research interest, and a recorder keeps a written record of the discussion session. A topic guide developed in advance is used as a framework for discussion. As with in-depth interviews and survey research, focus group research has advantages and disadvantages. It is especially useful to discover or confirm the existence of broad patterns. It is not useful for measuring or quantifying patterns. Since it is not based on a random sample, its findings cannot be projected to a larger population.

In Manica, we conducted five FGDs, two focused exclusively on AIDS and STIs. They were conducted in villages or in the compounds of traditional healers in order to help participants feel relaxed and unintimidated by any of the trappings or symbols of allopathic medicine or the government. Nevertheless, many healers tended to adopt a polite, accommodating, deferential manner they had learned to present to government officials. There seemed to be pressure during FGDs for healers to conform to a unified view, in line with the views of health authorities. In-depth interviews held in private yielded far more useful information.

Findings

According to our research, healing knowledge is passed along within families, often from a paternal or maternal grandparent. There are two basic types of healers, herbalists and diviner-mediums. Diviner-mediums claim to gain diagnostic and healing knowledge directly from ancestral spirits, or through dreams. While apprenticeship was acknowledged to occur, little information was gathered on the extent and nature of the empirical training (e.g., learning about curative herbs and diagnostic techniques) that healers undergo.

Manica healers recognize two broad categories of illnesses believed to be sexually transmitted: *siki* and *nyoka*-related.

Siki *Illness.* In several Shona dialects a generic term, *siki*, designates the more serious sexually transmitted illnesses. A few older healers suggested that the term *siki* may derive from the English "sick" and may have been borrowed from the Shona of neighboring Zimbabwe, where English is the official language. This derivation might lend credence to the local belief (found elsewhere in Africa) that syphilis and gonorrhea were introduced by Europeans. Some Shona healers said that *siki* can result when people whose "blood doesn't mix" have intercourse. In several neighboring societies, STIs are sometimes conceived as illnesses involving blood that becomes "bad," "dirty," or "impure" from excessive "mixing" or contact with "strange blood" through having many sexual partners (Schapera, 1940).

The specific *siki* illnesses known as *chimanga, chicazamentu, mula, songeia, chikeke,* and *gobela* seem roughly equivalent to the categories of more serious biomedically recognized STDs such as syphilis, gonorrhea, chlamydia, and chancroid—the STDs that are cofactors of HIV infection. *Siki* illnesses were uniformly described as "adult diseases," meaning they are not found in children before the age of intercourse. At the risk of generalization, *siki* illnesses are characterized either by painful urination and a milky discharge (*chicazamentu, songeia*) or by various types of genital sores or boils (*chimanga, chikeke, gobela*). Healers report that *siki* illnesses are more common in men than women (Green et al., 1993). They also explained that if a woman remains untreated for *siki* illnesses, especially the one resembling gonorrhea, she can become infertile. This was mentioned often, reflecting the concern with fertility throughout most of sub-Saharan Africa. There was also recognition that *siki* can infect newborn infants.

Shona healers believe that *siki* illnesses are caused by *khoma*—a common tiny, invisible, animate agent—or by direct contact with pus or other genital discharges that contain *khoma*. *Khoma* was sometimes described by healers as a tiny worm or insect. One healer conversant in biomedical concepts explained that *khoma* was like a "microbe," or germ. Different illnesses are carried by different *khomas*, so the word must be regarded as generic.

Manica healers are not unlike biomedical physicians in their treatment of *siki* illnesses: they introduce a medicine into the body to kill or neutralize the specific illness-causing *khoma*. In one type of medicine, special roots are boiled, after which the liquid is cooled and given to the patient to drink. In another type of medicine, certain leaves are crushed or ground, then the resulting juice is drunk. There are also medicines applied directly to genital sores. Healers also advise *siki* patients to refrain from intercourse and from drinking alcohol until cured. Treatment is usually conducted in the patient's home over the course of several days (Green et al., 1993). Some healers reported locating and treating recent sexual partners of a *siki* sufferer. There were said to be different medicines for men and women to prevent *siki*. These were described as always effective if taken before intercourse with someone carrying the illness.

Healers reported that women with the *siki* illness *chimanga* will contaminate their babies. In the words of one healer, "The reason the baby dies inside a woman with *chimanga* is that there is something dirty inside her uterus, and the fetus eats this dirt and then dies." Another healer explained that if *songeia* (a *siki* illness) remains untreated, the "impurity goes inside the stomach and causes internal abscesses." Healers also report that menstruating women will contaminate their sexual partners; that physical contact with "tiny animals" from a "contaminated person" will make another person sick with the same illness; that treatment of *chimanga* requires medicines to make both the mother and father "clean" so that they won't contaminate the fetus in the mother's womb; that the *nyoka*-related sores of a contaminated baby are difficult to cure; that *chicazamentu* results when someone has contact with the clothes of the contaminated person, or steps in that person's urine, or steps on that person's "little animals."

What we see here is evidence of pollution belief, or a mixture of what Murdock (1980) called naturalistic infection with pollution (which he called mystic contagion). Examined closely, pollution belief is actually not so mystical. The basic premise is that when one comes into physical contact with an essence considered unclean or ritually impure, one becomes sick. "Contaminated" individuals—to use the Shona term—believed to be in an unclean or polluted state are often kept apart from other people, since they are considered contagious until ritually "purified," a process that might involve therapy with herbal medicines.

Note from these examples the link between *khoma*/germ and pollution ideas. In fact, pollution illnesses are conceived as being highly contagious in southern Africa (Hammond-Tooke, 1989; Ngubane, 1977). This is not so with illnesses caused by witchcraft, sorcery, or spirits, in which only a specific individual—not others in the area—is thought to be targeted for illness or misfortune by a super-human being or force. Indeed, the defining characteristic of both "naturalistic infection" and pollution theories is that they are impersonal: one has contact with a "germ" or *khoma*, or with a dangerous essence, therefore one becomes ill. These ethnomedical theories are not "personalistic" (Foster, 1983) or supernatural.

Some Manica healers reported that they remove a *siki* illness and bury it. A person passing over the spot where the illness is buried can become infected. Burying the source of illness is a common health-related practice in Africa, and it implies belief in contagious illness and specifically in pollution (according to Douglas, 1992).

Nyoka-*Related Illness.* In parts of southern Africa there is a belief in the existence of an invisible, internal snake, often described as a power or force that dwells in a person's stomach but that can move throughout the upper body, from the area of the heart to the abdomen. It is designated by the local term for snake: *nyoka* in Shona and Tsonga. Shona healers described the *nyoka* as a protective force that requires that the body it inhabits be kept free of impurities or contaminants lest the *nyoka* react with displeasure, causing pain and discomfort. The *nyoka* itself can be angry or calm. *Nyoka* may be thought of as a personified immune system or a "guardian of health" or "guardian of bodily purity" (Green, 1997; Green et al., 1994).

All people are believed born with a *nyoka*, which remains in the body until death. It is not visible, even if one cuts open a body. Its existence is confirmed through bodily sensations when it is disturbed. For example, if "dirt" or spoiled food or bad medicine enters the body, *nyoka* may contract and cause cramps, or it can make noises of complaint in the stomach. *Nyoka* cleanses the body of impurities by means of discharges such as diarrhea, vomiting, menstruation, or pus, all of which are seen as natural purifying functions.

Manica healers described two sexually transmitted illnesses associated with this concept: *nyoka kundu*, which affects men, and *nyoka dzoni*, which affects women. A woman who has sex with a man who has *nyoka kundu* is said to contract the female disease *nyoka dzoni*, and vice-versa, through a process described as "contamination." *Nyoka dzoni* can also be caught by stepping in urine or feces contaminated by the male disease. Some healers also described congenital transmission.

If a man does not treat his *nyoka kundu* with indigenous medicines, not only will he remain sick, but at the moment of conceiving a son, the son's *nyoka* will be "contaminated." Contaminated sons will not only have symptoms of the illness *nyoka kundu*, but will also be susceptible to various other illnesses. A mother also passes *nyoka dzoni* on to her unborn daughter if she is not treated.

The symptoms of *nyoka* illnesses are diverse and may approximate a variety of genitourinary infections and conditions such as nonspecific urethritis, yeast infections, prostate infections, and trichomoniasis. Among these are conditions that, according to biomedicine, are probably not sexually transmitted but affect the genital or lower abdominal area. The *nyoka* STIs are treated by applying a topical herbal medicine in the genital area and having the patient drink a liquid from boiled roots. Treatment for *nyoka dzoni* is aimed at regulating menstruation and preventing infertility.

Other Syndromes with Genitourinary Symptoms. There are other syndromes with genitourinary symptoms recognized in Manica province, which are regarded neither as *siki* nor as *nyoka* illnesses. Syndromes of this sort, which healers consider less serious than *siki*, include *chitheta*, *iumanga*, *mugarapadima*, and *sikumbe*. Symptoms include menstrual irregularities, vaginal inflammations and discharges, sores in the groin or elsewhere, hydrocele, miscarriage, and infertility. Some of these are regarded as adult diseases but not as sexually transmitted.

Only one STI was related to sorcery. *Rikawo* is believed to be caused directly by contact with a dangerous medicine used by men to "protect" their wives and lovers from sexual contact with other men. The deeper cause of *rikawo* is adultery or infidelity.

Healers' Understanding of AIDS. Although all traditional healers interviewed had heard of AIDS in 1991, most claimed to know little about it beyond what they had heard on the radio or from other people: that it is incurable, fatal, and sexually transmitted, for example. Our findings about AIDS are supportive of findings from KAP surveys of general populations in Mozambique and elsewhere in Africa. Some healers reported that AIDS is highly contagious and is characterized by progressive weakness, sores on the body, appetite loss, prolonged diarrhea, emaciation, and coughing. There was little understanding, however, of how AIDS is transmitted, beyond the role of sexual intercourse. Several forms of casual contact, such as sharing eating utensils, were mentioned as means of transmission. About 10% of healers mentioned extramarital sex as a cause of AIDS and noted its increase in modern times. About 10% of healers commented that it is better to prevent than try to cure AIDS, even mentioning the use of condoms.

A majority of healers believed that they had neither seen nor treated this disease and that it was new to Mozambique. A few healers associated AIDS with familiar STIs—even referring to it as a *siki* disease—perhaps because they had heard that it is sexually transmitted. These healers claimed that AIDS is not really a new disease—it is the familiar disease *songeia*, or perhaps *chimanga*. Therefore, they believed, a variety of familiar medicines can cure or prevent the disease, a belief also found elsewhere in Africa (Ingstad, 1990; Scheinman et al., 1992; Staugaard, 1991). A few healers thought that although AIDS is different from familiar STIs, there are nevertheless indigenous medicines to cure it. In short, some healers claimed they could cure—and had cured—what they believed to be AIDS.

There were several factors favoring development of an STI strategy for Manica healers. It seemed unnecessary to accommodate our message to complex magico-religious beliefs since *siki* illnesses are thought of in a manner similar to the "germ" medical model of STD. To the extent that *siki* illness relates to pollution beliefs including *nyoka*, even these are essentially naturalistic (impersonal) and fundamentally compatible with the medical model. Furthermore, several existing practices relating to STI prevention were biomedically sound: avoiding adultery and intercourse with strangers; avoiding intercourse during menstruation; refraining from intercourse and from drinking alcohol until *siki* was cured; and healers locating and treating recent sexual partners of patients.

There are other parallels with biomedicine, such as recognition that STIs can infect newborn infants and that STI symptoms can become latent. Shona healers also recognize that untreated STIs, especially the disease resembling gonorrhea, lead to infertility.

The question, however, remained: What to advise about treatment? Healers were convinced that only their own medicines could treat *khoma*, the causal agent of *siki* illnesses. Some healers even said that *khoma* "retreats" in the presence of hospital medicine and so may become impossible to cure. Even if it seemed feasible to advise healers to send their patients to a hospital for treatment of STDs, hospitals in Manica and elsewhere in the provinces and districts would run out of antibiotics, at least for emergencies that are not life threatening. Assuming the availability of antibiotics in hospitals in the future, we hoped it would be possible to build on the growing trust and cooperation which had developed since the first workshop and to persuade healers to allow at least their *siki* patients to benefit from both hospital and indigenous medicines.

Once research provided a base of ethnomedical information, common ground was identified, and specific areas of existing beliefs and behavior were targeted for encouragement or discouragement, we developed a strategy for communication with traditional healers that embodied these elements. Specifically, we promoted educating clients who might engage in risky sexual encounters about condom use; sterilization of razor blades used in treatment; and appropriate referrals of STI patients with persistent symptoms. We wished to reinforce the existing belief that it is dangerous to engage in sexual intercourse outside of marriage (however defined), with strangers, with many partners, and with a person showing symptoms of *siki*. We also encouraged the belief that there is a force within people that requires bodily purity, and we pointed out that *nyoka* is similar to what Western doctors call the immune system. We discouraged healers having direct, unprotected contact with the blood of patients.

Workshop Process and Content

Thirty participants were invited and planned for in the 1991 workshop for traditional healers. Participant selection was handled by AMETRAMO (the national traditional healers' association, Manica branch). The GEMT provided selection criteria with a view toward (1) male–female balance; (2) geographic representation; and (3) attracting participants who were specialists in STIs (or child diarrheas). Eighteen traditional healers appeared for the workshop, and one elderly man dropped out after the first day. The remaining 17 healers completed the workshop. The lower-than-expected turnout may have been due to internal AMETRAMO differences or lack of coordination. Moreover, traditional healers from outlying areas may have been suspicious of government motives. This has occurred in other countries during initial efforts to attract healers to a workshop. (A year or two after the GEMT pilot program, the problem became one of accommodating the large number of healers who wished to participate.)

The workshop lasted a week and basically consisted of give-and-take discussion between healers and government health personnel, with each group trying to learn from the other. The Shona language was used, even though government policy and practice at the time was to overcome "tribalism" through exclusive use of Portuguese, the national language. Most workshop participants spoke Portuguese poorly, if at all. The first few hours of each new topic was devoted to listening to healers explain their understanding of the topic.

Discussion of AIDS occurred without use of scientific terms such as "virus." AIDS and HIV transmission were explained in terms of healers' existing understanding of *siki* illnesses and their general beliefs about contamination. We explained that AIDS, like *siki*, is transmitted by an invisible *khoma*. However, the

AIDS *khoma* is not transmitted in familiar ways, such as touching, sharing eating utensils or blankets, or stepping in a sick person's excrement or discharges. It is carried in sperm, blood, and in a woman's vaginal fluids. The AIDS *khoma* needs to get into the blood to infect someone. If there are sores or wounds on the genitals of men or women, the AIDS *khoma* can enter the blood more easily. It may help if the *nyoka* is strong because the body is pure and free of any illness or contamination.

We also informed healers about another opportunity for the blood of a sick person to infect or contaminate another's blood through traditional use of razor blades in vaccination or scarification. Unless new razors are used with each patient and/or used razor blades are properly sterilized, small amounts of blood—or even the invisible *khoma* of AIDS or other illness (we described tetanus and hepatitis)—can cling to the blade and enter the bloodstream of the next person on whom the same razor is used.

Condom promotion was part of the GEMT program. Due to many factors, there was and is great resistance to using condoms on the part of Mozambicans, and our research clearly showed that condoms were held in low regard. As a means of STI prevention, traditional medicines were believed far superior to condoms. Our approach was to find an opportune entry point among traditional healers, upon which we could build a more ambitious program of condom promotion. Since many healers already advised their patients with *siki* illnesses to avoid intercourse during treatment, we tried to persuade healers to provide their clients with condoms to better ensure their compliance with healers' advice. We suggested that healers adopt some "modern technology" used in other countries to help them accomplish what they were already advising. Healers seemed to find this proposition reasonable, and, in any case, healers appreciated the government's gesture of trust in wanting to share medical devices with them.

Discussion

In their review of the challenge of AIDS prevention in Africa, de Zalduondo et al. (1989:165) conclude that "the complex nature of AIDS points to the need for small-scale projects geared toward culturally homogenous communities where trained staff can translate the information into locally meaningful terms." "Trained staff" from biomedical backgrounds are rarely as skilled in culturally appropriate approaches to behavior change as indigenous healers who already share—and strongly influence—the health beliefs of those who consult them. Regarding cultural homogeneity, the strategy developed in the pilot program was for Shona speakers in central Mozambique; it may not be fully appropriate for other groups in Mozambique.

Our applied research showed that there was considerable common ground upon which to develop a collaborative program involving healers. The "fit" between what exists and the biomedical model is greater for STIs/STDs than it would be for other health domains (such as mental illness) where causation involving witchcraft, sorcery, and evil spirits prevails. Both models agree that the cause of sexually transmitted illness is impersonal and relates to conditions that may be modifiable, such as avoiding sex with strangers, or "contamination" (infection) with an unseen agent of illness that can be sexually transmitted. Both perspectives are concerned with prevention of contact with agents of illness, whether conceived of as agents of pollution or as microbes. Both agree generally on the role of blood: traditional healers sometimes referred to STIs as well as AIDS as a condition of bad or impure blood. Among the nearby Tsonga, Zulu, and Bemba, one's blood can become "bad" or "dirty" or "weak" from having sexual intercourse with too many partners, or through contact with the dead or other polluting influences (Green et al., 1995; Nzima, 1995; Schapera, 1940), propositions with which Shona healers are likely to agree. Certainly the admonition that people must avoid contact with the blood of a person with AIDS made sense to traditional healers. It therefore seemed feasible to develop safe-sex messages in which public health and traditional healers promote essentially the same program in similar terms for similar reasons, perhaps even using similar or compatible symbols and metaphors.

Designing an AIDS Workshop for Traditional Healers

How does knowledge of such details help in practical public health efforts? It seems logical that promotion of behavior change and of health-related technology would be more effective if based on knowledge of existing beliefs and behavior, even if it is difficult to measure this effect. As Airhihenbuwa (1990–91:56) put it, "While there is no single strategy that serves as a panacea for understanding the complex health problems in developing countries, an understanding of the complexity of the problem is a necessary prerequisite for proposing an effective solution." Our approach was to build on existing local beliefs and practices, rather than to ignore or challenge them. We were willing to accept existing beliefs and practices, yet without compromising public health principles. Our assumption was that ethnomedical practices can (by Western public health measures) be considered promotive of health, damaging to health, or of no direct health consequence but socially and psychologically useful. In simplest form, our behavior modification strategy was to encourage practices that promote health, discourage those that damage, and respect the rest while not interfering with them.[2]

Since syphilis, gonorrhea, and chancroid correspond to illnesses locally classified as *siki* rather than *nyoka*-related, the GEMT communications strategy focused on *siki* illnesses. It seemed probable that other STDs such as chlamydia and lymphogranuloma venereum were also classified as *siki* by local healers.

It was never our intention that "training" would be one-way, with traditional healers being the only ones to learn and change. We knew from experience that health workers knew (or pretended to know) little about indigenous medicine, and that many had negative attitudes toward healers. We also believed that clinic treatment could be improved in ways that would attract more STD patients to choose this option as a first choice for treatment. Hospitals and clinics are often regarded as busy, impersonal, and very public places to be seen waiting in line when one has an embarrassing condition. Africans with STDs often regard traditional healers as more sympathetic, more likely to keep confidences, and more accessible than modern health workers; in addition, healers' STD medicines are often believed to be more, or at least as, effective as biomedical treatments (Green, 1994; Green et al., 1993). During all phases of the pilot program (and subsequent projects) we tried to sensitize health care providers in the following areas: to appreciate that STD patients feel embarrassed and therefore need to be treated with special consideration; to be discreet and personal in their approach; and not to make patients feel ashamed if they have visited a traditional healer. However, given work and facility conditions in poor countries, along with entrenched attitudes regarding "obscurantists" or "witch doctors," it was idealistic to expect significant change in this area, at least on a wide scale.

A major question should be answered before attempting to influence STI/STD therapy choice among traditional healers: Can healers successfully treat any STDs? Limited in vitro studies of medicinal plants in Africa have shown that some exhibit antimicrobial activity against *Neisseria gonorrhoeae* (e.g., Chhabra and Uiso, 1991). Needed are in vivo clinical trials. For argument's sake, if healers in a given area cannot successfully treat STDs, then emphasis must be either on influencing healers to refer their patients to clinics, or thinking about involving healers in so-called syndrome-based treatment, at least on a pilot basis. This approach refers to treating common STDs based on symptoms alone, following a clinical flowchart to guide drug choice, without requiring laboratory tests (Dallabetta et al., 1996). This saves time and money, and it allows less-trained health personnel to treat STDs. Since publication of an influential study showing a 42% reduction in HIV incidence as a result of treating existing STDs in a rural area of Tanzania where condom usage remained low (Grosskurth et al., 1995), substantially more effort has gone into STD treatment as a way of combating AIDS in developing countries. Such results are likely to be improved if programs involve traditional healers who treat most patients with STDs.

If, on the other hand, healers can cure at least some STDs, we need to first determine which STDs. This outcome would obviously modify the general strategy of influencing clients of traditional healers to report to clinics instead of to healers—a difficult task under the best of circumstances. It was hoped from the time of the pilot program that simple research would be carried out to determine if at least some indigenous STD medicines are pharmacologically effective. This has not been done to date.

AIDS/STD Prevention Strategy

Prevention rather than treatment is the foundation of public health in general and AIDS programs in particular. Africans are often thought to be fatalistic and to believe that prevention of illness and misfortune is not possible. This characterization is only partially true in southern Africa. Hammond-Tooke (1989) proposed four categories of illness causation traditionally recognized in southern Africa: witchcraft (in which category he includes sorcery), ancestors, pollution, and Supreme Being.

I have found that healers in southern Africa, including Shona, tend to think of illness attributed to witchcraft, sorcery, spirits, or a Supreme Being as difficult or impossible to prevent because mere human effort cannot thwart superhuman will. On the other hand, illness attributed to "naturalistic infection" or pollution may be preventable; indeed, these appear to be among the most preventable illnesses. For STIs, prevention may involve use of protective medicines or change of behavior to avoid contact with *khomas* or pollution agents such as menstrual blood or corpses.

Behavioral prevention of STIs appeared to be so self-evident to traditional healers that they often failed to mention it in response to questions about STI prevention. Some took the question to refer only to medicinal prevention. But as most STIs involve the violation of rules governing sexual behavior, it follows (and healers readily agreed if asked) that one would not get these illnesses if one did not violate the rules in the first place.

Prevention involving indigenous agents of contagion (*khoma*, polluting essences) is probably the area we know least about, yet it is the area most closely relevant to successfully promoting use of condoms or other barrier methods. An important question in AIDS prevention is: Can contact with agents such as *khoma* or "dirt" or menstrual blood be avoided during sexual intercourse if a condom is used? *Khoma* are seen as physical, living entities, and as such they resemble microbes. Yet they might have superphysical or mystical attributes as well and therefore might not be contained or blocked by physical barriers. During a 1993 workshop in South Africa, the opinion of traditional healers was divided over whether condoms can block "heat," which in this sense refers to pollution related to sexual intercourse. In Mozambique, we simply suggested to healers that *khoma* and pollution can be blocked by use of condoms. I am not sure how much healers believe this, and I feel that more effective condom promotion strategies can be developed, based on a better understanding on our part of the attributes of various agents of contagion.

In any case, there is considerable common ground between indigenous and biomedical STD theory for the development of safe-sex messages. The only "concession" AIDS educators need to make to traditional beliefs is essentially in adoption of the language, symbolism, and metaphors of STIs already in local use. AIDS educators would not have to adopt the language, symbolism, and metaphors of witchcraft, sorcery, or evil spirits in preventive messages.

In both the pilot and subsequent programs in other provinces, workshop moderators and other participating health staff have tried to draw parallels between indigenous concepts and their biomedical counterparts. Both healers and their clients may already have drawn some such parallels, but AIDS educators assisted the process by reinforcing and sanctioning them and by drawing others. Once healers and AIDS educators feel they are both "talking the same language," there appears to be maximum chance for effective communication and behavior change. This may sound easy, but too often AIDS and other health educators pay lip service to indigenous beliefs and the importance of culture, then go ahead and teach about AIDS in language laced with concepts and terminology that are alien to healers and their clients.

Should Emphasis Be on Using Condoms or Reducing the Number of Sexual Partners?

Despite intensive promotion of condom use in some African countries (e.g., Uganda, Zambia, Zaire, Zimbabwe, Tanzania), there has been scant "payoff." For example, by late 1992, regular condom use among the general, sexually active male population in Uganda was only about 2% (Serawadda, 1992a, 1992b). And, according to the Demographic and Health Survey in Zambia, 1.4% of Zambian women 15–49 years of age were current condom users and 9.2% were "ever-users" (Brunborg et al., 1993). Therefore, by this time, the GEMT felt that it made more sense to put even more emphasis on where the payoff seems to lie: promoting avoidance of sex outside of marriage, with strangers, and with prostitutes. The message that AIDS and other STIs can be avoided by abstinence or fidelity to one partner is one that reinforces what Mozambican traditional healers—as well as local Christian and Muslim clergy—already believe and to some extent promote.

The last comment deserves explanation. It seems that Mozambican healers do not ordinarily offer gratuitous advice about preventing illness—their job is thought to be one of explaining and curing illness. Cynically, preventive advice could even be seen as bad for future business. Yet healers may be willing to promote fidelity or avoidance of indiscriminate sex more actively if they are made to feel that this puts them in partnership with their health ministry and government, which is often regarded as enhancing their prestige and bestowing a new, "modern sector" legitimacy (Fassin and Fassin, 1988; Ventevogel, 1996). The

GEMT is therefore developing a strategy to motivate and empower healers to take a more active role in "preaching" what they already believe to their patients and perhaps to others in their communities.

Preliminary evidence from Uganda, Zambia, and parts of Tanzania indicates that both STD and HIV incidence have declined markedly since about 1993. Male condom use rates remain too low to account for this apparent decline, although some might argue that condom use in high-risk encounters such as with commercial sex workers has contributed to the decline. Healers interviewed in Zambia in 1995 noted a decline in STIs and attributed it to a reduction in multiple or indiscriminate sex partners. This seems reasonable: with 25% or more of the sexually active populations of Uganda and Zambia HIV positive, it is safe to say that everyone knows someone who is dying, or has died, of AIDS. (This is not true in Mozambique, at least not yet.) Fear causes people to change entrenched sexual behavior. Yet most have not adopted condom use; instead they appear to change behavior toward reduction in the number of partners (Asiimwe-Okiror, 1995; Pool et al., 1996). Traditional healers as well as clergy and church leaders are well positioned to promote and reinforce this type of behavior change.

The Current Program in Mozambique

Since the initial pilot research and collaborative workshop in Manica in 1991, the pilot and workshop have been replicated in other provinces in Mozambique. From 1993 to 1995, ethnomedical research and collaborative workshops were carried out in Zambesia, Maputo, Inhambane, and Nampula. Workshops have continued in Manica itself, sponsored by UNICEF, the Mozambique Red Cross, and at least one foreign nongovernmental organization. In Manica, topics have expanded beyond diarrhea and AIDS/STDs to include tuberculosis, acute respiratory infections, asthma, mental health, and water/sanitation. The suspicion over government motives encountered in Manica in 1991 has diminished and there are now many more healers wishing to participate than can be accommodated. In some areas, the healers' association, AMETRAMO, has taken the initiative to train its members in what the GEMT has taught in its workshop, with no requests for outside assistance.

Although there has been no evaluation of the impact of the pilot Manica workshop, there has recently been an evaluation of workshop impact in Inhambane province. The programmatic strengths and weaknesses found there are probably representative of programs elsewhere in Mozambique. In this evaluation, 20 healers out of the 30 who participated in a workshop in June 1994 were reinterviewed in October–November 1995 (the other 10 were not available to interviewers at the time of the evaluation). We also interviewed an additional healer who had been trained by a healer who had been to the workshop, and a small sample (N=8) of diarrhea and STI patients of the 20 healers were also interviewed. Patient interviews provided a means of verifying healers' self-reported behavior and yielded valuable insights into the healing process and the reinterpretation and dissemination of information and advice presented at the workshop.

Among the most important findings relating to STIs were that 85% of healers had learned that AIDS is caused or transmitted by sexual contact with a person with the illness and that use of condoms or fidelity to one (uninfected) partner can prevent AIDS. The role of blood, or "contaminated blood," in HIV/AIDS transmission was well understood. Virtually all healers said they now use only one clean razor per patient, or boil a razor if they must reuse it, or sterilize the blade in bleach. Most (81%) claimed that they had promoted condom use with their STI (*siki*) patients. We were unable to verify this from interviews with former STI patients, since these patients were reluctant to identify themselves because of the stigma associated with STIs. (We were able to interview mothers of diarrhea patients, and we found corroboration of healer-derived information on diarrhea treatment.)

The condoms distributed by healers in almost all cases were those supplied by the GEMT in the 1994 Inhambane workshop; most healers had never been resupplied, nor had they taken their own initiative to find condoms. Among other weaknesses encountered, there was still confusion about transmission of HIV/AIDS through superficial contact, for example, using the same toilet, eating food touched by a sick person, using clothes of a person with AIDS, or kissing a sick person. There was also poor understanding about the role of STIs in increasing vulnerability to AIDS.

The GEMT program has been less active in developing workshops for traditional healers since 1995, due to personnel changes in the Ministry of Health. This is often the fate of programs operating in the public sector in Africa (Green, 1988). Collaborative programs involving healers have proven to be very fragile, and they are never high priorities in an African ministry. Nevertheless, the GEMT achieved its general objective of developing collaboration between traditional healers and a variety of agencies and organizations, in diverse areas of public health, and in most regions of Mozambique. Many nongovernmental organizations are currently working with Mozambican healers following the general model developed by the GEMT. The combined resources of these organizations is far greater than those of the GEMT, as is the public health impact of their programs.

Notes

1. STDs are defined as sexually transmitted diseases, STIs, as sexually transmitted illnesses. The former denote biomedical concepts, whereas the latter denote indigenous or "folk" concepts, (Hahn, 1984): syphilis is an STD; *chimanga* (discussed later) is an STI. "Biomedicine" refers to Western, cosmopolitan medicine, including its branch of

public health; it is distinguished from African "traditional" (although dynamic, adaptive, and changing) systems of "indigenous medicine."

2. Some health officials in Mozambique and elsewhere have only agreed to allow— or participate in—collaborative programs involving healers when assured that "discouraging the damaging practices" was an objective.

Acknowledgments

I wish to thank Annemarie Jurg and Amando Dgedge for their help in the original research upon which this analysis is based, as well as Josefa Marrato and Manuel Wilsonne for their help in the development and evaluation of the GEMT's later program.

References

Airhihenbuwa CO (1990–91) A conceptual model for culturally appropriate health education programs in developing countries. *International Quarterly of Community Health Education* 11:53–62.

Asiimwe-Okiror G (1995) Brief Report on Population Based Survey in Jinja District. Kampala: National STD/AIDS Control Programme, November.

Bannerman RH, Burton J, Wen-Chieh C (1983) Traditional Medicine and Health Care Coverage. Geneva: World Health Organization.

Bentley M, Pelto GH, Straus WL, Schumann DA, Adegbola C, de la Peña E, Oni GA, Brown KH, Huffman SL (1988) Rapid ethnographic assessment: applications in a diarrhea management program. *Social Science and Medicine* 27:107–116.

Bishaw M (1989) The implications of indigenous medical beliefs to biomedical practice. *Ethiopian Journal of Health Development* 3:75–88.

Brunborg H, Fylkesnes K, Msiska R (1993) Behavioral change related to the AIDS epidemic in Zambia. Paper presented at the International Population Conference, Montreal, Canada, August 24–September 1.

Chhabra SC, Uiso FC (1991) Antibacterial activity of some Tanzanian plants used in traditional medicine. *Fitoterapia* 62:499–503.

Dallabetta G, Laga M, Lamptey P, eds. (1996) Control of Sexually Transmitted Diseases. Arlington, Va: AIDSCAP/Family Health International.

De Sousa JF (1991) Traditional Beliefs and Practices Related to Childhood Diarrhoeal Disease in a High-Density Suburb of Maputo. BA thesis. Harare: Department of Sociology, University of Zimbabwe.

De Zalduondo BO, Msamanga GI, Chen LC (1989) AIDS in Africa: diversity in the global pandemic. *Daedalus* 118:165–204.

Douglas M (1992/1966) Purity and Danger. London: Routledge.

Fassin D, Fassin E (1988) Traditional medicine and the stakes of legitimation in Senegal. *Social Science and Medicine* 27:353–357.

Fierman S (1981) Therapy as a system-in-action in northeastern Tanzania. *Social Science and Medicine* 15B:353–360.

Foster G (1983) "Introduction to Ethnomedicine." In: Traditional Medicine and Health Care Coverage. R Bannerman, J Burton, C Wen-Chieh, eds. Geneva: World Health Organization, pp. 17–24.

Good CM (1987) Ethnomedical Systems in Africa. Patterns of Traditional Medicine in Rural and Urban Kenya. New York: Guilford Press.

Green EC (1988) Can collaborative programs between biomedical and indigenous health practitioners succeed? *Social Science and Medicine* 27:1125–1130.

Green EC (1994) AIDS and STDs in Africa. Bridging the Gap between Traditional Healers and Modern Medicine. Boulder, Colo, and Oxford, UK: Westview Press.

Green EC (1995) Commentary: Anthropologists as villains. *American Anthropologist Newsletter* May.

Green EC (1997) Purity, pollution and the invisible snake in Southern Africa. *Medical Anthropology* 17:1–18.

Green EC, Jurg A, Dgedge A (1993) Sexually transmitted diseases, AIDS and traditional healers in Mozambique. *Medical Anthropology* 15:261–281.

Green EC, Jurg A, Dgedge A (1994) The snake in the stomach: child diarrhea in central Mozambique. *Medical Anthropology Quarterly* 8:4–24.

Green EC, Nzima M (1995) The Traditional Healer Targeted Intervention Research Study in Zambia. Lusaka: Morehouse/Tulane AIDS Prevention Project, September 6 (Report).

Green EC, Tomas T, Jurg A (1991) A Program in Public Health and Traditional Health Manpower in Mozambique. Mozambique Ministry of Health and the European Community. Maputo, March 30 (Report).

Green EC, Zokwe B, Dupree JD (1995) The experience of an AIDS prevention program focused on South African traditional healers. *Social Science and Medicine* 40:503–515.

Grosskurth H, Mosha F, Todd J, Mwijarubi E, Klokke A, Senkoro K, Mayaud P, Changalucha J, Nicoll A, ka-Gina G, Newell J, Mugeye K, Mabey D, Hayes R (1995) Impact of improved treatment of sexually transmitted diseases on HIV infection in rural Tanzania: randomised controlled trial. *Lancet* 346:530–536.

Hahn RA (1984) Rethinking "illness" and "disease." *Contributions to Asian Studies* 18:513–522.

Hammond-Tooke WD (1989) Rituals and Medicines. Johannesburg: A.D. Donker.

Hanlon J (1984) Mozambique. The Revolution under Fire. London: Zed Books.

Ingstad B (1990) The cultural construction of AIDS and its consequences for prevention in Botswana. *Medical Anthropology Quarterly* 4:28–40.

Murdock GP (1959) Africa. Its People and Their Cultural History. New York: McGraw-Hill.

Murdock GP (1980) Theories of Illness. Pittsburgh: University of Pittsburgh Press.

Ngubane H (1977) Body and Mind in Zulu Medicine. London: Academic Press.

Nzima MM (1995) Preliminary Programmatic Considerations, Questions and Related Analysis of the Targeted Intervention Research (TIR) Conducted in Collaborative Programs Involving Healers, Chimwemwe, Kitwe (June 13 to 24, 1994). Lusaka: Morehouse/Tulane AIDS Prevention Project (Report).

Pool R (1994) On the creation and dissolution of ethnomedical systems in the medical ethnography of Africa. *Africa* 64:1–20.

Pool R, Maswe M, Ties Boerma J, Nnko S (1996) The price of promiscuity: why urban males in Tanzania are changing their sexual behavior. *Health Transition Review* 6:203–221.

Reis R (1994) Evil in the body, disorder of the brain. *Tropical and Geographical Medicine* 46(suppl):S40–43.

Schapera I (1940) Married Life in an African Tribe. London: Faber & Faber.

Scheinman D, Nesje R, Ulrich E, Malangalia E (1992) Treating HIV with traditional medicine. *AIDS and Society* 3:5.

Serawadda D (1992a) Church of Uganda AIDS KAP Survey (draft). Kampala: Makerere Medical School, November.

Serawadda D (1992b) Islamic Medical Association AIDS KAP Survey (draft). Kampala: Makerere Medical School, April.

Staugaard F (1991) Role of traditional health workers in prevention and control of AIDS in Africa. *Tropical Doctor* 21:22–24.

Ventevogel P (1996) Whiteman's Things. Training and Detraining Healers in Ghana. Amsterdam: Het Spinhuis.

Yoder PS (1997) Negotiating relevance: belief, knowledge, and practice in international health projects. *Medical Anthropology Quarterly* 11:131–146.

5

Anthropological Perspectives on Childhood Pneumonia in Pakistan

DOROTHY S. MULL

Acute respiratory infection (ARI) is the leading cause of child mortality in the world today, accounting for about 4 million deaths each year (Kirkwood et al., 1995). Almost all of these deaths are due to acute infection of the lower respiratory tract, mainly in the form of pneumonia. In developing countries, pneumonia case fatality rates range from 5% to 20% vs. 0.4% in the United States, and the incidence rate is much higher in such countries as well (Galway et al., 1987; Selwyn, 1990). Among 966 children under five years of age living in one Pakistani village, there were 442 verified cases of pneumonia over a six-month period in 1993 (Mehnaz et al., 1997). More than 90% of all pneumonia deaths occur in the developing world (Murray and Lopez, 1996), where crowding, undernutrition, and indoor air pollution contribute to the high incidence of the disease and increase its severity (Douglas and D'Souza, 1996).

Most children who die of pneumonia do so because they do not receive adequate medical attention early enough, either because of access problems or because the mother or other caretaker does not recognize the seriousness of the child's condition. Typically, a life-threatening pneumonia for which antibiotics are needed is mistaken for a self-limiting upper respiratory infection until it is too late to save the child's life. Since pneumonia can cause death very rapidly—even within three or four days after onset of symptoms—early detection of cases is essential.

Extensive research has shown that fast breathing is the single best clinical sign distinguishing pneumonia from a common cold (Shann, 1995).[1] Chest indrawing, or observable depression of the lower chest wall as the child tries to breathe in with lungs stiffened by infection, indicates that pneumonia is severe. If these two signs were recognized in a timely fashion, most pneumonia deaths in the developing world could be averted. Thus in the late 1980s the World Health Organization (WHO) launched a global campaign to promote recognition of fast breathing and chest indrawing by health care providers and, if possible, by mothers as well. The Government of Pakistan began its national ARI control program in 1989, using WHO diagnostic and treatment guidelines and focusing first on the training of physicians in government clinics.

The aim of these initiatives was not only to improve diagnostic accuracy and thus reduce pneumonia mortality but also to decrease the widespread use of antibiotics for viral illnesses such as the common cold, which not only wastes scarce resources but may produce strains of antibiotic-resistant bacteria.[2] In developing its training materials, WHO took the unprecedented step of involving anthropologists from the start. An anthropologically oriented manual for studying ARI in the developing world was produced (WHO, 1993), and preliminary versions were tested in 10 countries. Later the manual was used to carry out the Focused Ethnographic Study of ARI (FES) in six other field sites (Gove and Pelto, 1994).

During the first national workshop on ARI in Pakistan, plans were made to conduct a countrywide study of attitudes and behaviors related to respiratory illness, and it was hoped that a FES could be carried out in 1990. However, political events forced abandonment of the project.[3] Spending in Pakistan by the United States had decreased following Russia's withdrawal from Afghanistan, creating anti-American sentiment which was exacerbated when the Gulf War broke out in the winter of 1990–1991. Many Pakistanis saw the war as a religious conflict and sympathized with the Iraqi leadership vis-à-vis the United States. In this climate of mistrust and uncertainty, both international and binational agencies interrupted their programs in Pakistan, yet a need remained for baseline ARI data against which progress could later be measured.

In response to this need, between 1990 and 1992, my colleagues and I designed and conducted four anthropological studies of pneumonia in two different regions of Pakistan: Punjab Province in the north and the port city of Karachi in Sind Province in the south. Like the FES, these studies had an "applied" purpose: they were concerned with meeting practical objectives rather than theory-building. Our immediate aim was to make a contribution to the national ARI initiative by bringing to light local understandings, behaviors, and conditions having an impact on the accurate diagnosis and appropriate treatment of pneumonia in Pakistan. Beyond that, we hoped to develop methods that could be used as models by pneumonia researchers elsewhere in the world.

Pakistan, Community Healers, and Pneumonia

Founded as a homeland for Muslims in 1947, Pakistan remains a predominantly Islamic state. Its 135 million inhabitants, most living in rural areas, include 17 major linguistic and ethnic groups. Urdu is the official language, but large numbers of people—especially rural women—understand only regional languages such as Punjabi. English is widely used by the educated classes. The three dominant forces in Pakistan are religious leaders, large landowners, and the military, which has been in effective control of the government during most of the period since the country was formed. In recent years the annual rate of population growth has hovered around 3%, and spending on defense—mainly aimed at deterring an attack by India—has been eight times spending on education and health combined (World Bank, 1989).

The typical household structure in Pakistan would be described by anthropologists as "patrilocal." This means that when women marry, they typically move to their husband's place of residence. Often the husband's parents and brothers (and their families) also live in the home, that is, there is an extended family. If present, the mother-in-law is usually very involved in episodes of childhood illness as well as in other domestic matters. Continuing gender inequities are revealed by the fact that, in 1985, literacy was estimated at 43% for men and 18% for women; some progress has been made since then but a sharp disparity remains. The infant mortality rate, while officially about 100 per 1,000 live births, is twice as high in impoverished areas (National Institute of Population Studies, 1992). As in many developing countries, accurate disease-specific mortality rates in Pakistan are unavailable, but pneumonia is believed to account for at least 80,000 child deaths each year (USAID, 1988).

Pakistan's pluralistic health care system includes an array of practitioners without formal medical (MBBS) degrees. Besides the religious leaders (*pirs* or *moulvis*), who specialize in treating illnesses thought to have a spiritual cause, there are *hakims*, homeopaths, and self-trained allopathic practitioners widely known as *"chota* doctors." (*Chota* means "small" in Urdu, the implication being that these are "lesser" healers as compared with licensed physicians.) *Hakims* are practitioners of *hikmat*, a form of therapy based on the ancient theories of Hippocrates and sometimes referred to as *Unani* (literally "Ionian," i.e., Greek) medicine. Traditionally, they diagnosed by feeling the pulse and relied mainly on herbs for treatment. Homeopaths tend to specialize in chronic conditions, typically administering minute quantities of substances on the principle that "like cures like." In Pakistan, both *hakims* and homeopaths often break with tradition to make use of allopathy in ways of their own devising. Some use stethoscopes, dispense pills, and administer injections.

Chota doctors have usually been associated with hospitals, for example, as dispensers (similar to pharmacists' assistants), supply clerks, orderlies, or even janitors.

Many work in low-level positions in hospitals by day and moonlight as "doctors" at night. The one essential is that they have access to drugs, which are reportedly often purloined from their employers. The notion that the healing "influence" of a particularly eminent person such as a licensed physician can be absorbed via contact with that person underlies the patronage of such individuals. No one knows how many of these self-trained allopaths exist in Pakistan, but they certainly outnumber the 60,000 or so credentialed MBBS physicians. In India, a large-scale survey indicated that they outnumber licensed practitioners ten to one (Kakar et al., 1972). They are responsible for much inappropriate antibiotic therapy of illness, including pneumonia (Dr. A. Fozia Qureshi, personal communication, 1991).

The Research Setting

Our first study (Mull and Mull, 1994) was carried out mainly in mothers' homes. We chose two widely separated sites located in or near large population centers: villages in rural Punjab near the city of Rawalpindi in the north of Pakistan and squatter settlements in Karachi in the south. In Punjab, clay-daubed huts were surrounded by fields of yellow mustard (the cooked greens were a dietary staple); buffaloes and goats roamed dusty paths; women plastered dung patties on walls to dry them for later use as fuel. In Karachi, concrete-block houses abutted each other in congested enclaves; half-starved dogs foraged hungrily through garbage heaps; flies and raw sewage were everywhere. Most people in the villages spoke Hindko; in Karachi, all major languages of Pakistan were represented, including Punjabi, Kutchi, Baluchi, Pashto, Sindhi, and Hindi. In both sites, about two-thirds of the people lived in extended families.

The three subsequent studies were carried out in Rawalpindi General Hospital, a 507-bed government facility serving a poor population living in and around Rawalpindi in Punjab Province. The majority Punjabis spoke Punjabi and/or Hindko and some also understood Urdu as a second language; the minority Pathans spoke Pashto. Whatever their ethnicity, most lived in extended families. Although attendance at the outpatient clinics was virtually free and basic medicines were provided, the hospital had few of the amenities taken for granted in industrialized nations. More than once, we saw bleeding patients on gurneys trundled down crowded staircases (there were no elevators) on their way to the surgical suite. Electrical outages were common; bathroom facilities were few and basic; rudimentary patient records—mainly attendance and mortality figures—were kept stacked in enormous ledgers. Such figures were summed each day without benefit of so much as a hand-held calculator and were later reported to the government, as required by law.

As in many such facilities in the developing world, mothers of children hospitalized with pneumonia stayed in the ward, sleeping in the bed with the ill child or on a nearby wooden bench. Meanwhile, various other family members camped out in the corridors, going to the market to obtain medications or food for the mother and child as needed. Such items were purchased and paid for by the families. A hospitalized child who did not have family members in attendance would have been disadvantaged indeed, since nurses were few and usually too busy to provide much in the way of individual attention. There were no partitions or visual barriers between beds; the mothers and children all ate and slept in one crowded, noisy public space. Chaotic but colorful, the pneumonia ward was the site of the last of our studies.

Four Anthropological Studies of Pneumonia in Pakistan

I present here a broad description of the topics, methods, and results of our four studies; the papers as originally published provide additional details (Kundi et al., 1993; Mull and Mull, 1994; Mull et al., 1994; Cody et al., 1997). In interpreting our findings, one must remember that, because of the cumulative nature of anthropological research, not every informant was asked every question, so it is often possible to speak only of general results rather than of percentages. Where the questions had to do with such things as demographic features, patterns of health care seeking, or recognition of clinical signs, the results could be quantified.

The Community Study (Mull and Mull, 1994)

We began our research in 1990 by asking a community sample of mothers in Punjab and Karachi about common respiratory illnesses—what they were, what caused them, and what were the proper treatments. We also collected local words and phrases for the physical signs connected with those illnesses and explored maternal concepts of physiology. From this we developed a tentative "folk model" of pneumonia, that is, a representation of the disease as seen by mothers. Finally, we visited a government health center in rural Punjab and observed the activities of four *chota* doctors in Karachi squatter settlements. By selecting two research sites located at opposite ends of Pakistan, we hoped to improve the generalizability of our results. This is often a problem in the developing world, where there can be many ethnic groups within the same country. Traditional anthropologists often tolerate and even celebrate site-specific results, but applied researchers try to avoid them because they may be of limited practical utility.

Methods. In each locale, our first step was to identify and interview key informants—perceptive individuals knowledgeable about illness who were members of the cultural group being studied and yet, by virtue of having received some medical training, could stand back from that group to see local health beliefs and practices in relation to biomedical concepts. In Karachi our main key informant was a male community health worker; in Punjab we relied primarily on a female social scientist who had done research for international and binational health agencies. Both also served as interpreters. It was necessary to use interpreters in the homes because almost all of the mothers spoke only regional languages, although most of the government clinic personnel and *chota* doctors visited spoke at least some English.

After collecting basic information about local concepts of pneumonia from our key informants, we conducted in-depth interviews in mothers' homes. A pilot study of five women was followed by interviews of 35 women in Punjab and Karachi combined. We used a "convenience sample," essentially interviewing any woman who had a child under five years old. To enhance the generalizability of results, we sought out informants from many different ethnic groups.

We spent an hour or more in each home questioning mothers with the use of an interview guide, which is a basic list of topics to be covered. The interview guide was refined as more and more homes were visited. Closed-ended questions with a single answer were used to collect information on simple socio-demographic variables such as ages of children. Open-ended questions such as "What kinds of illnesses do children get around here?" and "What kinds of things can cause a cough?" were used to collect more complex cultural information. In the time-honored anthropological tradition of repeatedly asking "Why?," we used many follow-up questions to clarify what had been said, since the locations were often so remote that we knew we would not be able to return easily.

The process was repetitive and additive: we took results obtained from one informant and presented them to a second person (and third, and fourth) for validation. Our prior research experience had taught us that frequently the second person would add details that would not necessarily have been forthcoming if we had not shown some prior knowledge of the matter, since it is tedious to educate an outsider about all aspects of one's culture.

If children in the families had had a respiratory disease, we were careful to collect their illness histories. Real-life narratives show how basic cultural beliefs are modified by the particular situation in which the family finds itself (Yoder, 1997). Actions may be affected by the availability of money, for example, or by a family's experience with a child's prior episode of illness. For an applied anthropologist working in the field of international health, what people do is always more important than what they say.

Although it was more difficult and time-consuming to go to homes than to conduct interviews in a clinic, we did it because people who attend clinics often differ in important ways from people who do not. In addition, going to homes usually allows interviewers to develop better rapport, since informants are more relaxed. Then, too, in homes one can observe and converse about objects that may be related to health beliefs and practices, such as amulets tied to cradles or bunches of herbs drying. Family interactions can also be seen. In fact, in these households there were so many people present that they functioned as virtual focus groups engaged in lively discussions of respiratory illness.

As in our other three studies, we tried to emphasize areas not extensively covered by the FES. Thus in Karachi we asked our key informant to take us to the offices of several *chota* doctors so that we could observe and converse with them. These unlicensed allopaths are wary of being interviewed because, technically, they are violating the law by dispensing medicines; but by adopting the demeanor of naive but intensely interested observers we were able to gather information about their diagnosis and treatment of respiratory illness. To investigate a different facet of the health care system, we also visited a government-run rural health center in Punjab—and noted the lack of patrons. Such activities allowed us to see what is available to consumers of health care in Pakistan rather than focusing only on the beliefs and practices of the consumers themselves.

Results. Of the 35 mothers interviewed, 25, including all of those in rural Punjab, had had no schooling and were illiterate; the rest were literate and had a mean of 5 years of formal education. All of the major ethnic groups in Pakistan were represented in our sample: Punjabi, Kutchi, Baluchi, Mohajir, Pathan, Sindhi, and Hindu. All mothers knew the term "pneumonia" (in English) and said that the disease was greatly feared. Older women reported having seen many pneumonia deaths. However, case histories revealed that the word was used for any severe lower respiratory ailment and was not limited to clinical pneumonia. Also, the term "double pneumonia" was used to mean "severe pneumonia," not pneumonia involving both lungs.[4]

Maternal ideas about anatomy were very different from biomedical concepts. Most women thought that the heart was in the center of the chest between the two lowermost ribs (Figure 5.1). When they were asked where the lungs were located, half did not know and the other half said they were located to either side of the "heart" and extended down below it in an area referred to as the *pasli* area of the body (Urdu *pasli*, "rib"). Regardless of their native language, all mothers made a linguistic distinction between the upper and lower ribs. Some added that when a child had severe pneumonia, the *pasli* area showed abnormal movement (Urdu *pasli chelna*, "the lower ribs move"), that is, chest indrawing. They said that in such cases, "pits" or "hollows" (Urdu *tohay*) were visible below the lower ribs and sometimes also at the base of the neck, and they pointed to their own lower rib area with both index fingers when discussing this sign.

Breathing was not associated exclusively with the lungs. Although most women said that when a person breathes in, the breath goes into the lungs, some said that it goes "all over the body," others said that it goes "into the heart," and still

others said that it goes "into the stomach." There was no clear distinction between the heart, the stomach, and the lungs in this regard (traditional South Asian
medicine almost completely ignores the lungs and does not specifically relate
them to the breathing process; see Zimmer, 1948). These ideas are important
because they affect people's expectations about proper treatment of respiratory
ailments.

For example, some mothers said that it was important to "vomit up" the mucus or phlegm (Urdu *raysha*) that was thought to prevent the breath from reaching the lungs when a child had pneumonia. Reportedly the *hakims*, with their
emphasis on the digestive system, have popularized this idea of vomiting as treat-

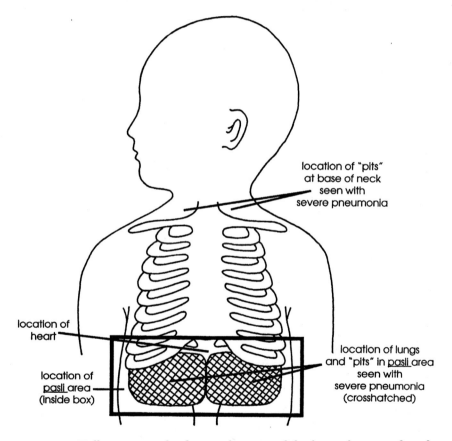

Figure 5.1. Folk anatomy of a disease: location of the lungs, heart, and *pasli*
(lower rib) area—and the "pits" or "hollows" (*tohay*) seen with severe pneumonia—as elicited from mothers interviewed in various parts of Pakistan, 1990–
1992, superimposed on a schematic diagram of basic skeletal structures. (Reprinted from Kundi et al. 1993:657. Used by permission.)

ment (Dr. M. Z. M. Kundi, personal communication, 1990). Concern about excess phlegm is central to Unani thought and is also consistent with the teachings of classical Hindu medicine (cf. Nichter, 1989:136). People worry that any phlegm that remains in the body after the episode of acute illness may cause chronic respiratory problems or even tuberculosis, and they are extremely anxious to get it *all* out. "Hot" allopathic medicines like penicillin are much sought after because they are thought to "burn the cold phlegm away."[5]

Although most mothers knew that fast breathing was abnormal, they judged it impressionistically rather than by counting breaths. Further, they usually did not recognize it as a sign of pneumonia, connecting it with fever instead; some noted that people and animals panted when they became overheated. In their descriptions of pneumonia, they put much less emphasis on fast breathing than on cough, fever, and the "difficult" breathing that they said accompanied the child's chest pain. Only 5 of the 35 mothers spontaneously named it as a sign of the disease. Further, about half the women had no way to time breaths because they had no watch or clock in working order, and in any case most said they were unable to count to 50.

Pneumonia was almost universally thought to be caused by various forms of "coldness." Three informants, all older women, said that pneumonia could be caused not only by coldness but also by an adverse supernatural influence, a "shadow" (Urdu *saya*), coming over the child. Overall, however, environmental influences—not sin, pollution, or contagion—were regarded as the main cause of pneumonia. Mothers' concepts of contagion were very limited. Although most knew that colds were spread by sneezing, as a practical matter we observed that they allowed their children to sneeze on each other without covering their mouths, and they routinely wiped infants' nasal secretions on their own clothing.

By "coldness," informants meant principally cold weather, including cold drafts, although some said that pneumonia could occur even in hot weather if a child took a cold bath or drank a cold drink when overheated. The phrase *garum-sard* (literally "hot-cold") was used to describe the resultant "shock" to the system caused by the clash of extremes. Both coldness and *garum-sard* could be transferred to the child from the mother through breastmilk. Children exposed to wetness along with coldness were thought to be at increased risk, for example, if they were carelessly bathed in cold weather. Though not as important as weather, cold foods were also mentioned as causing pneumonia. Some of these were foods actually cold in temperature such as ice cream and soft drinks served cold or with ice. Others were foods classified as "cold" in the humoral system such as citrus fruits, yogurt, bananas, and rice.

Home treatments of pneumonia were mainly aimed at creating "heat" to counter the "cold effect" in the body. All mothers said that ill children should be kept warmly dressed and protected from cold drafts; bathing them was out of the question. About half added that the child's chest should be rubbed with commercial ointments that give a sensation of heat or with beaten raw egg yolk (humorally very hot), and then wrapped with strips of cloth to keep the heat inside. Most of these remedies were designed to loosen up phlegm in the body so that it could be expelled. Coughing was considered to be a sign that the child was unable to do this by himself.

Virtually all mothers recognized that home remedies could not cure pneumonia and that "doctors' medicines" must be used. However, several added that only if they lacked other options would they take their children to community-based government facilities, expressing dissatisfaction with the medicines provided there. (These facilities, called Rural Health Centers or Basic Health Units, are staffed by young physicians fulfilling their government social service requirement. Such physicians commonly have no particular interest in the health of the local community, and they rarely stay on after their required service is completed.)[6]

As one woman put it, "The doctor is no good: his medicine is free but it doesn't cure the child so we spend [money] to go elsewhere." When asked to elaborate, she said, "Whatever the problem he gives the same tablets to the child." (Physicians interviewed in Rawalpindi speculated that she referred to cotrimoxazole tablets, since current treatment guidelines in Pakistan state that cotrimoxazole, an inexpensive antibiotic, should be given for most diarrheas as well as for nonsevere pneumonia. Further, private practitioners—unlike government physicians—frequently give cortisone injections, which lower fever in an immediate, dramatic way and are interpreted by mothers as curing the child, whereas the effect of cotrimoxazole is much more gradual.) Many mothers said that they preferred injections or pediatric suspensions to tablets, and one approvingly displayed liquids of three different colors, each of which, she explained, a private physician had told her to administer at a specific time of day.

Most women said that instead of patronizing government facilities, they turned to private "doctors," many of whom were almost certainly unlicensed. When asked how long she would wait before seeking medical care for pneumonia, one rural mother said, "I don't count days—I would just go if the cough and fever were really bad." Observers in the area (a government vaccinator and a physician) commented that week-long delays were not uncommon and that some rural women never brought the child to a health care facility at all because they failed to recognize the signs of pneumonia, because the child took a turn for the worse at night when transport was unavailable, or because of fatalism ("they surrender themselves to God").

When we visited four *chota* doctors in Karachi, we found that they were unable to diagnose pneumonia correctly and had built their practices around the indiscriminate use of antibiotics for ailments of every kind. They shared their patients' beliefs about respiratory illness. The only difference was that they wielded stethoscopes, antibiotics, and authority. None counted breathing rates or even observed them; none had any idea what the normal rate was. In fact, when we questioned them we found that a rapid pulse was more noted and considered more dangerous than rapid breathing—a possible carryover from the *hakims'* emphasis on diagnosis by pulsing. Although stethoscopes were much in evidence, they were used in a cursory, ineffective manner, serving as mere props. The practitioners did not check patients for chest indrawing. They gave one day's worth of antibiotics at a time, usually in the patient's own bottle, and dispensed those drugs for virtually all cases of sore throat, cough, and fever.

In short, treatment of respiratory illness was driven by perceived demand and local understanding of pathology, not by scientific precepts. As one practitioner said quite candidly, "What can I do? If I don't give patients the medicines they want for their children, they'll go somewhere else." Besides the fact that small doses of antibiotics can create drug resistance, often there was no follow-up. Women reported that "doctors" told them to try a particular medicine for one day and then to come back for more if the child was better or for a different medicine if he was not. However, they said that what usually happened was the reverse: mothers didn't return if the child was better and they went to some other doctor if he wasn't (cf. Faisel et al., 1990, for a similar finding). The myriad half-empty bottles of antibiotics observed in informants' homes attested to the extent of multiple drug use among the poor.

The Study of Mothers Attending a Pediatric Pneumonia Clinic (Kundi et al., 1993)

In this study, our goal was to validate the general model of pneumonia that had been elicited in the community study by collecting case histories from a random sample of 50 mothers in a clinical setting. We also developed a schematic diagram representing mothers' reported patterns of health care seeking during the illness episode. Finally, we tested the mothers' ability to diagnose pneumonia by comparing their perceptions of fast breathing in their own children with physicians' perceptions of the same sign. Data collection was carried out in the ARI outpatient clinic at Rawalpindi General Hospital near Islamabad by two experienced Pakistani pediatricians who were on the hospital staff and were fluent in the languages used by patients.

Methods. Over a two-month period (January–February 1991), the pediatricians evaluated every twentieth child waiting to be seen at the ARI clinic to assess the presence of fast breathing and chest indrawing. Children with chest indrawing (i.e., with severe pneumonia) were excluded and the next in line was evaluated until a sample of 50 children with non-severe pneumonia (fast breathing but no chest indrawing) had been reached. Children with severe pneumonia were excluded because we were interested in whether mothers could see fast breathing before the disease reached an advanced stage.

Mothers of the 50 children were interviewed before the pneumonia diagnosis was conveyed; fathers and/or other relatives were sometimes present as well. The mothers were asked for sociodemographic information and a detailed history of the child's illness. Then they were asked two open-ended questions: (1) "What symptoms does your child have today?" and (2) "What symptoms alarmed you enough to come to the hospital?" If mothers did not spontaneously mention fast breathing, the physicians asked them whether it was present. The results of the pediatricians' examinations were used as the "gold standard" for diagnosis of pneumonia signs and symptoms.

We were able to trust study results because, in collaboration with the US Centers for Disease Control, the hospital was conducting a large-scale double-blind test of the efficacy of cotrimoxazole as a treatment for pneumonia (Straus et al., 1998). In preparation for that test, hospital staff had been given refresher training on diagnosis of pneumonia, and respiratory rates were being counted with special care. Thus we could be sure that pneumonia diagnoses were being made according to strict WHO criteria—not always true in developing countries.

Results. Findings were consistent with those obtained in the first study. The types of home remedies used, the basic sequence of health care seeking, the infrequent use of community-based government facilities, the ideas about human anatomy, the recognition of fast breathing coupled with its general failure to cause alarm, and the pneumonia treatment preferences were the same in the two studies. What the second added was the representative sampling of mothers in a particular locale, the systematic elicitation of data, and the concreteness achieved by focusing on a current episode of pneumonia in a physically present child.

Of the 50 children studied, 29 (58%) were male and 21 (42%) were female. This approximates the percentage of males among all children brought to the ARI clinic during 1991 (55%). It is also consistent with much research indicating that medical care is sought more often for boys than for girls in impoverished areas of South Asia (MacCormack, 1988), including Pakistan (Hunte and Sultana, 1992; Khan et al., 1993). In this and the following study, there was a statistically nonsignificant trend toward lower levels of maternal education being associated with bringing a male rather than a female child to the clinic. Although the significance level of this association was only $\leq .07$, it is possible that mothers with less schooling (who tended to have lower incomes than mothers with more schooling) may have been more likely to direct household resources toward boys.

More than half the 50 mothers were illiterate; the rest—all literate—had a mean of seven to eight years of schooling. Almost all spoke Punjabi as their native language. In recounting the illness episode that had brought them to the hospital, they described a sequence of therapy that typically began with one or two days of home care involving home remedies, watchful waiting, or both. Most mothers gave the child herbal teas and humorally hot foods, but some also gave allopathic medicines that they had on hand from prior episodes of pediatric illness. The most dangerous of these was Piptal, which contains the sedative phenobarbital and is widely used as a cough suppressant in Pakistan. Although the package label states "To be dispensed on prescription of a Registered Medical Practitioner only," Piptal—like most other drugs—is readily available without prescription.

For 34 of the 50 mothers (68%), home therapy was followed by one to four days of consultation with various types of health care providers outside the hospital; 16 mothers (32%) went directly to the hospital (Figure 5.2). The mothers who did not go directly to the hospital said that they allowed only one or two days for each practitioner's treatment to work before moving on to the next practitioner or coming to the ARI clinic. For this group of 50 women—who were interviewed in a health care facility and thus presumably believed in its merits—the mean delay between onset of pneumonia symptoms and arrival at the ARI clinic was 3.8 days. Those mothers who went directly to the hospital delayed a mean of 2.8 days; those who used one practitioner delayed a mean of 4.1 days; and those who used two practitioners delayed a mean of 5.7 days. Mothers who had had prior experience with pneumonia came to the hospital about a day earlier than those who were inexperienced.

When the 13 mothers who did not go directly to a licensed doctor were interviewed, the case histories showed a clear progression from the less costly and often more easily accessible healers such as *hakims*, homeopaths, and *chota* doctors to licensed physicians. Only 2 of the 50 mothers had sought care from a physician in a community-based government clinic, and in neither case was the physician assigned to the clinic on the premises; both had been seen by auxiliary personnel. Every mother except two who were divorced or separated said that she had had to obtain consent from her husband (and mother-in-law, if she lived in the home) before coming to the hospital. The women explained that this was mainly because coming to the hospital impinged on their ability to care for their other children, cook, and do housework.[7]

When they were asked which of the child's symptoms had led them to come to the hospital, mothers emphasized cough, fever, and inability to sleep. Although, as noted above, all 50 children had fast breathing, that symptom was mentioned spontaneously by only three women; yet almost two-thirds affirmed fast breathing when they were asked about it. Those who had had prior experience with pneumonia were 1.5 times as likely to say that the child had fast breath-

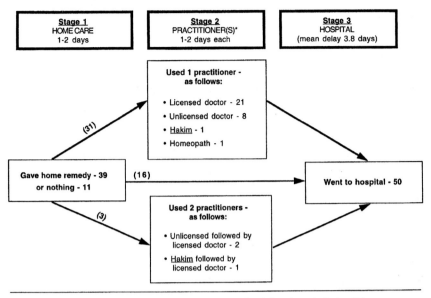

| Stage 1 HOME CARE 1-2 days | Stage 2 PRACTITIONER(S)* 1-2 days each | Stage 3 HOSPITAL (mean delay 3.8 days) |

Used 1 practitioner - as follows:

• Licensed doctor - 21
• Unlicensed doctor - 8
• Hakim - 1
• Homeopath - 1

(31)

Gave home remedy - 39 or nothing - 11   (16)   Went to hospital - 50

(3)

Used 2 practitioners - as follows:

• Unlicensed followed by licensed doctor - 2
• Hakim followed by licensed doctor - 1

* Sixteen of the 50 mothers used no practitioner, i.e., they went directly from home to the hospital.

Figure 5.2. Patterns of health care utilization for treatment of childhood pneumonia as reported by 50 mothers interviewed in a hospital in Rawalpindi, Pakistan, 1991. Numbers refer to number of mothers who engaged in each behavior mentioned. (Reprinted from Kundi et al. 1993:653. Used by permission.)

ing as were those who had not. In addition, 71% of the 35 mothers living in extended families said that their children had fast breathing, whereas only 47% of the 15 not living in extended families did so ($p \leq .01$), suggesting that family members' comments may have contributed to accurate recognition of this important diagnostic sign.

Most mothers held diagnostic and treatment preferences at odds with the national ARI guidelines. For example, the guidelines direct doctors to count breaths rather than relying on stethoscopes for diagnosis of pneumonia, since accurate diagnosis with stethoscopes is difficult, but 84% of mothers said that stethoscopes should be used, describing them as "mirrors" that reveal everything within the body. Still, we noted that they were satisfied with the quality of care at the hospital despite the fact that stethoscopes were never used. They said this was because the doctors showed interest in the children and took time to explain things. As one woman put it, "*These* doctors are so experienced that they don't *have* to use stethoscopes." Thus, in the actual therapeutic setting, a belief stated in the abstract was overcome by other factors judged to be more important.

The Case-Control Study of Mothers' Ability to Recognize Pneumonia Signs (Mull et al., 1994)

In January and March 1992, we expanded our research on maternal perception of pneumonia signs, implementing a simple case-control study to see whether a hospital sample of 320 mothers associated fast breathing and chest indrawing with pneumonia rather than with a common cold. In addition to doing the case-control study, we examined other relationships—for example, possible associations between a pneumonia diagnosis and membership in a particular ethnic group. Delay in seeking health care became a focus. Thus we attempted to bridge the gap between anthropology and epidemiology—an activity that is becoming increasingly common as each discipline realizes how much it can learn from the other (Hahn, 1995; Inhorn, 1995; Janes et al., 1986).

Our aim was to ascertain whether mothers not only recognize fast breathing and chest indrawing in cases of child pneumonia ("sensitivity") but also see these signs exclusively in pneumonia ("specificity"). If not, maternal overdiagnosis of pneumonia could overburden health care providers and cause needless anxiety among mothers. We recognized that the ideal would be to conduct a large community-based study, as Campbell et al. (1990) did in The Gambia, but our limited time and resources made this impossible. We did, however, retain that study's central concept: mothers' perceived prevalence of specific symptoms in children with pneumonia was compared with the perceived prevalence of the same symptoms in children with a cold or with no illness at all.

Methods. We used a case-control design in which the cases were 160 children with pneumonia, almost all with severe disease. Their mothers were interviewed, half in the outpatient ARI clinic prior to any discussion of a pneumonia diagnosis and half after the child was referred to the pneumonia ward for hospitalization. The controls were 160 children with no pneumonia. Half those children had a common cold, that is, an upper respiratory infection (the "URI" group), and half were well, having been brought to the hospital for routine vaccinations. Using the "pneumonia ward" children as the index group, cases and controls were matched for sex, age, and mother's education. The "pneumonia ward" and "pneumonia clinic" groups were also matched so that, in each group, all the children had fast breathing and 75% had chest indrawing.

What made our study "anthropological" rather than strictly epidemiological was that we went beyond the standard case-control design to note differences between responses elicited before and after the pneumonia diagnosis had been conveyed, between responses to marked fast breathing and borderline fast breathing, and between responses from mothers who did or did not have prior experience with pneumonia. In other words, we tried to understand the results in the light of conditions and circumstances surrounding the data gathering.

Interpreters were used in this study since the interviewing authors did not speak Punjabi, Hindko, or Pashto. First, each of the 320 mothers was asked an open-ended question: "What symptoms led you to bring your child to the hospital today?" Then a list of possible symptoms—cough, fever, difficult breathing, nasal flaring, chest pain, and so on—was read to her and she was asked whether she had noted the presence of any of these symptoms in the child. Finally, all mothers except those in the pneumonia ward were asked what the signs of pneumonia were. Every mother in the URI group who mentioned difficult breathing, fever, and/or feeding difficulty as a sign of pneumonia and who had also said that her child had these symptoms was asked whether the sign as it occurred in pneumonia was different from the sign as it occurred in her own child, and if so, how.

Results. When mothers were asked an open-ended question about what symptoms had brought them to the hospital, relatively few in the pneumonia groups spontaneously mentioned fast breathing (16% of mothers) or chest indrawing (6%); as in the earlier study, cough (74%) and fever (63%) were noted more often. Even so, significantly more mothers in the pneumonia group than in the URI group (19 vs. 6) mentioned fast breathing ($p \leq .05$). When the mothers were prompted with a symptom list, all symptoms—which I will refer to as "elicited"— were reported much more frequently than when mothers were asked to volunteer them. Again, cough and fever were the symptoms most frequently mentioned, and again, more pneumonia than URI mothers said there was fast breathing ($p \leq .0001$), with the increased significance level probably partly because the mothers agreed with items suggested by the interviewer.

A comparison between results for the pneumonia ward group and the pneumonia clinic group showed that mothers were more likely to say that their children had serious signs after the pneumonia diagnosis had been conveyed, suggesting that interaction with doctors had influenced their views (a form of recall bias). For example, although all children with pneumonia had fast breathing, 80% of mothers in the ward reported this sign vs. 58% of mothers in the clinic ($p \leq .01$). As would be expected, when fast breathing was marked, it was correctly diagnosed more often than when it was borderline. Mothers who had prior experience with pneumonia were significantly better able to diagnose fast breathing ($p \leq .01$) than those who did not.

Comparison of elicited responses from the pneumonia clinic group with those from the URI group showed that mothers' reports of fast breathing and/or chest indrawing predicted the presence of pneumonia with a sensitivity of 64% (51 of the 80 true pneumonia cases were diagnosed) and a specificity of 90% (72 of the 80 URI cases were excluded). These sensitivity/specificity figures are similar to those reported in other studies attempting to relate maternal diagnoses to clinically diagnosed pneumonia, all of which have been published in medical or epidemiological journals (Gadomski et al., 1993; Harrison et al., 1995; Kalter et al., 1991; Kambarami et al., 1996; Lanata et al., 1994). In our study, sensitivity was relatively low, not because fast breathing and chest indrawing are poor ways to diagnose pneumonia—in fact, they are very good signs of the disease (Shann, 1995)—but rather because some mothers had not noticed these signs.

Our study showed that chest indrawing was not recognized nearly as well as fast breathing, probably because it is a late sign of severe disease and hence relatively uncommon. However, we found that once their attention was directed to the indrawing, with very few exceptions even those mothers who had not initially diagnosed it could see it. Usually they referred to it as *pasli chelna* ("the lower rib area moves"), but about 10% of mothers described it as a *stomach* problem in which the stomach becomes "inflated" or "swollen" while the lower rib area "goes down" (cf. Chand and Bhattacharyya, 1994, Lanata et al., 1994, and Mishra et al., 1994 for similar findings in other countries). This may be related to a lack of differentiation between the lungs and the stomach in the folk model of pneumonia physiology (see Figure 5.1).

As noted earlier, we asked mothers in the URI group how the difficult breathing, fever, and feeding difficulty that they had reported in their own children differed from that seen in pneumonia. This simple question produced very useful data. Most mothers said that in pneumonia the difficult breathing was irregular and resulted from mucus in the chest, but in a cold the breathing was difficult only because of a blocked nose, and was otherwise regular. Also, in pneumonia the fever was high—which is probably true because most pneumonia in the developing world is thought to be of bacterial rather than viral origin (Shann, 1995)—whereas with a cold it was low or absent. Further, the feeding difficulty in pneumonia was not simply due to blocked nose, as in common cold, but because the child was very weak.

While the level of maternal familiarity with pneumonia symptoms reported here may seem impressive, it must be remembered that 75% of the pneumonia ward children were brought to the hospital very late, when chest indrawing was already present. Conversations with mothers made it clear that this was mainly because of lack of awareness that the child was seriously ill. Many said that they had first tried to cure the child by visiting practitioners who were conveniently located near their homes and could see the child fairly quickly. Coming to the hospital was described as an all-day proposition involving a long journey and long waits. Some women added that they had feared that if they came to the hospital, the child might be admitted and they would have to stay there for days.[8]

Still another reason for delay mentioned by mothers was the presence of a competing responsibility involving the welfare of the entire family. For example, one woman said she had put off coming to the hospital because her husband's buffaloes were sick; she had taken the child to a nearby practitioner because she had to stay home to nurse the animals. Other family crises included a grandmother's death, illness of a sibling, or the mother's own sickness or postpartum seclusion—events that had distracted everyone's attention from the ill child.

There were statistically significant findings on three demographic variables. First, a much higher percentage of mothers in the two pneumonia groups (18%) than in the URI and well groups (7.5%) belonged to ethnic minority groups in the area, that is, they were not Punjabis ($p \leq .01$). Most were Pashto-speaking Pathans. Only about 5% of the people in the hospital's catchment area belong to a minority group (Federal Bureau of Statistics, 1990:87); and overall, they tend to have fewer economic resources than the majority Punjabis. They live in worse housing with more indoor air pollution and have poorer nutrition. Thus the possible concentration of pneumonia morbidity in this "high-risk" group is not surprising (cf. Douglas and D'Souza, 1996).

The study also showed that a lower percentage of mothers in the two pneumonia groups (60%) than in the URI and well groups (78%) lived in extended families ($p \leq .05$). This may indicate that living in an extended family confers a health advantage on children because older family members are available to advise the mother and help her protect the child against environmental risk factors for pneumonia. Finally, there was a preponderance of males (60%) in the pneumonia ward index group. It is possible that the boys were more fragile, or were the focus of more parental concern, or both. There is considerable evidence that boys are in fact more susceptible to pneumonia (Glezen and Denny, 1973). However, the boys included in our study may have been less ill than the girls when they were brought to the hospital. It is noteworthy that although there were only 32 girls in the index group vs. 48 boys, the two children who died of the disease during the course of the study were both girls.[9]

The Study of Illness Histories of Children in a Hospital Pneumonia Ward (Cody et al., 1997)

In this fourth and final study, we collected very detailed case histories from mothers of 103 children interned in the pneumonia ward at Rawalpindi General Hospital—to our knowledge, the largest body of such histories collected to date in any country. We gathered information on traditional remedies and allopathic medications used during the illness episode. We asked about licensed and unlicensed health care providers consulted before the child entered the hospital, including the diagnostic and treatment practices of such providers and the cost of their therapies. In an attempt to understand the family dynamics involved in the process of health care seeking, we questioned mothers closely about decisions to seek medical treatment: who made the decisions, when, and why.

Methods. An effort was made to interview the mother or caretaker of every child admitted to the pneumonia ward during the seven-week period of the study

(January–March 1992). Although about half the mothers were missed for a variety of logistical reasons, we do not believe that they differed from those interviewed in any systematic way. Case following was done by the first author, who did not speak Punjabi, Hindko, or Pashto but sat in the pneumonia ward day after day reviewing records and interviewing mothers with the help of a skilled female interpreter. The interpreter, who also served as a key informant, had been trained as a biochemist and was married to a staff physician.

Each mother was asked to recount what happened from the time she first noticed that her child was ill to the time of the interview, including whom she had consulted and why. For each reported visit to a health care provider, mothers were specifically asked about the provider's use of a stethoscope and questioned about any activity indicating that the provider was trying to measure a respiratory rate (use of a watch, looking at the chest for a long time with the child's clothing pulled up, etc.). Informants were also asked to say what they thought had caused the child's illness.

Results. The 103 children hospitalized with pneumonia were 61% male and 39% female, once again illustrating the predominance of boys among patients at the hospital. Two-thirds of the children were less than a year old, the age group accounting for most pneumonia mortality in the developing world (Bang et al., 1994). As in the second and third studies, about half the mothers had had no formal education and were illiterate. The rest, however, had completed an average of seven to eight years of school, far more than the average of five years reported by community women interviewed in squatter settlements in Karachi during our initial research.

Consistent with our previous results, mothers reported overwhelmingly that exposure to "cold" caused pneumonia and that "heating" remedies should be used to treat it. Most remedies were harmless: ointments and oils used to massage the child, herbal teas, and humorally hot foods such as egg. However, two children had had their lower chests tightly bound with a cloth to limit movement in an effort to reduce pain associated with severe pneumonia. This practice, known as "tying the pain" (cf. Rehman et al., 1994), is especially common in the northern areas of Pakistan; it is possible that such binding may further increase respiratory distress (Yurdakok et al., 1990). Two other children had been given opium as a sedative and painkiller, which can depress the respiratory rate and decrease the level of oxygen in the blood; one of these children died in the hospital.

Many mothers responded to respiratory illness by wrapping the child in multiple layers of clothing even when ambient temperatures were mild. While not as hazardous as opium or chest-binding, such overwrapping conceals chest movement, reducing the chance that the mother will be able to detect fast breathing or chest indrawing. We saw many cases in which mothers were so fearful of cold that they could barely be persuaded to allow the doctors to pull up the shirt to examine the child, and we noted that attendance at the ARI clinic fell markedly on cool, rainy days.

An aura of maternal culpability surrounded many discussions of the cause of pneumonia, and occasionally a mother-in-law would openly accuse her daughter-in-law of some supposedly negligent behavior. Perhaps she was not careful to dry and warm her hands after washing dishes or clothes and before breast-feeding, or perhaps she exposed the child to cold drafts while changing the diaper, or did not keep the doors properly closed. Blaming the mother in this way is consistent with well-established cultural patterns in South Asia (Mull, 1992; Stewart et al., 1994). Mothers were relatively powerless in the household, some having to ask permission even to leave the premises, yet they were held almost wholly responsible for their children's illness.

Circumstances like these have led some anthropologists to focus on the *household* production of health rather than only on the mother's individual ability to recognize signs of illness (Clark, 1993; Santow, 1995). Our case histories clearly show the forces arrayed against a mother's taking a child directly to the hospital—distance, time, the need for a male relative or mother-in-law to give permission and accompany her, various pressures from family members—as well as the family's growing sense of urgency as the child's condition worsens despite attempts at treatment. Two representative histories are summarized below (in each case, the child was successfully treated in the hospital and then discharged).

Case 1: Asif. A 20-year-old mother of two boys noticed that her younger son, Asif, 10 months old, had a fever and cough. She had been born in Rawalpindi but was living with her husband and his parents in a village about 175 miles away. On her mother-in law's advice, she gave Asif herbal teas, but he only got worse. On the third day of illness, the young couple took Asif to an unlicensed, self-trained practitioner (*chota* doctor) in their village whom they had visited many times before; he gave an injection and a day's supply of a red syrup. They administered the syrup for a day but the child showed no improvement.

Because it was raining the next day and the practitioner's office was located at some distance from their home, the father decided to take Asif to a dispenser (similar to a pharmacist's assistant, also self-trained) who was within walking distance. In that way the child did not have to be exposed to the rain for a long period. The dispenser gave a one-day supply of a dark pink syrup and three crushed tablets. However, Asif still did not improve, so the mother-in-law began giving him throat massages with mustard oil, an egg yolk a day, and *joshanda*, a commercial tea.

On the eighth day of Asif's illness his maternal grandfather came to visit and suggested that he be taken to Rawalpindi General Hospital. The whole family agreed. The grandfather took Asif and his mother back to Rawalpindi that night and they brought the child to the hospital the next morning. More than a week had passed since his symptoms were first noticed.

Case 2: Nasreen. A 35-year-old mother of five living with her husband's extended family in Rawalpindi noticed that her 21-month-old daughter, Nasreen, was feverish and had phlegm (*raysha*) in her head and chest. She gave herbal teas in an effort to melt the phlegm so it could drain out the child's mouth, but there was no improvement. That night Nasreen's coughing and crying kept the entire family awake.

The next day Nasreen's father described her symptoms to a dispenser adjacent to the government office where he worked as a typist. Without actually seeing the child, this practitioner suggested that Nasreen's fever be treated with a powder dissolved in warm water. The following day the child was still ill, however, so one of Nasreen's older brothers took her to a licensed neighborhood doctor who gave one injection, three crushed tablets, and a yellow syrup.

That day and the next, Nasreen still failed to improve. The mother became angry at the second practitioner's failure to cure the child and argued strenuously that she should not be taken back to him. This caused an argument with her husband, who told her, "You are illiterate, you don't know anything, we must go back to the same doctor." Unaccompanied by his wife, he took Nasreen back to that doctor, who gave the same medicines as before but to no effect. The next day—the fifth day after onset of illness—the mother and her mother-in-law took the child to Rawalpindi General Hospital with the husband's permission.

As these cases suggest, many family members typically participated in assessing a child's condition and deciding to seek medical care outside the home. No one person made decisions alone; rather, there was a dynamic, engaged, and constantly changing "therapy management group" (Janzen, 1978). This is common in poor families in the developing world. Of note, mothers almost never visited practitioners on their own. They were usually accompanied by their husbands or other male relatives, less often by the mother-in-law or older sister-in-law. The second case history illustrates how a father might even obtain medicine for a child without the child or the mother being present, through a process of "second-hand" diagnosis common in Pakistan as elsewhere in the developing world.

Mothers reported that a mean of 6.7 days of illness elapsed between the time when they first noted the child's respiratory symptoms and the time when the child was admitted to the hospital. This is considerably longer than the mean of 3.8 days found in our second study, but that study excluded children with severe pneumonia, whereas in this one most of the children had severe disease. The number of days of delay was positively correlated at the $p \leq .01$ level with the age of the child (i.e., younger children were brought sooner) and with the number of children at home, the latter perhaps reflecting the mother's difficulty in securing child care. There was no statistically significant correlation between delay and family income, but the less educated mothers reported greater delay $(p \leq .01)$.

The 103 families made a total of 194 visits to health care providers between the onset of illness and admission of the child to the hospital. Some practitioners were seen more than once. Overall, 56% of the 194 visits were to private physicians described by mothers as licensed doctors, though some may in fact have been unlicensed. Another quarter of the visits were to self-trained allopathic practitioners, about evenly divided between *chota* doctors and dispensers. Only five visits were made to homeopaths or *hakims* and only two were to licensed doctors in a community-based government clinic. It seemed that both traditional medicine and government clinic medicine were considered inappropriate for childhood pneumonia. The remaining 15% of the visits were to staff doctors in Rawalpindi hospitals, including Rawalpindi General Hospital (some children who were admitted had previously received outpatient treatment at the ARI clinic).

Patronage of licensed physicians is certainly much higher in Rawalpindi than it is in Pakistan as a whole, since 70% of the nation's population lives in rural areas where access to such practitioners is very difficult. However, underutilization of government clinics is widespread and has been documented by the Government of Pakistan (Khan et al., 1990) as well as by ethnographic studies (Hunte and Sultana, 1984). Especially for life-threatening pneumonia, a public perception that appropriate medicines (and staff) might not be available in such facilities would naturally lead people to bypass them.

Mothers' comments revealed a far greater interest in medicines and rapid cure than in the credentials of any given health care provider. The medicine, in fact, seemed to be the crucial part of the transaction. Mothers could describe the medicines dispensed in exquisite detail (color, consistency in the case of a syrup, size in the case of a tablet, etc.). They almost never knew what those medicines actually *contained*, only that they were "good for pneumonia" or "good for cough." Mothers had little choice but to focus on appearance, however, since they said that health care providers had told them nothing about the medicines and in fact had barely communicated with them at all, spending an average of only two to three minutes with them.[10]

When mothers were asked what had happened in the various practitioners' offices, results indicated that 46% of hospital-based doctors and 12% of private physicians counted the child's respirations, but *chota* doctors, dispensers, homeopaths, and *hakims* never did. Almost all of the hospital-based doctors who counted breaths were Rawalpindi General Hospital doctors specially trained for the Centers for Disease Control study, so it appeared that few other practitioners knew how to take a respiratory rate or recognized its importance.

Most providers reportedly used stethoscopes, a symbolically powerful medical accoutrement in Pakistan (Mull and Mull, 1994). Only about a third, however, lifted up the child's clothing, which is essential both for accurate interpretation of chest sounds heard through the stethoscope and for observation of possible chest indrawing. Indeed, when we visited the private office of one licensed physician, we observed that he placed his stethoscope briefly on each child's fully clothed body in an essentially symbolic fashion without appearing to listen and without moving it around; in one case, he put it on top of the child's head. Virtually no conversation took place, but after a minute or two he scribbled out a prescription on a piece of paper and handed it to the mother, who then took it to his dispenser to be filled. We later learned that he (and many other licensed and unlicensed practitioners) routinely gave cortisone injections to children with pneumonia, a very dangerous practice that brings down the fever but inhibits the immune response needed to fight the infection.

Based on mothers' reports, the diagnostic and prescribing habits of private office-based licensed physicians were almost indistinguishable from those of *chota* doctors, though visits to *chota* doctors were 30% less expensive. More than half of both licensed and *chota* doctors gave injections, while hospital-based doctors rarely did so. Further, both licensed and *chota* doctors usually dispensed only a one-day supply of medicine. Mothers explained the reasons for this. If the medicine was not working, they said, why should we keep giving it? And if the medicine did work and the child was better, why continue? The need for sustained antibiotic therapy both to cure the child and to avert bacterial resistance was not recognized.

Discussion

The four studies produced a rich, integrated picture of local concepts and practices surrounding childhood pneumonia in Pakistan, many of which have clear applicability to the design of intervention programs. Researchers within Pakistan have made use of our findings and share our view that knowledge of these cultural concepts and practices is essential (Iqbal et al., 1997; Marsh et al., 1993). Although one could carry out a national pneumonia campaign in the absence of such knowledge, it would be like trying to drive across a country without a road map. To bring these local understandings of pneumonia to light, we relied primarily on what anthropologists refer to as the ethnographic method.

The Ethnographic Perspective

The ethnographic method emphasizes participation in and close observation of a culture being studied. In its purest form, it implies a personal commitment to approaching cultural ("ethnic") phenomena with an open mind, asking "why" until those phenomena are understood, and then communicating that understanding to others. Hypotheses are arrived at via the anthropologist's experience with the culture rather than being determined in advance (Foster, 1987), and qualitative rather than quantitative methods are given primacy.

To its credit, WHO recognized that designing appropriate pneumonia interventions would be very difficult without using ethnographic methods to understand local conditions affecting diagnosis and treatment of the disease. This was partly due to problems encountered during its Control of Diarrheal Diseases (CDD) program, which immediately preceded the global ARI initiative (see Nichter, 1993, for a discussion). The Focused Ethnographic Study of ARI, or FES, was an outgrowth of WHO's understanding of the importance of the ethnographic perspective.

"Focused" or "rapid" ethnographic methods were developed by applied anthropologists in the late 1980s in response to health planners' time constraints (see Bentley et al., 1988; Scrimshaw and Hurtado, 1988). While the traditional anthropological commitment to close observation of a culture remains unchanged, a key feature of the newer methodology is asking questions in a variety of ways to improve the validity of results. If carefully used, rapid ethnographic techniques can capture a large amount of useful information in a relatively short period. For example, case histories of illness are usually collected to ascertain how health decisions are made in real-life situations. Informants may be asked to provide diagnoses and recommend treatments in response to vignettes describing hypothetical illness episodes. Observation of health-related practices, such as storage of medicines, is often carried out in homes. People are brought together to discuss particular topics in so-called focus groups to verify results gathered from individual informants and to reveal possible intracultural variation. Visual prompts may be used to stimulate discussion; for example, a WHO video showing children with ARI (Shann, 1986) was used in the FES to investigate whether mothers could reliably recognize fast breathing and chest indrawing. Researchers may also conduct "confederate" studies in which they pose as parents of ill children, visiting pharmacies to determine what remedies are recommended by shopkeepers. All of these methods were included in the FES.

The Focused Ethnographic Study of ARI

The FES has been mildly criticized for being overly focused and for putting too much emphasis on cognitive responses to illness while neglecting the surrounding circumstances (Nichter and Nichter, 1994). It is obvious that people's beliefs are only part of the story when a child is sick. Political, social, and economic forces can influence the course of illness episodes and thus determine their outcome, and the FES virtually ignores such matters. For example, an impoverished village mother may recognize that her infant daughter is breathing too fast but be unable to convince her husband that time and money should be spent on going to a distant hospital. The developers of the FES, one of whom is an anthropologist and the other a physician, admit this but argue that theirs is an intentionally focused study aimed not at investigating large, intractable problems such as poverty but instead at describing *modifiable* factors influencing illness outcomes (Gove and Pelto, 1994).

A large body of valuable data has emerged from the FES effort, some of which was published in a special issue of *Medical Anthropology* (vol. 15, no. 4, 1994) along with the results of other rapid ethnographic studies of ARI.[11] A major achievement of the FES was the collection of local words and phrases for physical signs, sounds, and the like, that could be used in educational interventions aimed at helping mothers recognize pneumonia. Researchers were also able to identify safe traditional therapies that could be recommended to mothers for home care of children with respiratory illness as well as dangerous ones (such as rubbing the chest with kerosene) that should be discouraged. These findings have been of immediate practical use to health educators, who have incorporated local terms and remedies into home care messages displayed in clinic facilities (Hudelson et al., 1995). In addition, the FES of ARI provides a model that can be used to study other diseases such as diarrhea.

The Contribution of Ethnography to the Understanding of Pneumonia in Pakistan

Ethnographic research almost always helps us better understand the obstacles to implementing public health interventions. For example, health planners often lament the fact that people in the developing world demand antibiotics for simple coughs and colds, not only because inappropriate use of antibiotics creates drug resistance but also because it squanders scarce resources. Antibiotics are useless against colds and cannot prevent pneumonia (Gadomski, 1993). The popular demand for such drugs is commonly blamed on defective prescribing practices and the multinational pharmaceutical firms which relentlessly promote them (Nichter, 1989). But studies of licensed and unlicensed practitioners in Pakistan help us understand another important reason for this behavior. Who could be surprised if people insist on antibiotics for all cases of respiratory infection in a setting in which they cannot be sure of practitioners' diagnostic skills and virtually no communication takes place?

In the best case, ethnographic research may not only reveal obstacles but suggest ways to overcome them. For example, our studies show that mothers have the basic awareness of respiratory symptoms necessary for the development of pneumonia education campaigns. In all major ethnic groups there is an existing cultural focus on the lower chest as the perceived site of the heart and lungs, and there is a widely used phrase, *pasli chelna*, which corresponds fairly well to chest indrawing. Mothers also know that fast breathing is abnormal (though they do not always recognize it as a pneumonia sign) and most can see it in their own children.

What is needed is to build on this knowledge rather than depending exclusively on top-down strategies such as reeducating government physicians. Perhaps through a media campaign, people should be taught that good doctors count breaths and look at the child's chest. Simple timing devices should be developed for use in rural areas where ability to count is limited. This has already been done in India with a one-minute sand timer and an abacus requiring women to be able to count only to 10 (Bang et al., 1994). Since antibiotics are freely available from unlicensed practitioners all over Pakistan, there would seem to be no reason not to train village health workers to identify cases and dispense medicines—a strategy that has already reduced pneumonia mortality in several developing countries (Sazawal and Black, 1992). In response to these findings, the Government of Pakistan has announced plans to train 33,000 workers to provide such services in 50,000 villages in remote areas of the country (Mehnaz et al., 1997).

Our studies also reveal important demographic distinctions that are obscured by epidemiological reports on pneumonia characterized by aggregation of data. For example, children from ethnic minority groups were significantly more likely to be at the hospital for treatment of pneumonia than for a cold or routine immunization ($p \leq .01$), whereas the reverse was true for the majority Punjabis. To the extent that this disparity reflects ethnic differences in disease incidence and severity, it also hints at underlying economic inequities that produce risk factors for pneumonia (crowding, malnutrition, etc.) but may be glossed over by public health officials emphasizing curative measures. Anthropologists traditionally identify with those on the bottom of the socioeconomic pyramid (Bloom and Reid, 1984) and less often overlook such matters.

One must also keep in mind that, in the developing world, the majority of fatal episodes of pneumonia are never brought to the attention of biomedical practitioners. In Indonesia, for example, households were regularly visited over an 18-month period and "verbal autopsies" were carried out for the 139 non–trauma-related pediatric deaths occurring during that time (Sutrisna et al., 1993). It was judged that more than half of these deaths were due to pneumonia. In only 36% of the cases had a biomedical practitioner been consulted, even though such practitioners were accessible; in the other 64% of cases, either a traditional healer had been used (42%) or there had been no outside care at all (22%). In Bangladesh, a program evaluation showed that fewer than 20% of children who died of pneumonia in the year after a large ARI intervention was implemented had been seen by community health workers (Stewart et al., 1994).

It is clear from such studies that reduction of pneumonia mortality will not be easy and will depend not only on the availability of antibiotics but also on improvements in people's standard of living and expansion of formal education for women. In Pakistan, as elsewhere in the developing world, it has been shown that mothers with more years of schooling make more frequent and better use of biomedical facilities during ARI episodes (van Ginneken et al., 1996). Yet the effects of schooling are very long-range contrasted with the "quick fix" of an antibiotic. Anthropology does not evade such issues. Its promise is that it not only can contribute to specific public health interventions as described in this chapter but also can stand as a discipline uniquely attentive to the broad social, economic, and environmental factors underlying differential rates of pneumonia morbidity and mortality.

Notes

1. The World Health Organization currently defines "fast breathing" in several ways depending on the child's age, since the normal respiratory rate is higher for infants than for older children. Fast breathing is defined as a respiratory rate of 60 or more breaths per minute for infants under 2 months old, of 50 or more for infants 2 to 12 months old, and of 40 or more for children 12 months to 5 years old (WHO, 1990).

2. Research carried out in Pakistan prior to full implementation of the national ARI initiative exposed major problems in these areas. For example, in one study (Faisel et al., 1990), 25 doctors assigned to government health centers were observed for one full working day each. Of the 63 ARI patients that they treated, only 8 were checked for chest indrawing or had their respiratory rate counted (p. 14). Almost a third of the doctors admitted prescribing antibiotics when they knew there was no pneumonia (p. iv), and many were observed giving pneumonia patients two prescriptions: one for tablets from the health center and the other for more powerful drugs, usually antibiotic injections, to be purchased in the market. The doctors contended that patients *demanded* injections, viewing them as more effective than tablets, and some even discarded the latter when prescribed.

3. In 1994, WHO sponsored studies of pneumonia in two communities in North West Frontier Province, one Pashto-speaking and one Hindko-speaking. Techniques drawn from the FES manual were followed and an action plan for using the results was developed (Pelto, 1996:30–31).

4. This finding shows why researchers working in developing countries need to ascertain how "imported" words are defined in the community rather than assuming linguistic equivalence.

5. As used here, the words "hot" and "cold" do not refer to temperatures but rather to a "hot" or "cold" quality believed to be inherent in certain foods, medicines, or bodily states or substances. This concept is derived from the ancient Greek system of humoral medicine formulated by Hippocrates and Galen and transmitted to the Islamic world by Avicenna about A.D. 1000. In the humoral system, balance is believed to be vital to health, and therefore "cold" conditions are seen as properly treated with "hot" rather than "cold" therapies. As the system has been passed down through the centuries, actual temperatures have acquired more prominence, to the extent that classification of items in terms of humoral qualities has almost vanished in some parts of the world. Nevertheless, the idea that a hot–cold balance is essential to health remains strong in Pakistan as elsewhere in South Asia.

6. These physicians are usually well-intended, but they are often placed in remote locations without laboratory facilities or adequate supplies of medicines. With no support system, unable to diagnose and treat illness properly, many succumb to loneliness, frustration, and depression. Some cut short their hours at the community-based clinics or fail to complete their assignments.

7. For the same reason, obtaining consent for hospitalization was often difficult. In one case, a rickshaw driver refused to allow his son to be hospitalized with severe pneumonia because, he said, his wife would have to stay with the child and there would be no one at home to cook for him and the other children. We offered to pay him what he would have earned during the period of hospitalization so that he himself could stay home with the other children but he refused, saying that it was not his "place" to do so. (No one on the staff was surprised by this answer.)

8. In a recent pneumonia intervention in a village in Sind Province, most parents failed to follow the community health workers' recommendation that they bring their very sick children to the hospital, which was located about 25 miles away. Only 6 of 64 cases of severe and very severe pneumonia were hospitalized; the rest had to be treated at home (Mehnaz et al., 1997).

9. It is also important to note that the youngest child in the study was 1½ months old. Although many pneumonia deaths occur during the first month of life, Pakistani infants—like those in India (Bang et al., 1994) and Indonesia (Sutrisna et al., 1993)—are not usually taken out of their homes during this period (Khan et al., 1993). Studies carried out in hospitals are likely to miss this highly vulnerable group of children.

10. In 1993, in a city in Punjab Province, 69 licensed physicians were observed in their offices for two to four hours each to see how they managed cases of acute respiratory infection in children under five years of age; 255 such cases were seen. The doctors spent an average of 2 minutes and 23 seconds with each child. Virtually all used stethoscopes but very few counted respiratory rates or looked for chest indrawing. Most children diagnosed as having upper respiratory infections received oral antibiotics and those diagnosed as having pneumonia received injectable antibiotics. The average number of drugs prescribed per patient was 3.4. The authors of the study comment that in Pakistan, multiple drugs are considered better than single and injections are perceived to be more effective than oral medications (Iqbal et al., 1997).

11. Three particularly well-done ARI studies that did not rely on the FES format are Stewart et al. (1994), Chand and Bhattacharyya (1994), and McNee et al. (1995).

References

Bang AT, Bang RA, Sontakke PG, the SEARCH Team (1994) Management of childhood pneumonia by traditional birth attendants. *Bulletin of the World Health Organization* 72:897–905.

Bentley ME, Pelto GH, Straus WL, Schumann DA, Adegbola C, de la Peña E, Oni GA, Brown KH, Huffman SL (1988) Rapid ethnographic assessment: applications in a diarrhea management program. *Social Science and Medicine* 27:107–116.

Bloom AL, Reid J (1984) Introduction: Anthropology and primary health care in developing countries. *Social Science and Medicine* (special issue) 19:183–184.

Campbell H, Byass P, Greenwood BM (1990) Acute lower respiratory infections in Gambian children: maternal perception of illness. *Annals of Tropical Paediatrics* 10:45–51.

Chand AD, Bhattacharyya K (1994) The Marathi "taskonomy" of respiratory illnesses in children. *Medical Anthropology* 15:395–408.

Clark L (1993) Gender and generation in poor women's household health production experiences. *Medical Anthropology Quarterly* 7:386–402.

Cody SH, Mull JD, Mull DS (1997) "Knowing Pneumonia: Mothers, Doctors, and Sick Children in Pakistan." In: The Anthropology of Infectious Disease. M Inhorn, P Brown, eds. New York: Gordon and Breach, pp. 331–372.

Douglas RM, D'Souza RM (1996) Health transition research in the control of morbidity and mortality from acute respiratory infection. *Health Transition Review* 6(suppl): 245–252.

Faisel A, Shafi S, Mian UK (1990) Study of Implementation and Utilization of Standard Treatment Guidelines for Acute Respiratory Infections and Blood in Stools in Sindh, Pakistan. Islamabad: Primary Health Care Project.

Federal Bureau of Statistics (1990) Statistical Pocket Book of Pakistan, 1990. Karachi: Manager of Publications, Government of Pakistan.

Foster GM (1987) World Health Organization behavioral science research: problems and prospects. *Social Science and Medicine* 24:709–717.

Gadomski AM (1993) Potential interventions for preventing pneumonia among young children: lack of effect of antibiotic treatment for upper respiratory infections. *Pediatric Infectious Disease Journal* 1993:115–120.

Gadomski AM, Aref GH, Hassanien F, El Ghandour S, El-Mougi M, Harrison LH, Khallaf N, Black RE (1993) Caretaker recognition of respiratory signs in children: correlation with physical examination findings, X-ray diagnosis and pulse oximetry. *International Journal of Epidemiology* 22:1166–1173.

Galway K, Wolff B, Sturgis R (1987) Child Survival. Risks and the Road to Health. Columbia, Md: Institute for Resource Development at Westinghouse.

Glezen WP, Denny FW (1973) Epidemiology of acute lower respiratory disease in children. *New England Journal of Medicine* 288:498–505.

Gove S, Pelto GH (1994) Focused ethnographic studies in the WHO programme for the control of acute respiratory infections. *Medical Anthropology* 15:409–424.

Hahn RA (1995) Sickness and Healing. An Anthropological Perspective. New Haven: Yale University Press.

Harrison LH, Moursi S, Guinena AH, Gadomski AM, El-Ansary KS, Khallaf N, Black RE (1995) Maternal reporting of acute respiratory infection in Egypt. *International Journal of Epidemiology* 24:1058–1063.

Hudelson P, Huanca T, Charaly D, Cirpa V (1995) Ethnographic studies of ARI in Bolivia and their use by the national ARI programme. *Social Science and Medicine* 41:1677–1683.

Hunte PA, Sultana F (1984) Undernutrition among children in rural Baluchistan. BIAD/UNICEF Sociocultural Report 4. Quetta, Pakistan: UNICEF.

Hunte PA, Sultana F (1992) Health-seeking behavior and the meaning of medications in Balochistan, Pakistan. *Social Science and Medicine* 34:1385–1397.

Inhorn M (1995) Medical anthropology and epidemiology: divergences or convergences? *Social Science and Medicine* 40:285–290.

Iqbal I, Pervez S, Baig S (1997) Management of children with acute respiratory infections (ARI) by general practitioners in Multan: an observational study. *JPMA [Journal of the Pakistan Medical Association]* 47:24–28.

Janes CF, Stall R, Gifford SM, eds. (1986) Anthropology and Epidemiology. Interdisciplinary Approaches to the Study of Health and Disease. Dordrecht: Reidel.

Janzen JM (1978) The Quest for Therapy in Lower Zaire. Berkeley: University of California Press.

Kakar DN, Murthy SKS, Parker RL (1972) People's perception of illness and use of medical care services in Punjab. *Indian Journal of Medical Education* 11:286–298.

Kalter HD, Gray RH, Black RE, Gultiano SA (1991) Validation of the diagnosis of childhood morbidity using maternal health interviews. *International Journal of Epidemiology* 20:193–198.

Kambarami RA, Rusakaniko S, Mahomva LA (1996) Ability of caregivers to recognise signs of pneumonia in coughing children aged below five years. *Central African Journal of Medicine* 42:291–294.

Khan MA, Qazi SA, Rehman GN, Bari A (1993) A community study of the application of WHO ARI management guidelines in Pakistan. *Annals of Tropical Paediatrics* 13:73–78.

Khan MA, Rehman GN, Qazi SA (1990) Control of Acute Respiratory Infections in Pakistan. Present Status and Future Developments. Islamabad: Federal ARI Cell, Children's Hospital, Pakistan Institute of Medical Sciences.

Kirkwood BR, Gove S, Rogers S, Lob-Levyt J, Arthur P, Campbell H (1995) Potential interventions for the prevention of childhood pneumonia in developing countries: a systematic review. *Bulletin of the World Health Organization* 73:793–798.

Kundi MZM, Anjum M, Mull DS, Mull JD (1993) Maternal perceptions of pneumonia and pneumonia signs in Pakistani children. *Social Science and Medicine* 37:649–660.

Lanata CF, Quintanilla N, Verastegui HA (1994) Validity of a respiratory questionnaire to identify pneumonia in children in Lima, Peru. *International Journal of Epidemiology* 23:827–834.

MacCormack CP (1988) Health and the social power of women. *Social Science and Medicine* 26:677–683.

Marsh DR, ul-Haq I, Qureshi AF, Noorani Q, Noorali R (1993) Childhood acute respiratory infection in Pakistan. *JPMA [Journal of the Pakistan Medical Association]* 43:14–20.

McNee A, Khan N, Dawson S, Gunsalam J, Tallo VL, Manderson L, Riley I (1995) Responding to cough: Boholano illness classification and resort to care in response to childhood ARI. *Social Science and Medicine* 40:1279–1289.

Mehnaz A, Billoo AG, Yasmeen R, Nankani K (1997) Detection and management of pneumonia by community health workers: a community intervention study in Rehri Village, Pakistan. *JPMA [Journal of the Pakistan Medical Association]* 47:42–45.

Mishra S, Kumar H, Sharma D (1994) How do mothers recognize and treat pneumonia at home? *Indian Pediatrics* 31:15–18.

Mull DS (1992) Mother's milk and pseudoscientific breastmilk testing in Pakistan. *Social Science and Medicine* 34:1277–1290.

Mull DS, Mull JD (1994) Insights from community-based research on child pneumonia in Pakistan. *Medical Anthropology* 15:335–352.

Mull DS, Mull JD, Kundi MZM, Anjum M (1994) Mothers' perceptions of severe pneumonia in their own children: a controlled study in Pakistan. *Social Science and Medicine* 38:973–987.

Murray CJL, Lopez AD, eds. (1996) The Global Burden of Disease. Cambridge, Mass: Harvard University Press.

National Institute of Population Studies (1992) Pakistan Demographic and Health Survey 1990/1991. Islamabad: Demographic and Health Surveys, IRD/Macro International.

Nichter M (1989) Anthropology and International Health. South Asian Case Studies. Dordrecht: Kluwer Academic Publishers.

Nichter M (1993) Social science lessons from diarrhea research and their application to ARI. *Human Organization* 52:53–67.

Nichter M, Nichter M (1994) Acute respiratory illness: popular health culture and mother's knowledge in the Philippines. *Medical Anthropology* 15:353–375.

Pelto G (1996) Control of acute respiratory infections. *Practicing Anthropology* 18:28–31.

Rehman GN, Qazi SA, Mull DS, Khan MA (1994) ARI concepts of mothers in Punjabi villages: a community-based study. *JPMA [Journal of the Pakistan Medical Association]* 44:185–188.

Santow G (1995) Social roles and physical health: the case of female disadvantage in poor countries. *Social Science and Medicine* 40:147–161.

Sazawal S, Black RE (1992) Meta-analysis of intervention trials on case-management of pneumonia in community settings. *Lancet* 340:528–533.

Scrimshaw A, Hurtado E (1988) Anthropological involvement in the Central American Diarrheal Disease Control Project. *Social Science and Medicine* 27:97–105.

Selwyn BJ (1990) "The Epidemiology of Acute Respiratory Tract Infection in Young Children. Comparison of Findings from Several Developing Countries." In: Etiology and Epidemiology of Acute Respiratory Tract Infection in Children in Developing Countries. JR Bale, ed. *Reviews of Infectious Diseases* 12(suppl 8):S870–888.

Shann F (1986) ARI Training Film. Geneva: World Health Organization.

Shann F (1995) The management of pneumonia in children in developing countries. *Clinical Infectious Diseases* 21 (suppl 3):S218–225.

Stewart MK, Parker B, Chakraborty J, Begum H (1994) Acute respiratory infections (ARI) in rural Bangladesh: perceptions and practices. *Medical Anthropology* 15:377–394.

Straus WL, Qazi SA, Kundi Z, Nomani NK, Schwartz B, and the Pakistan Co-trimoxazole Study Group (1998) Antimicrobial resistance and clinical effectiveness of co-trimoxazole versus amoxycillin for pneumonia among children in Pakistan: randomised controlled trial. *Lancet* 352:270–274.

Sutrisna B, Reingold A, Kresno S, Harrison G, Utomo B (1993) Care-seeking for fatal illnesses in young children in Indramayu, West Java, Indonesia. *Lancet* 342:787–789.

USAID (1988) Pakistan Child Survival. Project paper no. 391-0496. Washington, DC: United States Agency for International Development.

Van Ginneken JK, Lob-Levyt J, Gove S (1996) Potential interventions for preventing pneumonia among young children in developing countries: promoting maternal education. *Tropical Medicine and International Health* 1:283–294.

WHO (1990) Acute Respiratory Infections (ARI) Case Management Charts. Geneva: World Health Organization.

WHO (1993) Focused Ethnographic Study of Acute Respiratory Infections, ARI/93.2. Geneva: World Health Organization Programme for the Control of Acute Respiratory Infections.

World Bank (1989) Women in Pakistan. An Economic and Social Strategy. Washington, DC: World Bank.

Yoder PS (1997) Negotiating relevance: belief, knowledge, and practice in international health projects. *Medical Anthropology Quarterly* 11:131–146.

Yurdakok K, Yavuz T, Taylor CE (1990) Swaddling and acute respiratory infection. *American Journal of Public Health* 80:873–875.

Zimmer HR (1948) Hindu Medicine. Baltimore: Johns Hopkins Press.

II

CANCER

6

Ethnography and Breast Cancer Control among Latinas and Anglo Women in Southern California

LEO R. CHAVEZ,
F. ALLAN HUBBELL, AND
SHIRAZ I. MISHRA

Breast cancer is a major health problem for women of all ethnic groups in the United States. Although Latinas (Hispanic women) have somewhat lower incidence rates of breast cancer than Anglo (non-Hispanic white) women, they are more likely to have larger tumors or metastatic disease (or both) at the time of diagnosis (Calle et al., 1993; Richardson et al., 1992; Vernon et al., 1985). A number of studies have found that the explanation for this pattern lies, in large part, with Latinas' low rate of medical insurance coverage, low incomes, limited English competency, and limited knowledge about available services (American Cancer Society, 1985; Bastani et al., 1991; Hubbell et al., 1991; Loehrer, 1993; Loehrer et al., 1991; Michielutte and Diesker, 1982; Robert Wood Johnson Foundation, 1987; Solis et al., 1990; Vernon et al., 1992).

As a result of such obstacles, Latinas may delay seeking care for a breast problem and often do not receive appropriate breast cancer screening (Chavez et al., 1997b; Hayward et al., 1988; National Center for Health Statistics, 1987). Although these barriers have been well documented, the influence of cultural beliefs on the use of health services by Latinas is less clear. It is possible that Latinas may have culturally based beliefs about illness and disease that could affect cancer control efforts. For instance, a recent study found that Latino and Anglo members of a health maintenance organization, populations that should have similar access to medical care, differed greatly in their beliefs about, and

117

responses to, the causes and symptoms of cancer (Pérez-Stable et al., 1992). Thus it is important not only to remove the economic barriers but also to understand the culturally based knowledge, attitudes, and behaviors that may influence the impact of cancer intervention strategies.

We conducted a three-year study to examine breast cancer–related beliefs among Latinas and the role of such beliefs in their preventive behavior (Chavez et al., 1995a). The first year consisted of ethnographic interviews of Latinas, Anglo women, and physicians in Orange County, California. In year two, we conducted a random telephone survey to test the generalizability of our ethnographic findings. In year three, we developed and tested an intervention to apply insights from our findings. This chapter describes the methodology and results from the ethnographic interviews and summarizes how these findings influenced the design of a breast cancer control intervention for Latinas in southern California. Some preliminary findings of the interventions are then presented.

In designing this study, we were careful to avoid the problems found in other research studies on cultural beliefs and medical care. We wished to avoid the "deficit knowledge" approach that compares respondents' knowledge with the current standard biomedical guidelines (Loehrer et al., 1991; Michielutte and Diesker, 1982). By definition, respondents must be less knowledgeable than the standard that is used. While this approach may successfully characterize how little or how much respondents vary from the benchmark, it does little to further an understanding of what women themselves believe about risk factors for breast cancer. Moreover, Latinas are often considered a homogeneous group, with little regard for the important distinctions between immigrants and Latinas born or raised in the United States. Differences may also exist among Latinas of different national/cultural origins. These differences could influence cancer-related knowledge, attitudes, and behaviors, and could require varying approaches to cancer control strategies. Consideration of these issues guided our design of a study that included ethnographic interviews as well as a telephone survey.

Ethnography is a research method that explores cultural beliefs and behaviors, usually through in-depth interviews and observations of behavior and social interaction. Ethnography focuses on shared cultural knowledge and does not assume that researchers are aware of all relevant questions and issues in the local setting. Thus this approach is useful for exploratory studies designed to improve understanding of culturally based beliefs and to generate hypotheses for future research. Quantitative researchers criticize the ethnographic approach because of the small sample sizes that are often used and because of the qualitative nature of the analysis. To address these concerns, we conducted a telephone survey of randomly selected respondents to test the generalizability of the ethnographic findings. The survey data are not presented here but are available (Hubbell et al., 1996, 1997). The survey results supported the ethnographic findings.

Research Setting

We conducted the research in Orange County, California. This county is the third most populous in the state, with the 1990 population estimated at 2.4 million (US Bureau of the Census, 1991). It covers an area of 786 square miles, is largely urban, and contains 31 cities and numerous unincorporated communities. Approximately 23% of Orange County's population is Latino. Most Latinos—both US-born and immigrants—in the county are of Mexican heritage. However, the Latino population is increasingly more varied as immigrants from throughout Latin America move to the county. The approximately 12,000 Salvadorans are currently the largest non-Mexican group.

A note on the terminology used in this study. "Latinas" refers both to US-born and immigrant Hispanic women. Three groups of Latinas were included in the study: Mexican immigrants, Salvadoran immigrants, and Chicanas, who are US-born Mexican-American women. "Anglos" refers to non-Latina white women.

Ethnographic Methods

For the ethnographic survey, we designed a semistructured questionnaire that contained more than 300 closed-ended and open-ended questions regarding cancer in general, breast cancer, cervical cancer, general access to medical care, access to cancer screening and treatment services, and demographic characteristics. We included a pretested acculturation index, which we refer to as the language/acculturation index since the six questions primarily concern language use (Marin et al., 1987). The closed-ended questions came from the Cancer Control Supplement of the 1987 NHIS (National Health Interview Survey, 1987). The open-ended questions were developed to examine respondents' views about breast cancer and preventive behavior, including the use of cancer screening tests. We also developed questions based on focus group encounters and advice from the study's advisory committee on cancer among Latinas, which included professional and lay Latino community members. We pilot-tested the questionnaire using Latinas who did not participate in the study. A group of health services researchers not involved with the project and the study's advisory committee reviewed the questionnaire for content validity. Bilingual investigators translated the final questionnaire from English to Spanish and back-translated it using well-established methods (Bernard, 1988). Interviewers trained in ethnographic methods conducted the survey between August 1991 and August 1992.

Organization-based network sampling (Bernard, 1988) served as the method to select the non-physician respondents, all of whom were women. Following this approach, one of the investigators made presentations to social, educational, and religious organizations and asked for volunteers. He assigned a code number to each volunteer and randomly selected volunteer subjects from each study site with the goal of obtaining a sufficient number of Mexican immigrants, Salvadoran immigrants, Chicanas, and Anglos for both qualitative and quantitative ethnographic analysis. Respondents' ethnicity was determined by self-report. Organization-based sampling does have its limitations. It is biased toward settled individuals and families, and it is therefore less likely to sample recent, temporary, and highly mobile individuals and families. The advantage of this sampling method is that it uses trusted community organizations to provide entry into a population, such as undocumented immigrants, which may be difficult to sample using other methods. All interviewers of these community (non-physician) respondents were Latinas.

Similarly, the investigator selected physician respondents from a sample of primary care practitioners in the community and at the University of California, Irvine, and asked them if they would participate in the study. Physicians were not randomly selected. They were asked questions similar to those asked the non-physician respondents, but not as many.

The interviewers conducted and audiotaped the interviews in either Spanish or English, depending on the respondents' preferences. Interviews lasted two to four hours with the non-physicians and approximately one hour with the physicians.

This chapter summarizes findings from the questionnaire's sections on beliefs about risk factors, knowledge about symptoms, and attitudes about prevention and treatment of breast cancer.

After obtaining demographic information, the interviewers began the survey with a series of open-ended questions. To ascertain beliefs about breast cancer risk factors, they employed a systematic data collection technique called free listing (Weller and Romney, 1988), in which they asked respondents to list everything that, for example, could increase the risk of breast cancer, and to discuss the reasons for the listings. To determine which beliefs were most common, we reviewed all risk factors listed by five subgroups of respondents (approximately one-third of each study population), and determined the 10 factors mentioned most frequently by each group. We then reviewed these 50 factors to ascertain the number of distinct risk factors listed by all groups. This last step was necessary because more than one group listed some of the same risk factors. This process yielded 29 different risk factors for breast cancer. Finally, to ascertain the relative importance of the risk factors, we printed each of them on an index card and asked the respondents to rank order them from most important to least important. For the initial group of respondents from whom we established the list of risk factors for ranking, we accomplished the ranking task during a second interview. For the remainder of the respondents, the interviewers included the ranking task during the first and only interview.

This rank-ordering procedure allowed us to determine the extent of agreement among interviewees concerning the relative importance of the risk factors. We could also examine variations within individual groups and determine differences between groups in the study. This method did not impose a set of beliefs on the interviewees, who listed the risk factors themselves; the risk factors were based on interviewees' own ways of thinking about breast and cervical cancers. These items, therefore, might vary according to the group studied.

We used qualitative content analysis to analyze the data. Trained research assistants transcribed verbatim the open-ended responses. Three investigators examined the frequency of citations using a text organizing program called AskSam (Seaside Software, 1984). They independently evaluated the free listings, the rankings, and the open-ended responses and identified broader themes which appeared to link together specific risk factors. Later, they met as a group and discussed the themes until they reached agreement. They tested the trustworthiness (validity) of the findings by presenting them to Latinas and Anglos not involved with the study and asking them to judge the soundness of the results.

We used cultural consensus analysis to test for the existence of cultural models that would explain the respondents' rank ordering of the risk factors (Weller and Romney, 1988). Cultural consensus analysis is a mathematical model that determines the degree of shared knowledge within groups and estimates the "culturally correct" answer where an answer was previously unknown. The analysis contains a measure known as competence, which assesses the individual's expertise in relation to a set of culturally correct answers, that is, those shared by others in their society. Cultural consensus analysis provides estimates of each individual's competency and the average competency level of the group.

Ethnographic Results

Respondent Characteristics

We interviewed 121 non-physician community members, all women over 18 years of age. Interviewees included 28 Salvadoran immigrants, 39 Mexican immigrants, 27 Chicanas (US-born women of Mexican descent), and 27 Anglos (Table 6.1). The respondents were similar in age, with the mean age of the Anglos, Chicanas, Mexican immigrants, and Salvadoran immigrants being 38, 39, 40, and 35 years, respectively. The Anglos had the most education with a mean of 14 years, followed by the Chicanas with 12 years, the Salvadoran immigrants with 8 years, and the Mexican immigrants with 6 years. The Salvadoran immigrants had lived in the United States for an average of 4.5 years, and the Mexican immigrants had lived in the United States for 10.4 years. As one might expect, immigrants scored the lowest on the language/acculturation index. Chicanas were closer to Anglos than immigrants in education and income.

Table 6.1 Demographic Characteristics of Women Respondents

VARIABLE*	MEXICAN IMMIGRANTS (N = 39)	SALVADORAN IMMIGRANTS (N = 28)	CHICANAS (N = 27)	ANGLOS (N = 27)
Age, years	40.3 (22–67)	34.9 (19–85)	39.0 (23–67)	38.2 (24–66)
School, years	6.0 (0–13.5)	7.6 (1–16)	12.0 (3–17)	14.1 (12–19)
Years in United States	10.4 0.5–41	4.5 0.1–12	NA	NA
Income/month, dollars	$944 (80–4,843)	$949 (140–2,000)	$1,762 (480–6,000)	$2,923 (800–5,000)
Language/acculturation index, 5-point scale†	1.13 (1–2.4)	1.15 (1–3)	3.6 (1.6–4.8)	NA

*Upper row give mean value; numbers in parentheses indicate range.
†See Marin et al., 1987, for description of acculturation scale.

Although few of the interviewees had had cancer, most knew a relative or friend who had (Table 6.2). Latinas age 40 or older were much more likely than Anglos never to have had a mammogram or not to have had one within the past two years. Salvadorans had the lowest rate of mammography of all the women studied. Some Latinas also had characteristics suggesting that utilization of and access to US-based medical care was problematic. A significant proportion of Mexican immigrants (39%) and Salvadoran immigrants (43%) did not have a regular physician or clinic compared with 7% of Chicanas and only 4% of the Anglos. Only 36% of Mexicans and 39% of Salvadorans had medical insurance of any type compared with slightly more than three-quarters of Chicanas and almost all of the Anglos. Mexican and Salvadoran immigrants were also more likely to report having trouble communicating with medical personnel than were Chicanas and Anglos. Chicanas (15%) and Mexican immigrants (15%) were twice as likely as Anglos (7%) not to have had a medical checkup within the last year. Many more Salvadorans (39%) had not had a recent medical checkup. Many Mexicans (28%), however, had sought medical care in Mexico. This may account for Mexican immigrants' greater likelihood of having had a recent checkup compared with the Salvadorans: the latter may not have felt comfortable seeking health care in Mexico, especially if they were of undocumented immigration status and therefore would have had to re-cross the US–Mexico border clandestinely.

We also interviewed 30 physicians providing services in the area where the non-physician respondents lived. Of these physicians, 14 were university-based and 16 had community-based practices (Table 6.3). Among the university-based physicians, 6 practiced internal medicine and 6 were family practitioners, with

Table 6.2 Health-Related Characteristics of Respondents, Positive Answers by Percent

	MEXICAN IMMIGRANTS (N = 39)	SALVADORAN IMMIGRANTS (N = 28)	CHICANAS (N = 27)	ANGLOS (N = 27)
Have had cancer	0%	0%	4%	7%
Have family or friend who has had cancer	77	43	96	96
Age 40 or older, have never had a mammogram or had a mammogram two or more years ago	38	88	38	11
Have no regular physician/clinic or other health provider	39	43	7	4
Had last checkup more than a year ago	15	39	15	7
Had sought medical care in Mexico	28	4	7	4
Had trouble communicating with health care providers	23	18	7	4
Had private or public medical insurance	36	39	78	96

7 females and 7 males. The 16 community-based physicians, 5 females and 11 males, included 12 obstetricians/gynecologists, 2 general internists, and 2 family practitioners. The physicians also varied by ethnic background; 3 were Latino.

Attitudes about Cancer Prevention and Treatment

Virtually all of the respondents believed that early detection of breast cancer was beneficial (Table 6.4). About the same proportion of each of the Latina groups believed that there was not much that they could do to prevent breast cancer, a view held by a higher proportion of Anglos. Similar proportions of all populations also believed that they were likely to get breast cancer in their lifetime. There was, however, variation on other attitudes. All Latinas were significantly more likely than Anglos to believe that a woman needed a mammogram only if a lump had already been found in the breast. About one out of three Latinas held such a belief; few Anglos shared this belief. All Latinas, but especially Latina immigrants, were more likely than Anglos to believe that having cancer is like having a death sentence. However, about one out of five Anglos also held that belief. Latina immigrants were more likely than Chicanas and Anglos to believe that God gives people cancer because they live "bad" lives. Latina immigrants were also much more likely than Chicanas and Anglos to believe that going to a hospital for breast cancer means that there is not much chance for survival.

Table 6.3 Characteristics of Physicians

VARIABLE	ALL PHYSICIANS (N = 30)	UNIVERSITY-BASED (N = 14)	COMMUNITY-BASED (N = 16)
Age (mean), years	41.9	37.8	45.5
Years practicing medicine (mean)	16.7	11.7	21.1
Females	12	7	5
Specialty			
Internal medicine	8	6	2
Family practice	10	8	2
OB/GYN	12	0	12
Training and birthplace			
Foreign-trained	7	1	6
Foreign-born	9	2	7
Ethnicity			
Latinos	3	1	2
Asians	6	3	3
African-Americans	1	0	1
East Indian	1	0	1
Iranian	1	0	1
Anglo	18	10	8

Freelisted Beliefs about Risk Factors for Breast Cancer

The interviewees suggested a wide range of possible risk factors for breast cancer, of which the most frequently cited are summarized in Table 6.5. Risk factors mentioned by only one or two interviewees are not listed in the table. The
following discussion examines the perceived risk factors for the various study
populations.

Latina (Mexican and Salvadoran) Immigrants

Mexican and Salvadoran immigrants offered a number of possible breast cancer risks, which we grouped into a number of themes.

Physical Trauma. Three-quarters of the Mexican immigrants (74.4%) and almost half (46.4%) of the Salvadoran immigrants mentioned at least one risk factor having to do with physical stress and trauma to the breasts. In discussing breast
cancer, Latina immigrants emphasized three main forms of physical stress and
trauma. First, they warned against blows, hits, and bruises to the breast. They
believed that accidental hits to the breast, especially when young, from falling
on something sharp or pointed (such as a table corner) or being hit by something hard, would possibly lead to cancer later in life. In addition, Latinas noted
that breasts are subject to bruising and rough handling during breastfeeding,

Table 6.4 Attitudes toward Breast Cancer Prevention and Treatment, Agreement by Percent

	MEXICAN IMMIGRANTS (N = 39)	SALVADORAN IMMIGRANTS (N = 28)	CHICANAS (N = 27)	ANGLOS (N = 27)
If breast cancer is found early, it can be cured.	97	93	100	100
I only need a mammogram when I have a breast lump.	26	32	32	4
There is not much that I can do to prevent breast cancer.	37	32	36	48
I am likely to get breast cancer in my lifetime.	43	25	44	37
God gives people breast cancer because they have lived a "bad" life.	29	11	4	0
If you go to a hospital with breast cancer, there's not much chance of survival.	34	36	4	0
Having cancer is like having a death sentence.	63	68	48	22

especially from older babies with teeth and strong fingers that would pinch the breasts, leaving them bruised. And finally, they suggested excessive fondling of the breasts, for example, during sexual relations, as a cancer risk factor. The comments of a 27-year-old Mexican immigrant are illustrative:

> I imagine that sometimes when a man and a woman have sexual relations that are very exaggerated it can cause cancer. There are some men that are very rough, brutes you could say. They grab the woman as if she were an object. They don't treat a woman delicately. You know that when a man has sexual relations with his spouse they like to bite them [breasts]. This is not good. That is, sometimes because of the bruises, or something from grabbing the woman badly can also cause illness.

Another Mexican immigrant captured all three forms of bruising and hitting:

> Bruises to the breast are bad. The breasts are very delicate. So when a child sucks on the breast and leaves a bruise, it's bad. Hits to the breast can also cause cancer. And when the husband massages or squeezes the breast or sucks on it, that, too, can cause cancer.

Behavior. The second dominant theme in the Latina immigrants' perceptions surrounds a number of behaviors which could increase a woman's chances of

Table 6.5 Most Frequently Freelisted Risk Factors for Breast Cancer among Study Populations and Percentage* of Respondents Listing Each Factor

SALVADORANS (N = 28)		MEXICANS (N = 39)		CHICANAS (N = 27)		ANGLOS (N = 27)		PHYSICIANS (N=30)	
RISK FACTOR	%	RISK FACTOR	%	RISK FACTOR	%	RISK FACTOR	%	RISK FACTOR	%
Blows, bruises	29	Blows, bruises	64	Chemicals in food	30	Family history	67	Family history	100
Problems producing milk in breasts	29	Never breastfeeding	33	Environmental pollution	26	Radiation	26	Obesity	37
Breast implants	21	Chemicals in food	28	Blows, bruises	26	Unhealthy diet	19	Hormone supplements	33
Disorderly, wild life	16	Excessive fondling	23	Lack of medical attention	26	Smoking	19	First child after 30	30
Excessive fondling	14	Problems producing milk in breasts	23	Family history	26	Birth control pills	19	High-fat diet	30
Smoking	14	Birth control pills	18	Never breastfeeding	22	Environmental pollution	19	Prior history of cancer	30
Never breastfeeding	14	Breastfeeding	15	Smoking	19	It just happens	15	Age	27
Lack of hygiene	14	Lack of medical attention	15	High-fat diet	11	Blows, bruises	15	No children	20
Family history	11	Smoking	13	Large breasts	11	Never breastfeeding	11	Smoking	17
Abortions	11	Too much alcohol	13	Too much caffeine	11	Fibrocystic breasts	11	Fibrocystic breasts	13
Illegal drugs	11	No children	13	Birth control pills	11	High-fat diet	11	Ethnicity	13
Dirty work environment	11	Lack of hygiene	8					Early menses	13
		Illegal drugs	8					Birth control pills	13
		Family history	8						

*Respondents often listed more than risk factor. Consequently, percentages do not add up to 100.

getting breast cancer. Mexican (53.9%) and Salvadoran (64.3%) immigrants were about equally likely to suggest that a woman's behavior or lifestyle resulted in a breast cancer risk. They often cited smoking, taking birth control pills, drinking alcohol, lack of appropriate hygiene, breast implants, and taking illegal drugs as risk factors for breast cancer. Although none of the interviewees directly stated the belief that "God gives people cancer" during the interviews, they sometimes spoke in a way that suggested these behaviors were morally questionable ("bad") behaviors, and that women who engage in such behaviors run the risk of ill health and cancer. One 32-year-old Mexican said: "God doesn't punish [by giving cancer] but cancer can originate from the bad life that one leads, sexually. I don't believe God sends it."

Another Mexican immigrant noted:

> Well, there are so many medicines that they take so as not to conceive, that I believe this damages them because I have seen various persons that take [birth control] pills have sore breasts, they have swollen legs, they have a lot of problems when they menstruate, some months they menstruate, another two or three months they don't. I believe that because of all this their whole body breaks down.

Lack of Postnatal Care. A number of behavioral risks were related to postnatal care. For example, Mexican and Salvadoran immigrants cited having sex sooner than 40 days after giving birth (8% and 21%, respectively), not taking proper care of oneself after giving birth (8% and 21%, respectively), and not following the proper diet after giving birth (25% of Salvadorans). These postpartum prohibitions are widespread in Mexico and are known as *quarentena*, which lasts for 40 days. As one 25-year-old Mexican explained: "We have the belief that when a woman delivers a baby she has to take care of herself, not do heavy housework because the womb can fall and you can catch infections during the 40 days after birth if you are not careful."

Breastfeeding and Milk Production. Mexican and Salvadoran immigrants listed as possible breast cancer risk factors not breastfeeding (33% and 14%, respectively) and problems in producing milk (23% and 29%, respectively). As one Mexican explained:

> They say that when one has children but does not breastfeed, the milk accumulates in the breast and this is bad. I have heard this, but I know old women who have not breastfed and they are fine, they have not been sick. But for most, they have to breastfeed. If a child does not take out the milk, where does it all go? It stays there, it gathers into clots.

Women who choose not to breastfeed and chemically stop milk production are also seen as engaging in potentially risky behavior. As one Mexican said:

"Maybe it's because, for example, when one has a baby and one doesn't want to breastfeed, there are women who get injections to stop the milk. Maybe this is one of the causes."

Fifteen percent of Mexican immigrants also listed breastfeeding as a risk factor for breast cancer, but only 4% of the Salvadoran women listed it. It was not clear why breastfeeding would be included as a risk factor by some women, except perhaps that it may be related to physical stress from nursing.

Pollution. Some Mexican women (28%) worried that the chemicals in processed food in the United States posed a cancer risk. Some Salvadorans (11%) mentioned the breast cancer risk posed by a dirty work environment. Mexicans contrasted life in the United States with life in Mexico, where they ate mostly fresh food. Some Salvadorans also spoke of the greater purity of the water and land in their country, compared with what they perceived as the ubiquity of chemicals in the United States:

> Pollution is a cause of cancer. Here in this environment we live in there is a lot of pollution from the factories, car exhaust, and cigarettes. All this can cause cancer, I say, including the food. This food is bad. I think that canned food is especially bad because it is canned so long. When you buy it, it doesn't have any nutrition left for the body. They are not healthy foods. . . . I think that in our environment [in El Salvador] fewer people die of cancer than here. Perhaps it's because life is different there. The food is more healthy, more natural. Maybe here they use more dangerous fertilizers.

Lack of Medical Attention. Fifteen percent of the Mexican women cited a lack of medical attention as a risk factor for breast cancer. Latina immigrants often realized that women should seek preventive care for breast cancer. As one Mexican said:

> I don't have insurance. In my opinion, if one doesn't have insurance, it's bad because, well, here cures are expensive and, well you know, sometimes for many people, what we earn is not enough even to eat and live. So when we have these types of illnesses, we don't go to the doctor because of a lack of money.

Another Mexican immigrant was clear about the risk posed by a lack of access to medical care, which could result in a late diagnosis of cancer:

> There is a good reason why we don't seek medical attention. If I should have cancer, how can I look for a clinic? I don't have a social security number. I am not in this country legally. What am I going to do? Let myself die here or return to my country? But either way it's the same. There [in Mexico] I would go to a general hospital where they'd give me pills, but I know I am going to die because they could not cure an advanced case of cancer.

Anglos

Anglos were closest to the physicians in their beliefs. They listed risk factors cited by physicians in the study, but they also listed risk factors that physicians did not commonly cite, such as pollution of food and the environment, highly stressful lives, and breast implants.

Family History and Other Biomedical Risk Factors. Anglos (67%) often cited family history of breast cancer when discussing breast cancer risk factors, a factor rarely mentioned by Mexican and Salvadoran immigrants. They also mentioned the influence of hormones, age at birth of first child, breastfeeding, smoking, diet, birth control pills, and fibrocystic disease as risk factors for breast cancer. For example:

> [A risk factor for breast cancer is] taking the [birth control] pill or other hormonal things. Having a hysterectomy because that really affects your hormonal level. I know that you have a higher chance of getting it if you have your first baby after you're thirty, I believe that's what they say. They also say that women who breastfeed have a lower chance of getting breast cancer.

Although Anglos listed biomedical risk factors, they questioned their validity:

> God, I don't know. There have been so many things tossed about. Cigarette smoking, of course. I don't know. You hear about all kinds of junk. Well, I stopped smoking five years ago. I believe that if it's in your family you have more likelihood to get it. That's probably it. I don't know that it really singles out anybody for any specific reason. My mother never smoked a single cigarette in her life and she has breast cancer.

Some Anglos also emphasized risk factors for breast cancer not mentioned by physicians, such as radiation from medical X-rays (26%). For example:

> I understand that it kind of runs in families. I really can't tell you if this is true, but I would suspect that sometimes a drug that we take may affect breast cancer, but I can't really tell you which ones. I'm kind of hesitant about X-rays, even on my teeth.

Pollution. Nineteen percent of the Anglos mentioned environmental pollution as a risk factor for breast cancer. Environmental pollution included a wide array of risks, some of which had to do with electromagnetic fields:

> Maybe depending on where she works, you know, there might be like, might be exposed to nuclear radiation. Not radiation but, just like waves, and like if she works on televisions or something. You know, it depends. Or maybe sitting at, like, at a computer. Maybe the computer gives off something.

Water pollution was also a concern, this Anglo noted: "I have a feeling about water. I just feel all the cancer here might have to do with people's water, treating the water. That's not going to stop me from drinking water."

Physical Stress and Trauma. Although few (15%) of the Anglos mentioned physical stress or trauma to the breast, this idea was once pervasive in Anglo-American society (Patterson, 1987). The view of a few of the Anglos concerning physical trauma is illustrated by this woman's comment:

> I used to think, this is really stupid, but when I was in grade school the boys used to think that it was the funniest thing to run up to a girl who was just developing and squeeze her boob. They thought it was so much fun. I had that done to me so many times, because I developed pretty early, that it would hurt me so bad. I used to sleep at night thinking that I am going to get breast cancer because they won't stop tweaking my boobs (she laughs). I know it is really funny, but that is what I've always had in the back of my mind. I would still put it as a possibility because no one has ever told me no, that would not happen.

Behavior. Most Anglos (67.9%) also mentioned behavioral risk factors. Anglos, however, emphasized diet, which can also be physically destructive, in contrast to the Latina immigrants, who tended to emphasize physically destructive behavior such as drinking and taking illegal drugs. Anglos stressed the importance of a healthy diet, especially the potential negative consequences of eating a high-fat diet. When speaking about the breast cancer risk factors, 30% of the Anglos mentioned something similar to: "Eating meat. Just not getting enough fruits and vegetables in your diet."

Chicanas

Chicanas consistently cited possible cancer risk factors that were similar in some respects to those expressed by Mexican immigrants and in other respects to those expressed by Anglos. For example, 26% of the Chicanas suggested risks posed by blows or bruises to the breast (physical trauma), which was more often than Anglos but not as often as Mexican and Salvadoran immigrants. The following statement by a Chicana is similar to those of Latina immigrants:

> My sister had cancer and they removed a breast. At first, when it was a little lump and it was growing, she said to me, "Well, why is this here if I never hit my breast?" But I think for sure that at some time she hit it on something, she hit the wall or something and she didn't realize it. It is the only thing I can think of that might have caused it.

On the other hand, Chicanas listed family history of breast cancer as a risk factor more frequently than Latina immigrants, but not nearly as often as Anglos.

Chicanas shared with Mexican women a belief that a lack of medical care posed a risk for breast cancer. They shared with the Anglos the view that environmental pollution and an unhealthy diet, especially one with a high fat content, posed risks for breast cancer. Thus the Chicanas were bicultural in their perceptions of risk factors for breast cancer.

Physicians

The physicians believed that biomedically recognized risk factors such as family history, early first menstruation, and not bearing children increased the risk of breast cancer. Their perceptions reflected their biomedical training and knowledge of the epidemiological literature. The following comment expressed many of the factors physicians saw as risks for breast cancer: "Family history, nulliparity [no children], children after age thirty; a woman who carries her fat or heaviness above the belt. Family history is probably the overriding [factor]."

Although physicians did exhibit a high degree of consensus in their views of breast cancer risk factors, there was some variation between university-based and community-based physicians, and between older and younger physicians (McMullin et al., 1995). For example, community-based physicians ranked fatty/greasy food at 4, whereas university-based physicians ranked it 11; university-based physicians ranked early menstruation at 6 and community-based physicians ranked it 11.

Models

After reviewing the data presented above, we concluded that there were two general cultural models regarding beliefs about breast cancer, a biomedical model shared by physicians and the Anglos and a Latina model shared by the Mexican and Salvadoran immigrants. Chicanas were unique in that they held beliefs that were found among both Latina immigrants and Anglos (but not necessarily physicians). We confirmed the existence of these models using cultural consensus analysis (Weller and Romney, 1988).

Table 6.6 presents the rankings of the breast cancer risk factors by each study group. With consensus analysis we were able to show quantitatively that Latina immigrants and Chicanas did, indeed, reach a consensus on the risk factors to a level sufficient to indicate agreement with a general model we are calling the Latina immigrant model (Chavez et al., 1995a, 1995b). Mexican and Salvadoran immigrants and Chicanas shared the beliefs which characterize the Latina immigrant model, stressing physical trauma to the breast and behaviors such as smoking, drinking alcohol, and illegal drug use as important risk factors.

Physicians and Anglos shared a general biomedical model that differed considerably from the Latina immigrant model. Physicians' beliefs, in particular, fit

Table 6.6 Order of Breast Cancer Risk Factor Rankings for All Study Populations

ITEM	MEXICANS	SALVADORANS	CHICANAS	ANGLOS	PHYSICIANS
Blows, bruises, hits to the breast	1	2	3	20	26
Lack of medical attention	2	5	8	12	11
Smoking cigarettes	3	7	6	5	10
Birth control pills	4	6	5	4	13
Breast implants	5	3	4	9	15
Excessive fondling of breasts	6	1	16	28	29
Heredity, family history	7	20	1	1	1
Illegal drugs	8	4	11	14	23
Chemicals in food	9	9	9	3	14
Exposure to radiation (i.e., medical X-rays)	10	12	2	7	7
Lack of hygiene	11	10	24	29	27
Disorderly, wild life	12	8	22	26	28
Drinking too much alcohol	13	15	12	16	16
Poverty	14	29	26	27	18
Problems with milk production	15	13	13	17	22
Hormone supplements	16	11	7	2	6
Obesity	17	22	19	15	5
Never breastfeeding	18	16	25	18	12
Polluted environment	19	14	10	6	20
Fatty, greasy foods	20	23	14	10	9
Having first child after age 30	21	18	20	19	3
Dirty work environment	22	17	21	24	25
Not having a baby	23	26	29	22	4
Medications	24	21	17	11	19
Getting older	25	19	15	13	2
High stress	26	28	23	8	21
Large breasts	27	24	18	23	17
Breastfeeding	28	27	28	25	24
Early menstruation	29	25	27	21	8

into a biomedical model that embraced epidemiologically determined risk factors and gave little credence to other considerations. Anglos shared enough of the physicians' views to be included in a general biomedical model, but they also believed that other factors were important risks, such as environmental pollution and chemicals in food. For this reason, we would argue that Anglos' views form an important submodel, the lay biomedical model, which only partially reflects the physicians' biomedical beliefs and includes beliefs found in popular culture concerning health.

Chicanas held a bicultural model that fit well with the beliefs of both the immigrants and the Anglos, but not with the physicians. It is interesting to note that, as a group, Chicanas show consensus on a single model of breast cancer risks despite incorporating elements from divergent cultural models (the immigrants' and Anglos' models).

Intervention

Findings from ethnographic interviews suggested that Latinas' levels of knowledge and attitudes about breast cancer differed greatly from those of Anglos and physicians. For example, the Latinas believed that physical trauma to the breast and "bad" behaviors, such as illegal drug use, were the most important risk factors for breast cancer. They also expressed more fatalistic attitudes about the disease, such as the belief that God gave women breast cancer to punish them for living bad lives (Chavez et al., 1997a). In addition, the Latinas were much more likely to believe that they needed a mammogram only if they had a breast lump.

Because the beliefs of the Latinas, particularly immigrants, diverged so much from those of the biomedical community, we believed that it was important to develop a specific intervention for them. Our findings provided the necessary foundation to design a culturally sensitive breast cancer control intervention aimed at improving Latinas' knowledge and attitudes about breast cancer and increasing their use of breast self-examination and mammography (Hubbell et al., 1995). The intervention took into account the relatively low levels of formal education of the population, low income levels, and the preference for the Spanish language. Moreover, we felt that it was imperative to incorporate the Latinas' beliefs into the intervention rather than dismissing them as silly or folkloric. In addition, we were sensitive to the concept that the separation of health problems from belief systems and daily routines of a target population can diminish the effectiveness of health education efforts (Bandura, 1982). Finally, we wished to design an intervention that would have the best chance to change not only knowledge and attitudes but also behavior among Latinas.

With these considerations in mind, we modeled the intervention on Bandura's theory of behavioral change (Bandura, 1977, 1982) and on Freire's empowerment pedagogy (Freire, 1970, 1971) (Table 6.7). In brief, Bandura's theory predicts that individuals will change their self-efficacy (beliefs about their own power or their own abilities) once they have experienced mastery of a task from effective performance of it. An increased sense of self-efficacy, then, leads to changes in behavior, which may then lead to improved outcomes. For example, a woman will be more likely to perform breast self-examination if she feels competent to do it and, if her findings are validated by a clinician, she will then feel more competent in routine self-examination.

Table 6.7 Empowerment Model Intervention: Educational Content*

MODULE 1: BREAST CANCER: SHARING KNOWLEDGE. This module focuses on procedural rules of the sessions, reasons for staying healthy, what each member already knows about breast cancer, and myths and facts regarding the disease. The establishment of procedural rules by the group is a major means for instituting empowerment early in the process. This module also initiates entry into the "problem-posing" pedagogy. By discussing knowledge and by learning myths and facts, the women begin to assess how much they know. This stage of the intervention assists each woman in establishing a baseline level of efficacy against which she can assess the extent to which she "owns" the problem of breast cancer control.

MODULE 2: BREAST CANCER RISK FACTORS AND SYMPTOMS. This module focuses on ways in which the women are in control of their own health, on learning about risk factors and symptoms of breast cancer, and on discussing three types of early breast cancer detection: clinical breast examinations, breast self-examination, and mammography. The women also set goals in relation to the information presented, another step designed to elevate their own expectations of themselves.

MODULE 3: BREAST SELF-EXAMINATIONS. This module addresses the reasons why clinical breast examinations and breast self-examinations may not be performed; how to perform self-examination correctly; goals related to breast self-examination; and a plan of action for breast cancer detection. The women also practice breast self-examinations with models.

MODULE 4: MAMMOGRAMS AND FOLLOW-UP. This module focuses on what a mammogram is and how it is carried out; obtaining access to mammography in the community through lists of doctors and clinics providing mammograms; role playing for requesting mammograms; and the importance of following up on abnormal findings.

*The intervention consists of four educational sessions lasting approximately two hours each and occurring twice weekly.

The intervention also employed lessons learned by Paulo Freire during his literacy campaigns in developing countries, based on Bandura's theoretical perspective. Latinas in our study share many cultural and socioeconomic attributes, such as low levels of formal education, with groups that have already been helped by his empowering pedagogy. Freire found that individuals with low educational attainment absorb new information best when it is presented in a way that relates to their current environment and life circumstances. Thus the educational process should allow students to introduce into the educational setting those issues related to their broader social context which affect their beliefs about the health problem, in this case breast cancer. The educator then empowers the students to make the issue (breast cancer control) their own problem instead of the educator's problem. Through this strategy, the educator and the participants become involved in an interactive process that leads to more information about breast cancer–related beliefs while at the same time allowing students to become actively involved in a problem-solving process that may lead to improved health.

The theoretical model for the intervention stresses the need for the student to "own the problem." Freire developed what he termed a "problem-posing" educational method. He contrasted the problem-posing method with the "banking" concept of education, wherein "knowledge is a gift bestowed by those who consider themselves knowledgeable upon those whom they consider to know nothing" (Freire, 1970). He explains that the banking concept reinforces the individuals' fatalistic perceptions of their situation and consequently does not allow students to shape their own actions to achieve needed change. By contrast, the problem-posing method presents a particular situation to students as a problem to be solved by the group. This model of learning encourages the individual to analyze the way she perceives reality. Within this framework, the educational process involves "give and take" communication. Students are able to internalize and to evaluate critically the information they receive in an open dialogue with the educator. Given such an educational environment, students become intimately involved in the subject, and the solutions that are developed will likely be applicable to their own lives.

Intervention Pilot Test

Method

We pilot-tested an empowerment model intervention in a university-affiliated community clinic in Orange County (Mishra et al., in press). During each session, a health educator posed questions to the participants—all Latinas—which were designed to encourage thought and discussion about the potential impact of breast cancer on their lives, about risk factors and symptoms of breast cancer, and about prevention and treatment of the disease. The educator then guided the group to come up with solutions to the problem of breast cancer control. We obtained measures of breast cancer–related knowledge, attitudes, and practices prior to, immediately following, and six weeks after the intervention in the experimental group and in a control group which did not receive the intervention. Results of this pilot test allowed us to determine the effectiveness of the empowerment methodology in improving breast cancer control among Latinas.

We used a quasi-experimental, cohort design with random assignment of participants into either the experimental or control group. Over a 10-week period, research assistants conducted an initial eligibility interview and administered a pretest and two posttest surveys to these groups. The research assistants were specially trained and bilingual in English and Spanish. The pretest and first posttest surveys were separated by about two weeks, during which the experimental group received the educational program. The first and second posttest surveys were separated by a period of about six weeks. Each of the pretest and posttest surveys lasted an average of 45 minutes and the women received $80 for all the interviews.

Women eligible for the intervention study included those who were Latinas (US-born or immigrants from Mexico or other Central or South American countries), were 37 years old or older, had not had a mammogram in the past two years, had never been taught breast self-examination (BSE), and had never had breast cancer. The study began with 108 eligible women. At the end of the study, complete data from all three assessments were available on 88 women, 51 and 37, respectively, in the experimental and control groups.

We used multivariate logistic regression analyses to examine the impact of the educational program on knowledge and attitudes, that is, pretest-to-first posttest changes. We modeled the analyses to uncover, after controlling for pretest scores, the main effects of the education program on subsequent (first posttest) knowledge and attitudes.

Results

Pretest to First Posttest. The educational program positively changed knowledge about breast cancer among women in the experimental group. The desired changes in knowledge were reflected in the increased proportion of experimental compared with control group women who endorsed medically recognized risk factors and symptoms. At the first posttest, after controlling for pretest knowledge scores, women in the experimental group were significantly more likely to endorse medically reasonable risk factors such as giving birth to the first child after age 30 (odds ratio [OR]: 12.8, confidence interval [CI]: 3.8–43.4, $p < .001$), early onset of menses (OR: 11.0, CI: 3.9–30.9, $p < .001$), and medically reasonable symptoms such as puckering of the skin over the breast (OR: 8.1, CI: 2.5– 26.4, $p < .001$). Women in the experimental group also showed positive changes in knowledge about other medically reasonable risk factors such as family history and age; the changes, however, were not statistically significant ($p > .05$).

More important, the educational program reduced belief in less medically recognized breast cancer–related risk factors and symptoms among the experimental group women. At the first posttest, experimental compared with control group women were significantly less likely to endorse risk factors such as breast trauma (OR: 0.1, CI: 0.0–0.1, $p < .001$), breast implants (OR: 0.1, CI: 0.0–0.3, $p < .001$), chemicals in food (OR: 0.3, CI: 0.1–0.8, $p < .05$), and fondling of the breast (OR: 0.1, CI: 0.0–0.3, $p < .001$). In addition, fewer women in the experimental group endorsed other risk factors which were medically less reasonable, such as worrying about cancer, fate, and ingestion of antibiotics, but the pretest-to-first posttest changes, after controlling for pretest scores, were not statistically significant. In terms of medically less reasonable symptoms, at the first posttest, fewer women in the experimental group endorsed painful breast as a symptom of breast cancer (OR: 0.2, CI 0.1–0.8, $p < .05$), but more of them believed changes in a woman's breast size was a symptom (OR: 3.7, CI: 1.4–9.7, $p < .01$).

Other findings from pretest-to-posttest include proportionally more experimental group women having ever heard about BSE, clinical breast examination (CBE), and mammograms, but these changes were not statistically significant. The educational program also positively affected a few attitudinal changes regarding breast cancer among the experimental group women. At the first posttest, more experimental than control women agreed with favorable (less fatalistic) attitudes. For instance, significantly more experimental group women agreed that they could protect themselves from getting breast cancer (OR: 6.6, CI: 1.7–25.4, $p < .01$). In addition, fewer experimental than control group women felt that there was not much that they could do to prevent breast cancer (OR: 0.3, CI: 0.1–0.9, $p < .05$).

First Posttest to Second Posttest. At the second posttest, controlling for the first posttest scores, there were no significant differences in knowledge and attitudes among women in the experimental group. The first posttest scores after exposure to the educational program appeared to have remained relatively stable over time. With one exception, a similar picture emerged for women in the control group. The only change among the control group was that from the first to the second posttest, more women did not agree with the statement that there was nothing they could do to prevent breast cancer.

We also tested the frequency of conducting BSE, CBE, and mammograms, and the skills and proficiency displayed when conducting BSE on a silicone model. At the second posttest, the positive gains made by women in the experimental group remained relatively stable. Based on within-group analyses of first-to-second posttest changes, with one exception, we found no significant differences on any of the indicators of breast cancer control practices. Between the first and second posttests, there were small positive changes among experimental group women on indicators of the frequency with which the women conducted BSE, had CBE, and obtained a mammogram. More important, the experimental group women appeared to have maintained their skills and proficiency in the conduct of BSE learned through the educational program. Compared with the experimental group women at the first posttest, significantly more of them were able to detect a half-inch lump at the second posttest.

Conclusions

The methodology and findings of this study have important implications for future cancer control research and interventions. First of all, by allowing respondents to express their own beliefs in an open-ended way, ethnographic interviews can lead to a better understanding of cancer-related knowledge, attitudes, and behaviors. Through a large telephone survey of 803 Latinas and 422 Anglo women in Orange County, we found the ethnographic results to be generalizable (Hubbell et al., 1996, 1997). We found the same pattern of differences in beliefs and attitudes among Latina immigrants, US-born Chicanas and other US-born Latinas, and Anglos.

Variation in beliefs about breast cancer were influenced by the interviewee's birthplace (immigrant vs. US-born), ethnicity (Latina vs. Anglos), and expertise (experts vs. laypersons). Latinas in general share many beliefs about breast and cervical cancer risk factors, but US-born Chicanas also shared beliefs found among Anglos. The extensive nature of the analysis also provided many different instances in which to observe the biculturalism of US-born Chicanas. Chicanas consistently expressed views similar to both Mexican immigrants and Anglos. This finding reflects the Chicanas' lifelong experience with American society and at the same time their exposure to beliefs found in Mexican culture. Importantly, Chicanas' views appeared to be integrated into a coherent view of the world, or at least a coherent and integrated view of risk factors for breast cancer. These findings suggest that we must be cautious when speaking in general terms of a "Latina."

Our findings suggest that some risk factors may be ranked low by non-physician interviewees because of their basic lack of biomedical knowledge. But our interviewees also have definite beliefs about behaviors that, in their view, constitute possible risk factors for breast cancer. These beliefs may derive from a multitude of sources: popular media, conversations with health practitioners, and a set of culturally based health beliefs. Importantly, for the women in our study, cancer risk factors were often entangled in the moral, gender, and material contexts of their lives. Such contextually based risk factors were paramount for Mexican and Salvadoran immigrants, for whom biomedical information may not have been readily available. These findings suggest that, for effective communication between health practitioners and patients, it is important to understand not only patients' knowledge of biomedical risk factors but also the risk factors they learn from their particular cultural background. This may be as true for Anglos, who varied in important ways from physicians, as it is for Latinas.

Investigators should consider the use of ethnography in future investigations of inadequately studied populations. Cancer control educational materials could be improved by addressing culturally based beliefs that differ from those of the Anglo population, by whom materials are commonly prepared. An empowerment intervention that, like the ethnographic interviews, allows interaction between Latinas and the educator, and incorporates culturally based beliefs into the educational process, appears to improve knowledge and attitudes about breast cancer and increase the use of cancer control procedures.

Acknowledgment

This work was supported by grants from the National Cancer Institute (5 R01 CA 52931), the California Policy Seminar, and UC Mexus. The contents of the manuscript are solely the responsibility of the authors and do not necessarily represent the views of the funding agencies.

References

American Cancer Society (1985) A Study of Hispanics' Attitudes Concerning Cancer and Cancer Prevention. Atlanta: American Cancer Society.

Bandura A (1977) Self-efficacy: Toward a unifying theory of behavioral change. *Psychological Review* 84:191–215.

Bandura A (1982) Self-efficacy mechanism in human agency. *American Psychologist* 37:122–147.

Bastani R, Marcus AC, Hollatz-Brown A (1991) Screening mammography rates and barriers to use: a Los Angeles County survey. *Preventive Medicine* 20:350–363.

Bernard RH (1988) Research Methods in Cultural Anthropology. Newbury Park, Calif: Sage Publications.

Calle EE, Flanders WD, Thun MJ, Martin LM (1993) Demographic predictors of mammography and Pap smear screening in US women. *American Journal of Public Health* 83:53–60.

Chavez LR, Hubbell FA, McMullin JM, Martinez RG, Mishra SI (1995a) Structure and meaning in models of breast and cervical cancer risk factors: a comparison of perceptions among Latinas, Anglo women and physicians. *Medical Anthropology Quarterly* 9:40–74.

Chavez LR, Hubbell FA, McMullin JM, Martinez RG, Mishra SI (1995b) Understanding knowledge and attitudes about breast cancer: a cultural analysis. *Archives of Family Medicine* 4:145–152.

Chavez LR, Hubbell FA, Mishra SI, and Valdez RB (1997a) Fatalism and the use of cancer screening services among Latinas and Anglo women. *American Journal of Preventive Medicine* 13:418–424.

Chavez LR, Hubbell FA, Mishra W, Valdez RB (1997b) Undocumented Latinas in Orange County, California: a comparative analysis. *International Migration Review* 31:88–107.

Freire P (1970) Cultural action and conscientization. *Harvard Educational Review* 40:452–477.

Freire P (1971) "Education as Cultural Action: An Introduction." In: Conscientization for Liberation. LM Colonnese, ed. Washington, DC: Division for Latin America, United States Catholic Conference, pp. 109–122.

Hayward RA, Shapiro MF, Freeman HE, Corey MA (1988) Who gets screened for cervical and breast cancer? Results from a new national survey. *Archives of Internal Medicine* 148:1177–1181.

Hubbell FA, Chavez LR, Mishra SI, Magana JR, Valdez RB (1995) From Ethnography to Intervention: Developing a Breast Cancer Control Program for Latinas. *Journal of the National Cancer Institute* Monographs No. 18:109–115.

Hubbell FA, Mishra W, Chavez LR, Valdez RB (1996) Differing beliefs about breast cancer among Latinas and Anglo women. *Western Journal of Medicine* 164:405–409.

Hubbell FA, Mishra W, Chavez LR, Valdez RB (1997) The influence of knowledge and attitudes about breast cancer on mammography use among Latinas and Anglo women: brief report. *Journal of General Internal Medicine* 12:505–508.

Hubbell FA, Waitzkin H, Mishra SI, Dombrink J, Chavez LR (1991) Access to medical care for documented and undocumented Latinos in a southern California county. *Western Journal of Medicine* 154:415–417.

Loehrer PJ (1993) Knowledge in cancer beliefs: obstacles to care? *Cancer Treatment Reviews* 19:23–27.

Loehrer PJ, Greger HA, Weinberger M, Musick B, Miller M, Nichols C, Bryan J, Higgs D, Brock D (1991) Knowledge and beliefs about cancer in a socioeconomically disadvantaged population. *Cancer* 68:1665–1671.

Marin G, Sabogal F, Marin BV, Otero-Sabogal R, Pérez-Stable EJ (1987) Development of a short acculturation scale for Hispanics. *Hispanic Journal of Behavioral Science* 9:183–205.

McMullin JM, Chavez LR, Hubbell FA (1995) Knowledge, power and experience: variation in physicians' perceptions of breast cancer risk factors. *Medical Anthropology* 16:295–317.

Michielutte R, Diesker RA (1982) Racial differences in knowledge of cancer. *Social Science and Medicine* 16:245–252.

Mishra SI, Hubbell FA, Chavez LR, Magana JR, Nava P, Valdez RB (In press) Breast cancer control among Latinas: evaluation of a theory-based educational program. *Health Education and Behavior.*

National Center for Health Statistics (1987) National Health Interview Survey: United States 1987. *Vital Health Statistics* 10 (118).

National Health Interview Survey (1987) National Health Interview Survey Supplement Booklet Cancer Control. Washington, DC: US Department of Commerce, Bureau of the Census.

Patterson JT (1987) The Dread Disease. Cancer and Modern American Culture. Cambridge, Mass: Harvard University Press.

Pérez-Stable EJ, Sabogal F, Otero-Sabogal R, Hiatt RA, McPhee SJ (1992) Misconceptions about cancer among Latinos and Anglos. *Journal of the American Medical Association* 268:3219–3223.

Richardson JL, Langholz B, Bernstein L, Burciaga C, Danley K, Ross RK (1992) Stage and delay in breast cancer diagnosis by race, socioeconomic status, age and year. *British Journal of Cancer* 65:922–926.

Robert Wood Johnson Foundation (1987) Access to Health Care in the United States. Results of a 1986 Survey (special report). Princeton, NJ: Robert Wood Johnson Foundation.

Seaside Software (1984) AskSam. Perry, Fl: Seaside Software Inc.

Solis JM, Marks G, Garcia M, Shelton D (1990) Acculturation, access to care, and use of preventive services by Hispanics: findings from HHANES 1982–84. *American Journal of Public Health* 80 (suppl):11–19.

US Bureau of the Census (1991) Race and Hispanic Origin. 1990 Census Profile. Washington, DC: US Department of Commerce.

Vernon SW, Tilley BC, Neale AV, Steinfeldt L (1985) Ethnicity, survival, and delay in seeking treatment for symptoms of breast cancer. *Cancer* 55:1563–1571.

Vernon SW, Vogel VG, Halabi S, Jackson GL, Lundy RO, Peters GN (1992) Breast cancer screening behaviors and attitudes in three racial/ethnic groups. *Cancer* 69:165–174.

Weller SC, Romney AK (1988) Systematic Data Collection. Newbury Park, Calif: Sage Publications.

7

A Policy Approach to Reducing Cancer Risk in Northwest Indian Tribes

ROBERTA L. HALL,
KERRI LOPEZ, AND
EDWARD LICHTENSTEIN

While reduction of personal use of tobacco and elimination of secondhand smoke in public buildings have received considerable attention from public health practitioners in the late twentieth century, few projects have specifically focused on the population that has a special relationship to tobacco—the American Indian population. Yet these are the people whose ancestors revered and domesticated the tobacco plant (*Nicotiana* sp.) many centuries before European contact with the Americas. Because American Indians have higher smoking rates than the general population (Sugarman et al., 1992; USDHHS, 1989; Warner, 1989), and because of their unique historic relationship with tobacco (Seig, 1971), intervention programs designed to reduce the negative health effects of personal tobacco use are particularly important and at the same time require particular cultural sensitivity.

This chapter discusses an intervention that used both public health and anthropological methods. Focusing on tribally controlled policies regarding tobacco use and on personal rather than sacred or ceremonial use, the Tribal Tobacco Policy Project (TTPP) worked within cultural boundaries of individual Indian tribes and recognized their autonomy.

Background

Tobacco has been an important commercial product throughout Europe and the Americas for the last four centuries; within the last century its use has be-

142

come a worldwide phenomenon, in remote and cosmopolitan areas alike. Health problems associated with habitual use of tobacco have been recognized for centuries (Goodman, 1993; Hall, 1992), but early in the history of the United States the tobacco industry became powerful, and tobacco use has long been socially accepted. In the last decades of the twentieth century, however, public health officials, armed with empirical evidence of associations between use of tobacco and risk of cancer and other diseases, made significant progress in their campaign to reduce tobacco use. This campaign moved from a focus on individual decision making to the public arena after studies showed that "secondhand smoke" puts nonsmokers at significant health risk (EPA, 1992; NIOSH, 1991; Rabin and Sugarman, 1993; USDHHS, 1986).

The history of tobacco (*Nicotiana* sp.) as a product that humans cultivated and used lies with the native American population. In part because the largest number of wild species of the genus are found in South America, it is believed that domestication began there. In North America at the time of contact with Europeans in the late fifteenth century, native populations were cultivating the plant as well as using wild varieties, but native use and domestication probably predated the arrival of Europeans by at least 8,000 years (Goodman, 1993). At the time of first European contact, Indian tribes in the Pacific Northwest were growing the plant, and archaeological evidence suggests it had been used for at least 2,000 years (Endzweig, 1989). Oral traditions indicating that tobacco was a revered substance that was used in ceremonies are supported by archaeological observations. For example, Seig (1971) cites a Mayan carving of a priest puffing a tubular pipe; the carving, called *The Old Man of Palenque*, is believed to have been produced about A.D. 400. While tobacco was used in many forms, for example, in snuff and as a chewing substance as well as being smoked in pipes, the ethnographic record indicates that its primary use has been in spiritual, political, and healing rituals. In most areas, the relative scarcity of tobacco probably helped to ensure that it was reserved for ceremonial occasions. As such, tobacco did not constitute a health threat within the native social ecology.

Native traditions were upset when Europeans arrived and adopted the tobacco plant as a product for commercial development on plantations (Crosby, 1986; Weatherford, 1988). It joined sugar, which had been developed as a plantation crop on Mediterranean islands just a few centuries before Columbus's voyage in the late fifteenth century, as a basis for economic expansion.

Political and Economic Environment

Federally recognized American Indian tribes play important political and economic roles within the three Northwestern states (Oregon, Washington, and Idaho; see Figure 7.1), in addition to the contributions made through their culture and history. Tribes constitute independent governmental units with offic-

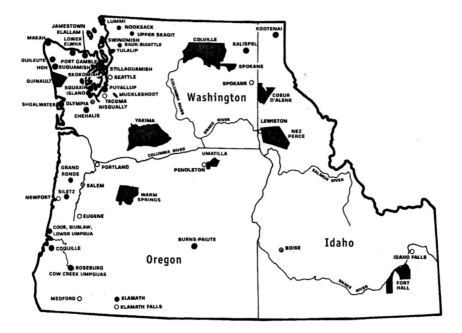

Figure 7.1. The 39 federally recognized Pacific Northwest tribes that participated in the Tribal Tobacco Policy Project.

ers elected by their members. Many Northwestern tribes have substantial business interests in addition to the economic impacts associated with governmental functions and social services. Businesses are diverse and include logging, lumber, construction, agricultural products, health care services, casinos, restaurants, and resorts.

"Tribal self-government" and "economic self-sufficiency" are common expressions that convey goals important to American Indian tribes in the last half of the twentieth century. These goals and the activities associated with them have replaced the federal policy in the first half of the twentieth century which tried to assimilate American Indian people into the general culture. Policymakers formerly believed that the very existence of tribes had negative economic and social consequences for the American Indian people and American society as a whole (US American Indian Policy Review Commission, 1976). In the late twentieth century, however, a different theory holds that economic disadvantages experienced by tribal members are the result of a variety of factors, among them lack of political empowerment, economic dependence, exploitation of reservation resources by non-tribal interests, and poor economic investment strategies, in addition to cumbersome federal bureaucracy. Remedies advocated include tribally based political, economic, and social control.

The Indian Health Service is the federal division of the Public Health Service specifically concerned with American Indian health needs. In many regions tribes have formed Indian Health Boards that represent local tribal issues to this federal service. The Northwest Portland Area Indian Health Board (NPAIHB) serves the 40 federally recognized tribes of Oregon, Washington, and Idaho;[1] its board consists of one representative from each tribe (NPAIHB, n.d.).

History of the Tribal Tobacco Policy Project

In 1987 the NPAIHB received a grant from the Indian Health Service to study the prevalence of smokeless tobacco use by Indian boys and girls. This project demonstrated that smokeless tobacco use was a serious health hazard to Indian youth (Hall and Dexter, 1988). In carrying out the study and presenting results to tribal health leaders, the board and researchers learned that many health workers in tribes were concerned about the health impact of tobacco use and believed that something should be done about it (Hall et al., 1995).

Rather than working one-on-one with potential tobacco users and attempting to convince them not to use commercial tobacco products, the Health Board, together with researchers from Oregon State University and the Oregon Research Institute, felt that changes in tobacco policy could be more beneficial in reducing the population's risk of cancer. Tribes exercise control over their own environments and thus tribal policies seemed a good place to start to reach both users of tobacco and potential users. In the 1980s, the health risks associated with second-hand smoke were becoming known; policies restricting the use of tobacco within tribal meeting rooms and businesses thus would have positive benefits for non-smoking tribal members including children and elders. Since the smokeless tobacco study had shown that children were being introduced to smokeless products at a very young age, it appeared that community elders needed to intervene to change community standards. It was felt that the Indian norm was one of tobacco use, and this had to be addressed by a policy-based approach; furthermore, this approach might be useful with youth (Pentz et al., 1989) and could enhance participation in smoking cessation programs (Rigotti, 1989).

Funding was sought and obtained from the National Cancer Institute, whose Special Populations Branch in the late 1980s developed a primary prevention and avoidable mortality program calling for intervention projects and their evaluation in native communities (Burhansstipanov and Dresser, 1993). This funding was used to carry out the Tribal Tobacco Policy Project (TTPP).

The Challenge: Develop a Culturally Sensitive Approach in a Region of Cultural Diversity

Geographically and culturally, the Pacific Northwest is a region of contrasts, including coastal, plateau, and mountain areas with densely populated cities and isolated rural areas. Similarly, the Northwest's American Indian tribes represent many separate and diverse cultures, language groups, and resource strategies. To add to the diversity among tribes, each has a unique history with the United States government. These historical, political, and social factors created a situation in which individual tribes have different approaches to self-government and decision making.

Tobacco Use and Health in Native American Communities. Studies of cancer in Native Americans, as well as surveys of health behaviors, indicate that smoking is a health problem that affects both men and women (Burhansstipanov and Dresser, 1993; Hampton, 1992; Horm and Burhansstipanov, 1992; Sugarman et al., 1992). Smoking rates among Indian people, particularly women, have not declined as much as smoking in other US populations in the past two decades (USDHHS, 1989; Warner, 1989). Given the high prevalence rates—which a 1987–1991 survey determined were 33.4% for native men and 26.6% for native women, compared with 25.7% for white men and 23.0% for white women (Burhansstipanov and Dresser, 1993:5–6)—leaders in Indian tribes and in Indian health agencies have moved to reduce tobacco smoke exposure within tribal offices and businesses.

In 1987 the Indian Health Service, following suggestions of Indian leaders, made its offices and clinics smoke-free; as a federal agency, hierarchically organized, it had the ability to do that unilaterally. Indian tribes, however, are organized in the opposite way; control goes up from individual members to elected officials. Tribal administration usually consists of a tribal council and elected officers, as well as a set of administrators. Much of the work of tribal governance and policy-making is invested in committees, which consist of tribal members with expertise or interest in particular issues. Clearly, for changes in tobacco policies to occur within tribal offices and tribal communities, the elected officers, committees, and administrators—and ultimately the entire tribal community—had to be involved.

Three Issues of Cultural Sensitivity. Even though the Northwest Portland Area Indian Health Board had sought and obtained approval for this project, the research team knew it had a formidable task with cultural dimensions and overtones. Its mission was to urge tribal leaders to enact policies to restrict the use of tobacco, without infringing on traditional values regarding tobacco, and in recognition of the fact that some Northwestern tribes derive income from selling tobacco. In the 1990s tobacco remains both a revered product, still used ceremonially, and a product that many individual tribal members use addictively. The solution came from two principles: (1) tobacco as used traditionally—sparingly and in special situations—does not present a health problem; and (2) tobacco used personally and addictively—as a "recreational" drug—produces health problems. It was essential for the research and intervention project to separate these two uses. The task was to propose clearly to tribal leaders and members that tribal leaders could control the personal consumer use of tobacco without infringing on sacred or traditional use. In practice, the research intervention team did not question tribal members concerning traditional use of tobacco but instead focused on personal consumer use, thus respecting rights of privacy regarding spiritual and traditional tobacco practices. This constituted the first aspect of cultural sensitivity with which the research project grappled.

A second set of cultural sensitivities existed in the diversity of governance practices within the area. In prehistoric times, people living in the three-state area of Idaho, Washington, and Oregon were organized in hundreds of political units in which many different languages were spoken. The European migration into the Northwest introduced diseases that led many individuals, and consequently some cultural traditions, to die out (Boyd, 1990). Many people were removed from their home areas and taken to reservations; in the process of relocation, other cultural traditions were lost. Some of the current federally recognized tribal units are confederacies of historic tribes; others are direct descendants of smaller groups of people who occupied villages in the same area in which tribal headquarters are located today. In the TTPP, each tribal unit needed to be respected as a unique cultural and political entity with its own history, social customs, and rules of governance.

A third, critical aspect of cultural sensitivity involved procedures governing publication of research results. Indian tribes in the past have felt that researchers used them as subjects but did not always fully involve them in the research or produced documents that did not accurately reflect tribal perspectives. To ensure that communication channels were open and that information concerning research with tribes represented tribal perspectives, the protocol for this project required that research papers, such as this one, be screened by an editorial committee consisting of an executive group at the Indian Health Service Institutional Review Board as well as at the NPAIHB. Although the process is time-consuming, it assures that conflicts of perspective are resolved and that the product is defensible within Indian communities as well as from a research perspective.

Methods

Choice of Approach

The decision to develop a program of culturally sensitive consultation interventions with tribal governments focusing on upgrading tobacco policies, rather than developing a tobacco use cessation program to offer to individual tribal members, derived from both theoretical and methodological considerations. Among direct effects, more restrictive policies could protect the health of nonsmoking tribal members at tribal offices and also could change social norms (Rabin and Sugarman, 1993). Over time, policies in which personal tobacco use is not seen as socially approved would give social support to smokers to stop smoking and could be more effective than cessation programs in discouraging youth from smoking or using snuff or chewing tobacco (Pentz et al., 1989). A program to change community norms would likely be much slower in reducing the number of smokers and snuff users, but, given enough time, it could produce much greater reductions.

The two approaches—cessation programs and policy change—involve different methods and different measures of success. A cessation approach would be directed at individuals; program completion and long-term cessation rates would offer measures of success. Interventions aimed at changing policies share with cessation programs the long-range goal of reduction in personal tobacco use, but this goal would be reached by changes in the social environment that, in turn, alter individual behavior (USDHHS, 1991). The project team chose tobacco policies enacted by tribal councils as the outcome measure of the intervention. In tribes that already had restrictive smoking policies, it was hypothesized that policies would become more stringent, and in those that lacked them, policies would be developed as a result of the program.

Because a secular trend of increased stringency of tobacco control was occurring throughout the country (Glasgow et al., 1990; Rabin and Sugarman, 1993; USDHHS, 1991), it was essential to have a control group as well as an experimental group. For the intervention trial, tribes were assessed on key variables, stratified, and then randomly assigned either to the "early treatment" (experimental) or "delayed treatment" (control) group. For ethical reasons, and to provide an additional assessment of the policy approach, the project provided the consultation intervention (delayed treatment) to control tribes after the intervention and its assessment had been completed for the early intervention (experimental) tribes. A baseline study of historical, cultural, and demographic features of the 39 tribes, along with the initial tobacco policy assessments, provided information needed in stratification. Attributes used to categorize groups of tribes for random assignment were number of members, comprehensiveness of the baseline tobacco use policy, and a consensus rating of each tribe's readiness to adopt a new tobacco policy or review its current policy.

A database called "Tribal Profiles" was developed to summarize key aspects of each tribe and its environment and to help staff of the TTPP understand and respond sensitively to each of the tribes. Key information was obtained by interviews with tribal officials: number of tribal members, location of offices and reservation lands; number of employees; history and governance structure; and current health programs. Geographic and demographic information about each tribe's setting included climatic indicators such as average temperature and annual precipitation, size and population of the cities and counties in which reservations and tribal offices were located, and principal industries. The tribal profiles served as an ethnographic sketch that helped team members develop an understanding and an effective working relationship with each tribe.

After tribes had been assigned to "treatment" and "control" phases of the study, we proceeded with (1) the interventions; (2) field observations at a subset of early and delayed treatment tribes and surrounding areas; and (3) postintervention assessment of policies in all tribes. All components included insights and approaches appropriate in native culture, and all three integrated approaches from public health and anthropology, but field observation methodologies emphasized anthropological methodology and the assessment of policies drew more heavily from public health.

The Intervention

A standardized protocol for the intervention was followed as much as possible, but individual characteristics of each tribe made it necessary to vary the routine. Concepts for the consultative process were adapted from worksite smoking policy projects (Glasgow et al., 1990). The delivery of the intervention by staff from the Northwest Portland Area Indian Health Board (NPAIHB) was in itself an exercise in cultural consideration.

Intervention consisted of a four-part process:

1. An introductory "kickoff" at the NPAIHB quarterly meeting, where representatives from tribes involved in the intervention were introduced to the project and were asked to identify staff or members to serve as the contact for the project.
2. A follow-up meeting at each individual tribal office, where a presentation was made of data relating to tobacco and the dangers of secondhand smoke, and there was a discussion of issues relevant to tobacco use and tribal tobacco policies. It was essential to offer available Indian-oriented resource materials at this and the next stage.
3. A working meeting where tribal people, using sample policies provided by the interventionist, developed their own draft tribal tobacco policy—a basic step. The draft usually was circulated for input from other tribal committees or staff members but in some cases it was taken directly to tribal council in resolution form to be passed, reworked, tabled, or denied.
4. Follow-up to the draft or resolution process, which was sometimes long and painful. It took numerous phone calls and sometimes a third or fourth visit to get closure on the policy. Closure was defined as having a copy of the final resolution from tribal council, or a copy of the draft policy that did not pass in tribal council.

In offering to consult with 19 or 20 tribes it is important to standardize procedures, while at the same time considering the degree of progress obtained in each tribe as well as particular health issues and rules of governance. In order to keep track of each tribe's progress, the interventionist kept a log of telephone and in-person contacts with each tribe. Summary data from these logs provide insights into the consultation process.

Materials used in the first three steps of the process included both educational materials developed for the general population and Indian-oriented materials developed for this project. At the first two meetings, the interventionist provided a factual presentation on the health risks of smoking and exposure to second-hand smoke and showed the video *On the Air*, which deals with worksite tobacco policy development (Wright, 1988). The interventionist also provided copies of the *Tribal Tobacco Policy Workbook*, developed for this project (NPAIHB, 1995). The workbook recommends that a tribal committee be formed to consider tobacco policy changes, lists key decisions in developing a tribal smoking policy, and suggests ways to publicize and implement a policy. It contains a sample tribal tobacco policy and smoking cessation resources available to tribes. The workbook and the interventionist emphasized that a tobacco policy should not be construed as "antismoker" but as an attempt to clarify where smoking could and could not occur; as such, it could open lines of communication among tribal members and make all of them more comfortable.

After baseline studies and assignment to the early or delayed treatment group, the intervention was provided to the early treatment group over an 18-month period. Assessments of all tribes at this point—when half had received the intervention and half had not—provided the strongest test of the intervention. After experimental (early) group intervention assessments were completed, and the intervention was offered to the delayed treatment group, a third assessment was conducted.

Adaptations to the Basic Intervention Procedure. Many adaptations to this protocol occurred. The identification of the contact or group for consultation for the tobacco policy varied. If the person or committee identified at the regional or quarterly board meeting was not appropriate or willing to work on policy, it took additional phone calls, requests to tribal council, and persistence with the NPAIHB delegate or the tribal health director to arrange for contacts and meetings. In different tribes, project staff worked with tribal health committee members, the tribal health director, public and community health nurses, the Indian Child Welfare Specialist, the Community Health Representative, tribal council members, the public health educator, and the environmental protection staff— a different mix of these officials in each tribal setting. All tribes selected to participate in the study eventually met with the project interventionist and drafted a policy, even though some tribes did not pass a policy.

The interventionist had to understand the various tribal cultural processes, as well as demographics and politics, in order to adapt the program to each tribe. Cultural factors, social organization, and the size and complexity of the tribe all affected the manner in which the intervention was delivered. In some of the smaller tribes, where communication among members and within the government appeared open and rapid, the interventionist was able to guide the tribe rapidly through the intervention protocol. In contrast, in some of the large tribes, representing confederacies of formerly independent bands or tribes, formal processes to assure that all segments of the membership have access to tribal government constrain the ability of tribal governments to make rapid changes in policy. Working in such settings, the interventionist had to patiently show respect for the individual governmental procedure of each tribe even when the pressures of completing a grant requirement within the allotted time period weighed on her.

One of the major problems the interventionist faced was simply getting on the agenda of the tribal councils. Because tribes serve diverse functions in areas such as health services, cultural activities, education, welfare, and economic development, it is difficult for any issue to be considered a priority. Justifying time and attention at tribal meetings and arranging appearances before committees and councils and with staff members created many hurdles. In addition, tribal offices are subject to lobbying by various people and agencies in both the Indian and non-Indian community, and as a consequence they tend to be wary of any requests presented to them.

Adding to logistical problems, elected officials and staff members changed positions frequently; when a change occurred, the interventionist had to begin negotiations once again with the new officers. Committee positions, occupied by tribal members who were not paid staff members of the tribe, also changed frequently. These volunteers, many of whom held other full-time jobs, had limited time available to discuss tribal policy with the interventionist or with other tribal members. For all of these reasons, the consultation intervention required many telephone calls. Visits were time-consuming as well as expensive, since the tribes occupy a wide geographic range throughout the three Northwestern states (Figure 7.1).

Cultural sensitivity was a constant in this project. In addition to Indian-specific cultural issues noted earlier, unanticipated considerations specific to Indian country were the traditional use of tobacco as opposed to the daily addictive use; lack of recognition of tobacco as a health priority in the Indian community, in part because of the enormity of other health issues; sovereignty issues; respect for elders, which precluded prohibiting them from smoking; and penalty issues, that is, identifying who is responsible for restrictions. It was extremely important to allow the work group in each tribe to identify its own "tobacco problems and areas" in order for the group to formulate its policy to fit its situation, including such topics as employee smoking policies, youth, elders, and consideration of who is affected by secondhand smoke.

Field Observations/Descriptive Assessments

Several anthropological methodologies were employed in the field observations (Kellehear, 1993). Traditional ethnographies (systematic field studies that record cultural behavior) examine all facets of a community's culture, but in this project briefer field studies known as rapid assessment procedures (RAPs), which focus on a specific issue or problem and employ a mix of objective descriptions and interviews, were used for descriptive assessment (Scrimshaw and Gleason, 1992). Reflecting the viewpoint and goals of anthropological studies, RAPs portray the viewpoint of the community—the insider's or "emic" viewpoint, and the social rules that govern a culture (Bernard, 1988); include direct field observations; are eclectic or multidisciplinary in the type of data they examine; use selective or convenience rather than random sampling of interview subjects; and make thematic rather than quantitative summaries of findings (Afonja, 1992). In addition to determining whether the environment encouraged or discouraged personal tobacco use, the descriptive assessments provided a qualitative sense of attitudes and approaches that tribes took toward tobacco control.

Because funding limitations prohibited descriptive assessments at all 39 sites, a subset of tribes was chosen to reflect the diversity of tribal settings with respect to size, rural or urban location, and other cultural and geographic characteristics. At the beginning of the study the Northwest tribes ranged in size from 124 to 7,783 members, with a median of 665. Full-time employees varied from 8 to 874, with a median of 55. Tribes chosen for field visits varied in size from 250 to 7,308 members. In the first pre-intervention round in 1991, the observer visited 11 tribes, 6 that were early intervention tribes and 5 in the late intervention mode. In the early intervention follow-up early in 1993 the same observer visited 12 tribes—the original 11 plus an additional late intervention tribe. In the late intervention follow-up in 1994, the same observer visited the same 12 tribes.

Field observations provided an understanding of how tobacco was used and controlled within tribal agencies. Artifacts such as ashtrays and cigarette butts were indicators of places where personal use of tobacco occurred (and was presumably sanctioned), while the absence of ashtrays, with or without the presence of no-smoking signs or educational posters about tobacco, provided important communications about negative attitudes and policies regarding personal use of tobacco.

Observations of these indicators were conducted in each of three periods over the course of three years by a single research staff member (a college student who was a member of one of the Northwest tribes and had experience in cultural surveys and management of tribal archives). When the observer entered a tribal office she identified her participation in the Tribal Tobacco Policy Project to tribal employees and asked simply to look around.

The observation protocol had two components: (1) a checklist (Hall et al., 1995:158) recording presence or absence of tobacco-related artifacts (ashtrays, cigarette butts, no-smoking signs, anti–tobacco-use posters, etc.); and (2) field notes recording observations of tobacco-related behaviors, artifacts, and conversations with tribal members concerning tobacco issues. The goal of observations was to portray the tribal setting and to determine whether and how tobacco use was encouraged or discouraged.

Observational assessments were made at tribally owned sites such as tribal government offices, health clinics, community centers, schools, and businesses. In addition, observations were made at non-Indian government buildings and public and commercial settings in adjacent communities that were part of the social environment of tribal members. In each round of observations, the observer spent an average of half a day with smaller tribes and up to 4.5 days with larger tribes, which maintain offices in several cities. The specific number of places observed varied from 3 to 51 per tribe in the first set of observations in 1991, from 8 to 48 per tribe in the second set in 1993, and from 7 to 76 per tribe in 1994. Tribal locations were sampled in proportion to their size and activities, but more checklists were completed in 1993 and 1994 than in 1991; there were 693 locations in 1994 and 653 locations in 1993, compared with 382 in 1991. In all three sets of visits the number of observations corresponded to tribal size.

Given the diversity among tribes, a standardized protocol of site selection was not possible, but every attempt was made to observe the same types of locations in each tribe—offices, agencies, businesses, and community centers, for example. While some of the Northwest tribes have large reservations where tribal members predominate, other tribes have offices in cities that are largely inhabited by the general population. Some tribes operate public sector businesses such as restaurants, resorts, and casinos, while others do not. The uniqueness of each tribal location precluded quantitative comparisons across tribes but permitted qualitative comparisons within each tribe between observation periods. In addition to comparisons from the first visit to the second and third visit within each tribe, observations of tribal environments were also compared with non-tribal environments.

Assessing Tribal Tobacco Policies

Assessing policies of these very diverse tribes required adapting standard social science methodologies. Ideally, we would have liked to make line-by-line comparisons of written policies, but this option was not valid because procedures for adopting policies, as well as the policies produced, varied among tribes.

Policies ranged from single-line resolutions or a memorandum passed at council meetings to extensive documents. Because of privacy and sensitivities to tribal governance processes and sovereignty, standardized assessment instruments not only could not be expected but, from a culturally sensitive standpoint, should not be expected.

Instead, the primary assessment of the policy came from a standardized phone interview administered independently to two key representatives from each tribe who were knowledgeable about tribal tobacco policies and health promotion activities. The 20-minute telephone interview was conducted by a staff member of the NPAIHB who did not work for the Tribal Tobacco Policy Project and who was blind as to the "treatment" or "control" status of each tribe. Topics in the interview included existing tobacco policy, policy adherence, tribal council characteristics, whether or not tribes received income from tobacco sales, and smoking cessation services. One representative was considered "primary" for the purpose of resolving potential discrepancies. Most primary representatives were tribal health directors (44%) or general managers (28%). Secondary representatives varied in roles, partly because of the diversity of tribal organizations, but included tribal council members (33%) and community health representatives (26%). Median percentage of agreement between informants was 82% with a range of 63%–92% (Glasgow et al., 1995; Lichtenstein et al., 1995). Based on these interviews, policies within each of three settings common to all tribes (staff offices, council rooms, and common work areas) were classified in one of three categories: lenient (0), moderately restrictive (1), and smoke-free (2). A composite stringency score was computed for each tribe by summing the scores for the three settings.

Results

The understanding that NPAIHB staff developed over a number of years assisted the interventionist in this proactive consultation. Although one member of each tribe served on the governing board of the NPAIHB, and the board had approved of the TTPP, the interventionist at no time could consider that full acceptance of tobacco policy programs had been given. Permission had been given for the project to consult with each tribal group, but the tribe's ultimate decision had to be made by its own membership through its own rules of governance. Thus the interventionist knew that each council member involved in the decision as to whether or not to change (or institute) a tobacco policy had to be personally convinced that doing so would be good for the tribe—no council member was likely to agree to it just because the interventionist was an Indian professional or was working for an organization to which the tribe belonged.

Variation in tribes' responses to the observer went from an (unusual) incident in which she was not invited to go beyond the reception area into tribal offices, to situations in which she was led by a staff member through offices and introduced to the staff. In the former case, although she did not leave the reception room, she could see ashtrays on a conference table and the absence of signs or posters related to smoking. By contrast, many of the tribes in which the observer was given a tour of the building indicated their concern about tobacco by displaying posters with titles such as "Smoking and Pregnancy" and "Snuff and Its Poisons." While many of the posters had quiet messages, some were bold, such as a poster showing a skull and stating, "If you don't chew—don't" and a humorous one showing three men with clothespins on their noses and the caption, "Thanks for not smoking."

While three-quarters of the tribes sent representatives to the kickoff meeting held at the NPAIHB, representatives of one-fourth of the tribes could not attend, so the interventionist provided a separate kickoff meeting at tribal headquarters. The median number of planning meetings was two, and some tribes had as many as five. Phone calls arranging appointments for consultations varied from 3 to 15, with a median of 6 in the first round of interventions and a median of 8.5 in the delayed interventions. In addition, the interventionist made up to six other personal contacts with each tribe, primarily at regular NPAIHB events attended by the interventionist and tribal representatives.

Changes in Tobacco Policies

Following study design, baseline assessments indicated an equivalent range and type of policies between the 19 treatment (early intervention) and 20 control (late intervention) tribes; 11 of the early intervention tribes and 11 of the late intervention tribes had lenient policies, while 8 of the early intervention and 9 of the late intervention tribes had some restrictions on smoking. Assessments following the first round of interventions indicated that treatment tribes had more stringent policies. At the beginning of the study, the mean composite score (on a 6-point scale in which 0 indicates no control and 6 indicates a totally smoke-free environment) was 2.8 for early intervention tribes and 2.9 for late intervention tribes. At the early intervention follow-up it was 4.7 for early intervention tribes and 3.7 for late intervention tribes; the difference is statistically significant ($p < .05$). Statistically significant differences also were found between intervention and control tribes concerning whether council meetings were smoke-free and concerning the existence of sanctions for violations of tobacco rules (Lichtenstein et al., 1995).

Measurement of changes occurring as a result of the delayed interventions was more difficult, because there no longer was a control group; we used a paired t-test to compare the mean composite scores of the 20 delayed intervention tribes before and after their interventions (Lichtenstein, 1996:Table 2). There are highly significant differences on all three primary dependent measures: the policy stringency composite (from 3.7 to 5.2), the percentage of tribes smoke-free in all three common areas (from 30% to 76%), and the percentage of tribes banning smokeless tobacco (from 25% to 62%).

Findings of Field Observations

Quantitative comparisons between checklist data gathered at baseline and early intervention follow-up visits indicate that smoking was occurring in substantially fewer indoor tribal areas in 1993 than in 1991. Most notable were changes in policies regarding smoking in reception areas of tribal offices: in 1991, ashtrays and cigarette butts were observed in 20% of reception areas visited, but these were evident in only 3% of the reception areas observed in 1993 (Hall et al., 1995). In the 18 months between early intervention follow-up visits in winter of 1993 and delayed intervention follow-up visits in the summer of 1994, the trend toward no-smoking areas within tribal buildings continued, though an abundance of data confirmed that considerable tobacco use was occurring in outdoor areas adjacent to tribal buildings. Field notes describing smoking in places where artifacts such as ashtrays and cigarette butts were seen—and the absence of tobacco use in areas lacking ashtrays and butts—confirmed that these artifacts are valid indicators of tobacco use.

Observations and conversations also gave insights into the processes of change and their perception by tribal members and visitors at tribal offices. While discussions with tribal employees at one site included some comments equating freedom with smokers' rights, the vast majority of discussions with employees indicated an acceptance of changing norms on indoor tobacco use. Employees also reported they complied with policies by taking smoke breaks outdoors. These reports were substantiated by observations; for example, field notes reported visitors to tribal and non-Indian government offices extinguishing cigarettes as they entered. The presence of large standing ashtrays at building entrances—sometimes with explicit signs about "snuffing it out"—indicated the continuing use of tobacco, although usually not in proscribed areas.

Intermediate levels of control were exemplified by a large tribe that had many buildings and offices, in which varying degrees of control were observed. In addition, the project observer was told that exceptions to the rule of no smoking were made for older smokers at wakes and funerals. This exception accords with the respect that Indian communities feel toward their elders. At this site, signs forbidding smoking were common in many rooms and appeared to be obeyed, but one exception observed was a tribal employee smoking in a tribally owned grocery store.

Posters concerning use of smokeless tobacco products—snuff and chew—were often directed at young people. At one of the tribal health clinics, the observer saw a bulletin board along a wall with the theme "Strike Out Tobacco." It included a collage of photos of baseball players in action, along with facts about snuff and chew. Detailed descriptions of posters and signs made it possible for project staff to speculate about the attitudes behind the change in behavior and in signs. One sign, for example, provided explicit evidence of a change in policy and suggested also that the regulation about smoking was recent and tentative. This official sign on an employees' lounge had read "smoking permitted," but the meaning had been reversed with the addition of the hand-written word "no" in front of the word "smoking."

In the third and final round of observations of the early and delayed intervention tribes, a number of tribal offices exhibited signs showing respect for tobacco traditions in the past and implying that casual consumer use of tobacco is especially inappropriate for Indian people. One of these signs, distributed by the California Department of Health Services, shows an Indian man, seated before a fire and holding a traditional, long-stemmed Indian pipe. Above the smoke rising from the fire is an eagle, and the poster's caption is: "Tobacco: use it in a sacred way." Such signs were found in 5 of 12 tribes observed. At the almost 700 spaces observed in this final period, instead of the three cigarette vending machines noted in the early intervention follow-up, only one was seen, and it was not plugged in to the wall outlet. All 12 tribes selected for field observations prohibited smoking in most locations, but 2 tribes permitted smoking indoors in designated areas of office buildings, and 2 others permitted smoking in their commercial businesses (bingo, gambling, and restaurants). In three others some infractions were observed, whereby smoking occurred in areas not designated for it, but these were minor exceptions to the rule of not using tobacco for personal or consumer purposes; over the period of the project, tremendous changes in the culture of personal tobacco use were reported.

In addition to less indoor smoking, there were new developments, such as the posters described above, that indicated proactive discouragement of personal smoking. Other changes that occurred between the second and third observation periods included the appearance of nonsmoking areas in one bingo hall and one casino—settings long associated with personal tobacco use. Other examples include subtle changes observed in an Indian smoke shop run by a tribal member. In the second round of visits, there had been single cigarettes for sale, but they were not for sale in the third round; cartons of cigarettes were held behind the counter instead of in front of it; and smokers' rights posters were no longer in evidence, as they had been 18 months earlier. Although none of these prevents the sale of tobacco products, they all signify reduced access to tobacco products, especially for youth, who may not be able to afford cartons and who may be questioned about their age.

Field observations provided evidence of compliance with policy changes. Smoking was most often observed on porches and in parking lots. Exceptions to compliance included a situation in which the observer smelled cigarette smoke within an office building and traced it to a rest room, with the smoker remaining elusive. Although exceptions signify infractions of rules, reports of this nature indicate awareness by smokers of policies prohibiting smoking. Infractions as well as compliance indicate awareness of tobacco control policies and, in general, acceptance of changing social norms that ultimately should lead to lower rates of personal tobacco use among Indian people.

Examination of non-Indian areas adjacent to Indian areas by the same procedures as those used in the Indian population showed that considerable similarity existed between sites under Indian control and those controlled by the neighboring non-Indian population. Field observations made in non-Indian commercial and public areas (restaurants, parks, gas stations, etc.) as well as in governmental offices (county courthouses, post offices, schools, libraries, and city halls) confirmed that in non-Indian as well as Indian-controlled areas, the greatest amount of tobacco control existed in official government offices and the least in tourist and recreational areas (Hall et al., 1995).

Generally speaking, more signs about tobacco control, and the most explicit messages about problems of tobacco use, were found in the largest tribes and the fewest signs in areas open to the general public (such as restaurants and other businesses). For example, in the patio of one of the larger tribes was a big standing ashtray and a large, bold sign showing a cigarette butt and asking visitors to "snuff it out." Discussions with tribal employees at large and small tribes suggested that the greater frequency of explicit messages in larger tribes did not mean that the smaller tribes were not equally concerned, however. In the smaller tribes, most of the visitors to tribal offices were aware of tribal rules, so the staff felt it was not necessary to put up signs. We believe that, in some cases, tribal officials felt it would be impolite to remind people of what they already knew or did not want to bring up controversies best left unspoken.

Discussion

The cooperative interaction of agencies with different administrative histories, cultures, and rules is a likely consequence when the approaches of anthropology and public health are integrated. This project also represented a cooperative effort among an organization representing Indian tribes (NPAIHB), a private health research organization (the Oregon Research Institute), and an anthropology department at a university (Oregon State University). These three groups, with their individual goals and methodologies, were brought together to solve a problem for which each had one portion of the requisite expertise.

Cooperative arrangements among the three organizations and with the National Cancer Institute (NCI) entailed logistical problems because each of these institutions is headquartered in a different city. These three organizations all were equidistant—both geographically and operationally—from NCI headquarters in Rockville, Maryland. In addition, the cultures, perspectives, and operational procedures of the institutions differ markedly. As a private institution, the Oregon Research Institute had the greatest flexibility in its operations, while Oregon State University, as a state university, had to respond to state directives and, as a teaching institution, was governed by the academic calendar. NPAIHB, whose administrative functions are funded largely by the Indian Health Service, is necessarily most responsive to its constituents, the federally recognized tribes in the Northwest. NCI was driven by complementary yet sometimes diametrically opposed directives: to offer substantial health initiatives to minority populations and be culturally sensitive to them, while at the same time conducting research that would be sufficiently rigorous to meet conventional scientific standards.

Considerable overlap exists in the goals as well as the methodologies of anthropology and public health. The anthropological and tribal perspectives were valuable in providing field data as well as historical background; the public health data regarding the epidemiological aspects of personal tobacco use as well as cancer risks were important in defining the problem and in developing a strategy to deal with it and rigorous tools to measure it. Understandings of tribal culture were essential in structuring the project so that activities not only emanated from members of the community but involved their membership in every step of the process: from approving the proposal to seek funds to reviewing research findings. In contemporary jargon, this process is known as "empowerment," but these methods of involving community members are standard in anthropology and have been accepted in public health. They also are a sine qua non for working with American Indian tribes in the 1990s.

Long-term benefits of the project are as yet unknown, but the project, which was officially completed in May 1995, already has one offspring. A grant made by the Centers for Disease Control and Prevention to the NPAIHB for tobacco education and control provides for an intervention project in the Greater Northwest (the original three states plus Alaska and Montana); the project includes primary tobacco use prevention in addition to education and resource information and technical assistance training. The development and implementation by NPAIHB staff offers testimony in support of the goals of the TTPP in that it demonstrates a desire by Northwestern tribes for a continuation of projects aimed at tobacco control and the reduction of tobacco-related deaths from cancer and other diseases.

Notes

1. The fortieth tribe was recognized after this project began; the project is involved with the 39 federally recognized tribes that existed in 1990.

Acknowledgments

This study was supported by Grant U01 CA 52230 from the National Cancer Institute. We appreciate the work of colleagues Bryson Liberty, G. Bruce Myers, Suzanne McRae, Cynthia Viles, and Russell Glasgow.

References

Afonja SA (1992) "Rapid Assessment Methodologies: Application to Health and Nutrition Programmes in Africa." In: RAP. Rapid Assessment Procedures. Qualitative Methodologies for Planning and Evaluation of Health Related Programmes. NS Scrimshaw, GR Gleason, eds. Boston: International Nutrition Foundation for Developing Countries, pp. 81–94.

Bernard HR (1988) Research Methods in Cultural Anthropology. Newbury Park, Calif: Sage Publications.

Boyd RT (1990) "Demographic History, 1774–1874." In: Handbook of North American Indians, Northwest Coast, vol. 7. W Suttles, ed. Washington, DC: Smithsonian Institution, pp. 135–148.

Burhansstipanov L, Dresser C (1993) Documentation of the Cancer Research Needs of American Indians and Alaska Natives. Washington, DC: National Cancer Institute. NIH Publication No. 93–3603.

Crosby AW (1986) Ecological Imperialism. The Biological Expansion of Europe, 900–1900. Cambridge: Cambridge University Press.

Endzweig P (1989) "Of Pots, Pipes, and People: Prehistoric Ceramics of Oregon." In: Contributions to the Archaeology of Oregon 1987–1988. R Minor, ed. Portland: Association of Oregon Archaeologists Occasional Papers No. 4, pp. 157–177.

Environmental Protection Agency (EPA) (1992) Respiratory Health Effects of Passive Smoking: Lung Cancer and Other Disorders. Publication No. EPA/600/6–90/006F.

Glasgow RE, Lichtenstein E, Wilder D, Hall RL, McRae SG, Liberty B (1995) The Tribal Tobacco Policy Project: working with Northwest Indian tribes on smoking policies. Preventive Medicine 24:434–440.

Glasgow RE, Sorensen G, Corbett K (for the COMMIT Research Group) (1990) Worksite smoking control activities: prevalence and related worksite characteristics from the COMMIT study. Preventive Medicine 21:688–700.

Goodman J (1993) Tobacco in History. The Cultures of Dependence. London: Routledge.

Hall RL (1992) "From Blackstrap Molasses to Smokeless Tobacco: A Chronicle of Assaults on the Dental Health of Native Americans of the Northwest." In: Biological Approaches to Health and Lifestyle Change. R Huss-Ashmore, J Schall, M Hediger, eds. Philadelphia: University of Pennsylvania Museum. MASCA Research Papers 9:43–50.

Hall RL, Dexter D (1988) Smokeless tobacco use and attitudes toward smokeless tobacco among native and non-native adolescents in the Northwest. American Journal of Public Health 78:1586–1588.

Hall RL, Viles CA, Lichtenstein E, Glasgow RE, Lopez K (1995) Rapid assessment procedures to describe tobacco practices at sites managed by Indian tribes. *Tobacco Control* 4:156–161.

Hampton JW (1992) Cancer prevention and control in American Indians/Alaska natives. *American Indian Culture and Research Journal* 16:41–49.

Horm JW, Burhansstipanov L (1992) Cancer incidence, survival, and mortality among American Indians and Alaska natives. *American Indian Culture and Research Journal* 16:21–39.

Kellehear A (1993) The Unobtrusive Researcher. St. Leonards, Australia: Allen and Unwin.

Lichtenstein E, Glasgow RE, Lopez K, Hall RL, McRae SG, Myers GB (1995) Promoting tobacco control policies in Northwest Indian tribes. *American Journal of Public Health* 85:991–994.

Lichtenstein E, Lopez K, Glasgow RE, Gilbert-McRae S, Hall RL (1996) Effectiveness of a consultation intervention to promote tobacco control policies in Northwest Indian tribes. *American Journal of Community Psychology* 24:639–655.

National Institute of Occupational Safety and Health (NIOSH) (1991) Environmental Tobacco Smoke in the Workplace: Lung Cancer and Other Health Effects. Current Intelligence Bulletin 54, DHHS (NIOSH) Publication No. 91–108.

Northwest Portland Area Indian Health Board (NPAIHB). n.d. Informational brochure about the Northwest Portland Area Indian Health Board. Portland: NPAIHB.

Northwest Portland Area Indian Health Board (NPAIHB) (1995) Workbook: Tribal Tobacco Policy Project, rev. ed. Portland: NPAIHB.

Pentz MA, Brannon BR, Charlin VL, Barrett EJ, MacKinnon DP, Flay BR (1989) The power of policy: relationship of smoking policy to adolescent smoking. *American Journal of Public Health* 79:857–862.

Rabin RL, Sugarman SD, eds. (1993) Smoking Policy. Law, Politics, and Culture. New York: Oxford University Press.

Rigotti NA (1989) Trends in the adoption of smoking restrictions in public places and worksites. *New York State Journal of Medicine* 89:19–26.

Scrimshaw NS, Gleason GR, eds. (1992) RAP. Rapid Assessment Procedures. Qualitative Methodologies for Planning and Evaluation of Health Related Programmes. Boston: International Nutrition Foundation for Developing Countries.

Seig L (1971) Tobacco, Peace Pipes, and Indians. Palmer Lake, Colo: Filter Press.

Sugarman JR, Warren CW, Oge L, Helgerson SD (1992) Using the Behavioral Risk Factor Surveillance System to monitor year 2000 objectives among American Indians. *Public Health Reports* 107:449–456.

US American Indian Policy Review Commission (1976) Report on Terminated and Nonfederally Recognized Indians. Washington, DC: US Government Printing Office.

US Department of Health and Human Services (USDHHS) (1986) The Health Consequences of Involuntary Smoking. A Report of the Surgeon General. DHHS (CDC) Publication No. 87–8398. Washington, DC: US Government Printing Office.

US Department of Health and Human Services (USDHHS) (1989) Reducing the Health Consequences of Smoking. A Report of the Surgeon General. DHHS Publication No. 88–8406. Washington, DC: US Government Printing Office.

US Department of Health and Human Services; Indian Health Service (USDHHS) (1991) Trends in Indian Health. USDHHS/300–165/50070. Washington, DC: US Government Printing Office.

Warner KE (1989) Smoking and health: a 25–year perspective. *American Journal of Public Health* 79:141–143.

Weatherford J (1988) Indian Givers. How the Indians of the Americas Transformed the World. New York: Fawcett Columbine.

Wright R (1988) On the Air: Creating a Smoke-Free Workplace [videotape]. Santa Monica: Pyramid Film & Video.

III

PHARMACY AND NUTRITION

8

The Rational Basis of "Irrational" Drug Use: Pharmaceuticals in the Context of Development

NINA L. ETKIN,
PAUL J. ROSS, AND
IBRAHIM MUAZZAMU

International health programs that promote pharmaceuticals frequently encounter difficulties when local patterns of drug use are different from those intended by manufacturers/distributors. Typically, health development planners interpret this as "irrational" drug use and/or "noncompliance" with health "authorities." This view reveals the failure of outsiders to understand that differing cultural premises and concepts may yield different—but internally consistent and fully rational—modes of drug use. Drawing on our research on Hausa ethnomedicine, we illustrate how anthropological methods can uncover the cultural basis of local preventive and therapeutic modalities and, in this way, help us to understand (even to predict) how indigenous patterns are influenced by the introduction of new medical paradigms and technology. This research can help to illuminate problems related to the introduction of pharmaceuticals and to shape culturally appropriate interventions.

Research Setting

Since the mid-1970s, we have conducted research in a rural Hausa village (Hurumi) in northern Nigeria, including two extended in-residence field sessions: 18 months during 1975–1976 and 12 months during 1987–1988. Between those periods, and since, the Nigerian member of our team (I.M.) revisited Hurumi on a regular basis to extend observations, conduct follow-up interviews, and generally ensure that the research represents current reality. The introduction of pharmaceuticals in the context of indigenous medicine is one element of our comprehensive investigation of medicine, diet, and health in rural Hausaland (e.g., Etkin, 1994a, 1994b, 1996, 1997a, 1997b, in press; Etkin and Ross, 1994, 1997; Etkin et al., 1990; Ross, 1987; Ross et al., 1991, 1996). Our ongoing laboratory investigations (in the United States) further illuminate the pharmacologic potential of Hausa medicinal plants.

Located east of Wudil town, 50 kilometers southeast of urban Kano, Hurumi is part of the Kano Close-Settled Zone (Mortimore, 1967), an area of much dispersed settlement but primarily characterized by the high population density and intensive land utilization that have defined this area for hundreds of years (Hill, 1982). More broadly, Hurumi falls within the Sahel, a region defined as savanna (i.e., scrubby and scattered shrubs and small trees) and subject to encroaching desertification. The marked seasonality of rainfall influences disease patterns and affects the full range of human activity, from subsistence to the timing of marriage property exchanges and religious training.

A scant 26 inches or less of rain falls between late May and early September, sufficient to support one harvest per year by rain-fed cultivation. Hurumi's subsistence base is intensive, nonmechanized agriculture (featuring sorghum, millet, cowpeas, and groundnuts) supplemented by small-scale livestock production (sheep, goats, fowl, cattle), gathering of wild plants, and some cash-cropping (typically groundnuts and cowpeas, recently small amounts of sorghum and millet). This is supplemented by trade in locally manufactured items (plant-fiber mats, leather handcrafts, prepared foods) and imports (kola nuts, cigarettes, botanical and other medicines, sugar). A small number of specialists—midwives (traditional birth attendants), scholars of the Qur'an (Muslim *malams*), and barbers (who perform ritual shaving, cupping/bloodletting, and other minor surgeries), and others—generate income in cash and goods.

Hurumi's center is a core settlement of 400 residents; the broader administrative area also includes outlying hamlets, with a total village population of approximately 4,000. The village still is not served by paved roads, electricity, or piped water. The basic living units, "compounds," have from 2 to 40 occupants and typically include a compound head, his wife or wives, his sons and their wives, and children. The presence of unmarried or divorced daughters and sisters of the compound head contributes an element of fluidity to the compound occupancy. Each compound is surrounded by a three-meter-tall grain-stalk fence; inside, sleeping huts, cooking hearths, granaries, and animal shelters are organized to define both common areas and space allocated to each nuclear family unit.

A compound commonly is home to more than one "household," or people who "eat from the same pot"—for example, the compound head's sons and their respective wives and children. Household composition shifts when members (typically young men) leave to seek temporary employment elsewhere, married women and their children return to parents' compounds for visits, divorced women move into their brothers' homes, and so on. Together with this fluidity of occupancy, the co-residence of several households raises the potential for intracompound variability in resources such as farm output, opportunity for wage labor, earnings from craft production, and the like—all of which can contribute to health differentials. As the number and character of residents change, household resources are differently distributed and can result in dissimilar disease experiences, uneven knowledge of medicines, and differential access to traditional and biomedical healers.

Methods

We first compiled data on Hausa medicine, diet, and health during 1975–1976, when preventive and therapeutic medicine in Hurumi was defined almost exclusively by an extensive traditional botanical pharmacopoeia. The principal objective was to comprehend Hausa explanatory models, which include disease etiology, means of diagnosis, pathophysiology and symptom progression, prognosis, prevention, and therapeutic strategies. These baseline data revealed a Hausa way of classifying diseases, including how discrete symptoms and diseases are related to one another. By paying careful attention to the expression and order of appearance of symptoms, we have been able to document similarities and differences between Hausa and biomedical classifications of disease.

We invited the participation of select respondents who were identified by others, and also perceived themselves, as most conversant in health issues. Extensive interviews were conducted with 14 principal respondents—5 women and 9 men—including a woman whose district-wide reputation and clientele reflected her comprehensive knowledge of botanical medicines. Another 12 respondents (6 women and 6 men) represented more narrow areas of medically related knowledge: a barber-surgeon, three midwives, and specialists in jaundice, venereal diseases, weaning medicines, witchcraft, sorcery, and religious (Muslim) healing. These individuals embodied specialized knowledge that reflected the unique experiences of their lives. An additional 50 respondents (20 women and 30 men) were identified by "snowball sampling" (one respondent recommending others, who in turn recommended others, and so on) and observations conducted throughout the village illuminated household health practices: "self-care" and "home-care" are common, and most adults know at least a few remedies for a variety of common disorders, including fevers, gastrointestinal complaints, children's illnesses, and skin conditions. This broader sample underscores the diffuse nature of medical and botanical knowledge, allowing us to comprehend intracultural diversity and to appreciate that for Hausa, prevention and therapeutics are community-wide phenomena.

Open-ended interviews with principal and specialist respondents were organized around (1) a catalogue of 808 diseases, symptoms, and related terms for which respondents described commonly used medicines, including source, preparation, additional constituents, approximate dose and schedule of administration, therapeutic objectives, and alternatives for circumstances in which that medicine was not available or did not produce the expected results; and (2) an inventory of 637 medicines (predominantly plants) that individuals identified by physical attributes, availability, and therapeutic, preventive, and other uses. Our observations are similar to those recorded for other parts of Hausaland, with differences that are understandable in view of ecologic variability and the time span over which information was collected, compounded by the varying methodologies, and especially ethnographic depth, of other researchers (e.g., Adam et al., 1972; Busson et al., 1965; Dalziel, 1937; Oliver, 1986; Stock, 1980, 1985, 1987; Wall, 1988).

A few plants were collected in bulk, air dried in the field, and shipped to our laboratory in the United States for phytochemical assessments. Rather than sample across the entire pharmacopoeia, we used cultural data to focus investigation on two subsets of plants related to conditions that were locally regarded to be important, with respect to both morbidity and prevalence—those used in the treatment of gastrointestinal disorders and malaria (Etkin and Ross, 1982, 1997).

A total of 231 voucher specimens were prepared for plants discussed in the interviews (fewer than the 637-item inventory, which includes synonyms and plants not available for local collection, as well as products of animal, mineral, and other composition) and later identified by botanical taxonomists at the Missouri Botanical Garden (St. Louis) and the Kew Royal Botanical Gardens (London). Vouchers are the basic specimen unit of all ethnobotanical inquiry, providing the only irrefutable link between local and bioscientific knowledge. Taxonomic identification allowed us to take advantage of published phytochemical data for those plants, as well as to design comparisons of the interpretation and use of particular species cross-culturally. In the analysis, we related the specific physiological actions and constituent chemistry of medicinal plants to that of pharmaceuticals, in order to comprehend the physiological implications of their combined or serial use.

The 1987–1988 follow-up study expanded our understanding of Hausa plant use and was the basis for additional plant collections to advance the laboratory component of our investigation (Etkin and Ross, 1997). Plants still predominated in Hausa preventive and therapeutic medicine, but during the intervening years there had been a dramatic incursion of biomedicine. Most significant was the markedly increased and widespread use of pharmaceuticals bought through the formal biomedical clinic and chemists' shops or, more commonly, from market vendors and itinerant herbalists who traditionally embellished their inventories with botanical exotics and now add pharmaceuticals as well (Etkin et al., 1990). To the catalogues of plants and symptoms from the earlier study we added the names of what had become commonly used pharmaceuticals (Table 8.1), as well as several biomedical terms that had entered the vocabulary as a result of people's (still extremely limited) experience with a new biomedical clinic eight kilometers from Hurumi—for example, treatment for high blood pressure, vitamin supplementation, diabetes, and the management of pregnancy. Especially interesting was the combination of plants and pharmaceuticals in the same therapeutic regimens.

Extensive open-ended interviews were combined with observations of therapeutic and preventive activities, to record the details of therapeutic objectives and medicine selection, preparation, and administration. The three principal respondents were a general healer (male) and two nonspecialists (a man and a woman) who were widely regarded as the most generally knowledgeable both in plant identification and in the rationale and substance of preventive and therapeutic medicine. These interviews were supplemented by a semistructured interview administered to an additional 52 respondents (20 women and 32 men); based on our ethnographic knowledge of the setting, these individuals represented the range of variability within the village adult population with respect to age, access to resources, education, disease experience, and familiarity with biomedicine.

In addition, we documented shifts in availability and cost of plants and pharmaceuticals at local and market sources, which eventually allowed us to argue that, in Hurumi, selection of a particular medicine is guided by specific criteria including biologic action, texture, source, and other qualities—and not simply by ease of access.

To capture an overview of disease prevalence and periodicity, we conducted a monthly village-wide health survey to record all disease episodes for all members of all households. In addition, we carried out a two-month investigation at the clinic during ordinary operating hours: randomly selected patients (approximately every third in line) and the staff who attended them participated in entry and exit interviews that explored, among other topics, reasons for clinic attendance and prior treatments, patient–physician interactions, diagnosis and prognosis, and "compliance" with clinic prescriptions and other instructions. These data allowed us to consider similarities and differences between local and biomedical assessments of a variety of physiological complaints.

Since 1988, regular follow-up research in the study community confirms the villagers' continued use of plants and pharmaceuticals and gradual increase in use of the biomedical clinic.

Table 8.1 Pharmaceuticals Commonly Used in Hausa Medicine

PHARMACEUTICAL*	INTENDED BIOMEDICAL APPLICATION (MODE OF ADMINISTRATION)†	HAUSA USE (RATIONALE)†
Andrews liver salts ($NaCO_3$) *Gishirin Andris*	Indigestion, peptic ulcer	Intravaginal diagnostic for obstructed childbirth (some obstructions are caused by dietary salt accumulation in the womb)
		Indigestion (physically resembles potash)
		Lower back pain (flushes the body of fluid/phlegm)
		GI disorders (belching, flatulence)
Antitussives *Kofta, Tom Tom*	Cough	Cough
		Spirits, sorcerers, witches (aromatic, sweet)
APC and other aspirin preparations compounded with caffeine *Kafenol, Fensik, Daga, A Fi Si, Fengo*	Headache, fever, pain, rheumatic diseases, musculoskeletal disorders	Fever
		Malaria
		Headache
		Stomachache (gastric irritation)
Chloramphenicol capsule *Farin Kafso*§	Various bacterial infections	Measles, chickenpox (bitter; grainy)
		Abortion (bitter)
		Spirits, sorcerers, witches (bitter)
		GI disorders (diarrhea)
		Various (itching)

Chloramphenicol ointment *Kwantsa*[§]	Eye infections (topical)	Eye disorders
Chloroquine tablet *Tab*[§]	Malaria, musculoskeletal disorders	Measles, chickenpox (bitter; itching) Abortion (bitter) Malaria Spirits, sorcerers, witches (bitter) Various (itching)
Clinoquinol ointment *Kwantsa*[§]	Skin inflammation (topical)	Various (rash)
Codeine tablet *Bi Kodin*	Pain, cough	Energy, strength
Dapsone tablet *Tab*[§]	Leprosy	Various (itching; rash)
Erythromycin capsule *Kafso*[§]	Respiratory infections	Measles, chickenpox (grainy; rash) GI disorders (gastric irritation)
Ferrous sulfate tablet *Tab*[§]	Anemia, malnutrition, pregnancy	Blood tonic (red) Jaundice/hepatitis (dark stool) Schistosomiasis (dark stool)
Methocarbamol tablet *Tab*[§]	Muscle relaxant	Pediatric malaria (discolored urine)

(continued)

Table 8.1 (*Continued*)

PHARMACEUTICAL*	INTENDED BIOMEDICAL APPLICATION (MODE OF ADMINISTRATION)[†]	HAUSA USE (RATIONALE)[‡]
Penicillin solution *Allura Mai Mai*[§]	Systemic infections (injection)	Eye disorders, by drop Sores, topical Earache, by drop Abortion (bitter)
Phenazopyridine tablet *Tab*[§]	Pain with urinary tract infection	Jaundice/hepatitis (red-orange urine) Schistosomiasis (red-orange urine)
Phenolphthalein tablet *Tab*[§]	Laxative	Jaundice/hepatitis (red-brown urine) Schistosomiasis (red-brown urine)
Providine iodine ointment *Mai*[§]	Surface wounds (topical)	Sores, topical
Rifampin capsule *Fuka*	Tuberculosis	Cough Jaundice/hepatitis (red-brown urine and feces) Schistosomiasis (red-brown urine and feces)
Sloane's liniment *Gashin Baki*	Muscle pain (topical)	Spirits, sorcerers, witches (aromatic)
Sulfonamide tablets *Tab*[§]	Urinary tract infections	Various (itching; rash)

Tetracycline capsule *Kala Biyu*	Bacterial infections	Measles, chickenpox (grainy; phototoxicity) Various (phototoxicity)
Tetracycline ointment *Kwantsa*§	Eye infection (topical)	Eye disorders, topical
Triamterene capsule *Kapso*§	Diuretic	Pediatric malaria (blue-green urine)

*Hausa name appears in italic type.

†Taken orally, if not otherwise noted.

‡Rationale, other than that the medicine has proven, or is reputed to be, efficacious.

§Hausa terms overlap because some drugs are identified by general appearance: *tab* = tablet, *kafso* = capsule, *kwantsa* = ointment, *mai* = solution.

Therapeutic Strategies and Pharmaceuticals in Hausa Medicine

Contrary to what health development planners anticipated, in Hausaland pharmaceuticals do not replace, but rather become part of, the existing pharmacopoeia. Moreover, pharmaceuticals are incorporated on *local* terms: they are subjected to the same dynamics of selection and outcome assessment that have been traditionally applied to new plants discovered in the vicinity or imported from elsewhere (Etkin et al., 1990) (Table 8.1). Hausa use of pharmaceuticals can be understood only in light of local therapeutic objectives.

For Hausa, healing is a process, not an event. While the ultimate objective is getting better, immediate goals include diagnosis, making the body receptive to treatment, and confirming the expulsion of disease agents. Hausa seek evidence that each of these stages of healing has occurred.

Ridding the Body of Disease

One of the central concepts that drives Hausa therapeutics is *disease egress*—ridding the body of disease. Disease is thought to be caused by reactions to the physical environment (e.g., heat, moisture); accumulation of body fluids (e.g., phlegm, blood); the presence of disease agents (e.g., dirt, intangible essences); object intrusion (e.g., of bone or animal fur) or soul loss caused by witches; or the malfeasance of sorcery. Thus treatment is directed in part to dispelling these morbid elements and aspects; vomiting, salivating, sweating, and rashes are among the common signs that disease has exited (Table 8.1).

Hausa therapies for gastrointestinal disorders typically include purging. Thus in the selection of pharmaceuticals, sodium bicarbonate is chosen because its "side effects," belching and flatulence, are taken as tangible evidence that disease agents are leaving the body. On the other hand, the constipating "side effects" of calcium carbonate and aluminum phosphate are reason to reject these antacids. For stomachache, traditional combinations of Hausa plants are both mucosal irritants and antimicrobial. These plants are used today in conjunction first with salicylates or erythromycin to provoke abdominal distress, and later in the therapeutic sequence with tetracyclines, chloramphenicol, and other antimicrobials that cause diarrhea (but also resolve gastrointestinal disorders of microbial origin).

Disease egress is further indicated by the color of the secreted or excreted matter. Most commonly, red or brown feces and urine evidence the exit of causative agents of *shawara* (jaundice/hepatitis) and *tsagiya* (schistosomiasis). Alone or in combination with plants administered with the same objective, pharmaceuticals that contribute to such (dis)coloration are rifampin, an antitubercular; phenazopyridine, a nonnarcotic analgesic; and phenolphthalein, a laxative. For pediatric malaria, egress is signaled by green diarrhea or urine. The desired effects are accomplished by the administration of certain botanical medicines and/ or pharmaceuticals such as laxative magnesium salts, the diuretic triamterene, and the muscle relaxant methocarbamol.

Egress is demonstrated as well by skin spots and itching, which indicate the externalization of disease. In addition to the numerous plants that effect this outcome, Hausa use several pharmaceuticals, principally because of their "side effects"—for example the antimalarial chloroquine (for itching), the topical antimicrobial clioquinol (for rash and irritation), tetracycline (for phototoxicity), and dapsone, sulfonamides, and chloramphenicol (for itching rash) (Table 8.1).

Choosing Pharmaceuticals: Signs of Efficacy

Some physical attributes of medicines are interpreted as signs of therapeutic efficacy. For fevers and nausea Hausa traditionally selected sour or acidic plants, and they now use this characteristic for the identification of pharmaceuticals that may indeed have antipyretic action as well as a broad range of other activities. Similarly, since many Hausa blood fortifiers include red plants, the color of capsules, tablets, and the like, is a stronger predictor of efficacy for Hausa health objectives than are, for example, labels that catalogue iron among the ingredients. Hausa regard very bitter plants as dangerous during pregnancy; they use this taste principle to identify potential abortifacients among pharmaceuticals: chloramphenicol, penicillin, and chloroquine. Medicines that affect spirits, sorcerers, and witches—all of whom cause a wide variety of physiological problems—are either palatable or repugnant, to appease or repel the offender and so remove the source of illness. In view of the importance of sensory qualities, Hausa regard elixirs and aromatic balms as the most efficacious types of pharmaceuticals for some disorders. One could thus predict that whatever taste- or smell-altering side effects a particular drug may have would dissuade Hausa from using it—for example, phenformin, an antidiabetic that produces a persistent metallic taste.

Balance of Opposites

Another principle in Hausa therapy is "balance of opposites." For Hausa, the most salient opposition is hot–cold, where, especially, lost heat results in disease. This occurs through exposure to cold air and cold water, or when a passage is created between the outside and the vulnerable body interior—the circumstances of childbirth and surgery constituting the most pronounced risk. Cold diseases are treated with hot medicines, and vice versa. Pharmaceuticals are easily assimilated into this paradigm: yellow and red capsules, tablets, and liquids are more likely to be labeled hot; silver-wrapped, white, and green drugs, cold. Hausa reject the leprosy medicine clofazimine because its itching side effects identify it as hot, and leprosy requires cold treatment. Other opposites include wet–dry, sweet–salty, and astringent–oily; but there is no consensus regarding the significance of these pairs for disease etiology, or the particular substances that can be manipulated to achieve balance. Nonetheless, individual perspectives—among which there exists considerable variability—on these opposites direct the selection of both medicinal plants and pharmaceuticals.

The Incremental Resolution of Complex Disorders

In the Hausa cultural perspective particular plants and pharmaceuticals are identified for one or more phases of treatment, which include confirmation of etiology, effecting disease egress, and the incremental resolution of symptoms. The Hausa treatment of *kyanda* (measles) illustrates both the incremental nature of therapeutics and the use of healing metaphors. Environmental heat and spirits are both thought to play a role in the etiology of *kyanda*. Early symptoms include spots inside the cheek, cough, and night fright (the latter is understood to mark the moment when the disease agent enters, or is inserted into, the body). When the measles spots are evident on the skin, bitter medicines are taken orally to externalize any residual spots inside. In a subsequent stage, cold and aromatic medicines encourage the rash to mature; the disease entity *kyanda* "likes the cold" and so is encouraged to develop. Next, the external spots are treated by topical application to the skin of bitter and astringent medicines that are understood to promote healing of the skin lesions. The internal/external treatment cycles are repeated as many times as necessary; finally, astringent and emollient medicines are applied topically to ensure full symptom resolution. Increasingly, pharmaceuticals replace and combine with plant medicines for measles. Penicillin for administration by injection is astringent and bitter, and so is taken orally for the internal aspect and applied topically to the spots. Pharmaceuticals that enter the therapeutic progression later are aromatic and cold. Abatement of internal signs and diminished lymphatic inflammation indicate that all spots have been externalized. Skin spots then are treated with a variety of astringent and emollient pharmaceuticals.

Of the 62 traditional Hausa medicines for measles (involving 49 plant species), disease egress is the objective of 47 (76%). Pharmaceuticals that are identified as substitutes/complements are primarily bitter (to drive the spots out). A small number (8, or 13%) of the traditional measles medicines entail crushing "seedy" plants (principally grasses), a metaphor for bursting internal and external spots. Pharmaceuticals selected as substitutes tend to be capsules, the granular contents of which physically resemble their botanic counterparts.

Is Hausa Pharmaceutical Use Safe?

Whereas clinical investigations of pharmaceutical use have been concerned chiefly with "compliance" (e.g., Donovan and Blake, 1992; Pratt and Jones, 1995; Trostle, 1996; Wright, 1993), anthropological studies of pharmaceutical use have largely centered on diverse cultural versions of medicine; assessments of efficacy; pharmacists' recommendations and self-medication; and the nature of prescription in the light of patients' expectations (Etkin and Tan, 1994; Nichter and Vuckovic, 1994; van der Geest and Whyte, 1988). The present discussion of Hausa pharmaceutical use contributes to this literature; it underscores both the tenacity of local traditions and their transformation as new elements of medical culture are combined with existing and evolving pharmacopoeias.

Further, we address the physiological implications of combining plant medicines and pharmaceuticals, a topic that has received little attention (e.g., Bedi et al., 1989; Dandekar et al., 1992; Etkin et al., 1990). The potentially harmful effects of concurrent use of pharmaceuticals and plants makes this an urgent public health issue.

Potentiating and Antagonistic Interactions between Medicinal Plants and Pharmaceuticals

Potentiation refers to the enhancing effect of something (typically another drug) on the activity of a drug. Potentiation can occur between the constituents of a single plant, between constituents of more than one plant, between plants and pharmaceuticals, and between pharmaceuticals. Iron absorption is enhanced by ascorbic acid, a common constituent of a wide range of medicinal plants. This is relevant when clinic and chemist shops promote iron supplements for pregnant women, and when individuals self-prescribe the same for general strengthening effects. Similarly, various antipyretic–analgesic drugs manifest intensified action when they are consumed at the same time as cruciferous plants. Both examples suggest that in prescription and labeling of pharmaceuticals more attention be directed to proper dosage, taking into account concurrent medications and diet.

As the term implies, drug *antagonists* are substances that impede the action of a drug. Tannins, found in most plants, bind some classes of pharmaceuticals, thus reducing their bioavailability. Diarrhea treatment is one context in which this antagonism is likely, when high-tannin plants—readily identified by their astringent taste—are selected for constipating action (e.g., *Acacia arabica*, *Adansonia digitata*). Tannins may diminish the bioavailability of some antibiotics that are routinely prescribed at the clinic or otherwise identified by patients for the treatment of diarrheas. Tannins impede iron absorption as well. Fruit juices, especially from *Citrus* and *Capsicum* species, interfere with the activity of some penicillins; and calcium, an important constituent of plant medicines (e.g., *Hibiscus sabdariffa, Momordica charantia*), has an antagonistic effect on tetracycline. Drug action may also be diminished by the high calcium content of milk, which is a popular vehicle for the administration of some Hausa medicines. Pectin, a common constituent of fruits, reduces the activity of some antibiotics. Plant constituents that have diuretic (e.g., *Cola nitida*) and anticoagulant (e.g., *Balanites aegyptica*) actions complicate antibiotic therapy as well.

Both potentiating and antagonistic interactions may occur as a result of the routine inclusion of *kanwa*—potash, impure sodium and potassium carbonates—in medicines and food. The culinary uses of this alkaline salt increase the palatability and digestibility of foods. Medicinally, *kanwa* is used in the postpartum and to diminish the accumulation of phlegm. In combination with pharmaceuticals, it increases the solubility (thus bioavailability) of oral sulfonamides and many other drugs, and it reduces the absorption of oral antibiotic tetracyclines. Like the foregoing examples, this too has implications for proper dosing of medicines.

Conclusions and Applications

The mixed and interchangeable use of plant medicines and pharmaceuticals is by no means unique to Hausa; the conclusions drawn here are applicable cross-culturally and have far-reaching implications regarding appropriate dosage in view of drug potentiation and antagonism. Our discussion has illustrated that pharmaceuticals are selected because of locally perceived and locally interpreted characteristics, rather than to conform with physicians' prescriptions. This can have far-reaching implications for people's health, generally—for example, when pharmaceuticals are used in nonprescription, even in contraindicated, modes. It also indicates the need for anthropological study of local cultures to predict the use of introduced materials.

Further, as one comes to appreciate the pharmacodynamic potential of plant medicines, it becomes apparent that these botanicals may have physiological effects no matter how they come into contact with the body. Thus the picture is complicated further by the multiple uses of these plants—for food, cosmetics, and other ends as well. On some level, then, the issue is exposure: How often and to what extent do people come into contact with pharmacologically active plants? and How is health influenced by interactions among plant constituents and other medicines (pharmaceuticals)?

The significance of drug interactions is already recognized in biomedicine, where patients typically are asked about prior and concurrent use of prescribed and over-the-counter medications. Especially in developing countries, and increasingly in the West, medical staff must appreciate not only the extent to which nonpharmaceutical medicines are used but also their potential influence on pharmaceutical therapy. At minimum, medical staff must be educated in local medical culture, prepared to describe plant–pharmaceutical interactions to patients, capable of warning about potentially deleterious combinations in a culturally sensitive manner, and—where appropriate—ready to modify the dose in which pharmaceuticals are prescribed in order to adjust to potentiating and antagonizing influences from plant medicines and foods.

Designs for culturally sensitive and otherwise appropriate "interventions" that educate health personnel and the community about pharmaceutical use already exist (e.g., Ross-Degnan et al., 1992). Successful programs have been based on local medical paradigms and include substantial community input and personnel. This needs now to be developed and implemented in a more systematic, cross-culturally applicable manner.

Our investigation of how biomedicine is embraced in a local Hausa context expands the understanding of how populations seek solutions to health problems. It is possible to specify when a particular pharmaceutical is introduced and to chart the course of its distribution, testing, adaptation, and evolving use. In a sense, then, we can document the creation and transformation of medical knowledge and practice within communities. This appreciation for how medical technology really enters the public domain better equips development planners and international health efforts to introduce biomedicine in an effective manner.

Acknowledgments

This research was supported in part by grants from the National Science Foundation (BNS-8703734), the Committee on African Studies of the American Council of Learned Societies, the Social Science Research Council, the Fulbright Senior Research Scholars Program, the Bush Foundation, and the University of Minnesota. Additional support was provided by the Social Science Research Institute of the University of Hawaii; and in Nigeria by Ahmadu Bello University, Wudil Local Government, and the Kano State Department of Health. We thank the people of Hurumi, who continue to inspire our reflections on the meanings and measures of health.

References

Adam JG, Echard N, Lescot M (1972) Plantes médicinales Hausa de l'Ader (République du Niger). *Journal d'Agriculture Tropicale et de Botanique Appliquée*. 19:259–399.

Bedi KL, Zurshi U, Chopra CL, Amla V (1989) *Picrorhiza kurroa*, an Ayurvedic herb, may potentiate photochemotherapy in vitiligo. *Journal of Ethnopharmacology* 27: 347–352.

Busson F, Jaeger P, Lunven P, Pinta M (1965) Plantes Alimentaires de l'Ouest Africain. Paris: Ministère de la Coopération.

Dalziel JM (1937) The Useful Plants of West Tropical Africa. London: Crown Agents for Overseas Governments and Administrations.

Dandekar UP, Chandra RS, Dalvi SS, Joshi MV, Gokhale PC, Sharma AV, Shah PU, Kshirsagar NA (1992) Analysis of a clinically important interaction between phenytoin and Shankhapushpi, an Ayurvedic preparation. *Journal of Ethnopharmacology* 35: 285–288.

Donovan JL, Blake DR (1992) Patient non-compliance: deviance or reasoned decision making? *Social Science and Medicine* 34:507–513.

Etkin NL (1994a) Consuming a therapeutic landscape: a multicontextual framework for assessing the health significance of human–plant interactions. *Journal of Home and Consumer Horticulture* 1:61–81.

Etkin NL (1994b) "The Negotiation of 'Side' Effects in Hausa (Northern Nigeria) Therapeutics." In: Medicines: Meanings and Contexts. NL Etkin, ML Tan, eds. Amsterdam: University of Amsterdam Press, pp. 17–32.

Etkin NL (1996) "Ethnopharmacologic Perspectives on Diet and Medicine in Northern Nigeria." In: Médicaments et Aliments: Approche Ethnopharmacologique. E Schröder, G Balansard, P Cabalion, J Fleurentin, G Mazars, eds. Metz, France: Société Française d'Ethnopharmacologie, pp. 58–62.

Etkin NL (1997a) Antimalarial plants used by Hausa in northern Nigeria. *Tropical Doctor* 27(suppl 1):12–16.

Etkin NL (1997b) Medicinal cuisines: diet and ethnopharmacology. *International Journal of Pharmacognosy* 34:313–326.

Etkin NL (in press) The pharmacologic implications of conserving biodiversity through indigenous models of plant utilization. *Journal of Ethnopharmacology*.

Etkin NL, Ross PJ (1982) Food as medicine and medicine as food: an adaptive framework for the interpretation of plant utilization among the Hausa of northern Nigeria. *Social Science and Medicine* 16:1559–1573.

Etkin NL, Ross PJ (1994) "Pharmacologic Implications of 'Wild' Plants in Hausa Diet." In: Eating on the Wild Side. The Pharmacologic, Ecologic, and Social Implications of Using Noncultigens. NL Etkin, ed. Tucson: University of Arizona Press, pp. 85–101.

Etkin NL, Ross PJ (1997) "Malaria, Medicine and Meals: A Biobehavioral Perspective." In: The Anthropology of Medicine. 3rd ed. L Romanucci-Ross, DE Moerman, LR Tancredi, eds. New York: Praeger, pp. 169–209.

Etkin NL, Ross PJ, Muazzamu I (1990) The indigenization of pharmaceuticals: therapeutic transitions in rural Hausaland. *Social Science and Medicine* 30:919–928.

Etkin NL, Tan ML, eds. (1994) Medicines: Meanings and Contexts. Amsterdam: University of Amsterdam Press.

Hill P (1982) Dry Grain Farming Families. Cambridge: Cambridge University Press.

Mortimore M (1967) Land and population pressure in the Kano Close-Settled Zone, northern Nigeria. *Advancement of Science* 23:677–688.

Nichter M, Vuckovic N (1994) Agenda for an anthropology of pharmaceutical practice. *Social Science and Medicine* 39:1509–1525.

Oliver B (1986) Medicinal Plants in Tropical West Africa. Cambridge: Cambridge University Press.

Pratt JH, Jones JJ (1995) Noncompliance with therapy: an ongoing problem in treating hypertension. *Primary Cardiology* 21:34–38.

Ross PJ (1987) "Land as a Right to Membership: Land Tenure Dynamics in a Peripheral Area of the Kano Close-Settled Zone." In: State, Oil, and Agriculture in Nigeria. M Watts, ed. Berkeley: Institute of International Studies, University of California, pp. 223–247.

Ross PJ, Etkin NL, Muazzamu I (1991) The greater risk of fewer deaths: an ethno-
demographic approach to child mortality in Hausaland. *Africa* 61:502–512.

Ross PJ, Etkin NL, Muazzamu I (1996) A changing Hausa diet. *Medical Anthropology*
17:143–163.

Ross-Degnan D, Laing R, Quick J, Ali HM, Ofori-Adjei D, Salako L, Santoso B (1992)
A strategy for promoting improved pharmaceutical use: the international network
for rational use of drugs. *Social Science and Medicine* 35:1329–1341.

Stock R (1980) Health Care Behavior in a Rural Nigerian Setting, with Particular Refer-
ence to the Utilization of Western-Type Health Care Facilities. PhD dissertation.
Liverpool: Department of Geography, University of Liverpool. Ann Arbor, Mich:
University Microfilms.

Stock R (1985) "Islamic Medicine in Rural Hausaland." In: African Healing Strategies.
BM du Toit, IH Abdalla, eds. New York: Trado-Medico Books, pp. 29–46.

Stock R (1987) "Understanding Health Care Behavior: A Model, Together with Evidence from Nigeria." In: Health and Disease in Tropical Africa: Geographical and
Medical Viewpoints. R Akhtar, ed. London: Harwood, pp. 279–292.

Trostle J, ed. (1996) Inappropriate distribution of medicines by professionals in developing countries. *Social Science and Medicine* 42:1117–1202.

Van der Geest S, Whyte SR, eds. (1988) The Context of Medicines in Developing Countries. Studies in Pharmaceutical Anthropology. Dordrecht: Kluwer.

Wall LL (1988) Hausa Medicine: Illness and Well-Being in a West African Culture.
Durham, NC: Duke University Press.

Wright EC (1993) Non-compliance: or how many aunts has Matilda? *Lancet* 342:
909–913.

9

Cultural Tailoring in Indonesia's National Nutrition Improvement Program

MARCIA GRIFFITHS
MICHAEL FAVIN

From 1972 to 1989, moderate and severe underweight among Indonesian children under five years of age fell from 17% to 11.4% (Soekirman et al., 1992). This important national achievement contributed to the decline in child mortality from 216 to 75 per 1,000 children between 1960 and 1995. The situation in Indonesia was unusual because those at the highest political levels understood the contribution of nutrition to national development and implemented programs designed to improve nutrition rather than waiting for it to improve as a by-product of other economic and social changes. At the program level, the focus was on actions to improve child growth, not only to eliminate severe undernutrition. The appropriateness of this focus and the active pursuit of nutrition improvement have been borne out; recent analyses of nutrition and mortality indicate that not only severe malnutrition, but also mild and moderate malnutrition, increase a child's risk of death (Pelletier et al., 1993).

The achievement of improvements in growth can be explained by examining three key factors (UNICEF, 1992):

1. *Food security*: Beginning in the 1950s, Indonesia moved from being a rice-importing nation to one with rice surpluses, enabling nutrition programs to change their focus from increasing food quantity to improving diet quality.

182

2. *Health*: A nationwide effort to make health services more accessible led to an increase in the number of professionals and facilities and to establishment of community-based programs in family planning and nutrition that delivered basic services such as immunization and oral rehydration therapy.
3. *Child care*: National programs recognized the importance of community and family education to improve key health and nutrition practices for children.

The program at the center of many of these improvements is the Family Nutrition Improvement Program (UPGK). In the mid-1970s, a careful analysis of the earlier Applied Nutrition Program, which had focused on supplementary feeding of the undernourished, led to UPGK's focus on self-reliance at both the family and the community levels and on intersectoral collaboration among the Ministries of Health, Planning, Religion, and Agriculture and the National Family Planning Board and women's programs. The premise is that there is enough food for the majority of families and that, with education and support, families can better feed and care for their children.

Although adapted and implemented locally, the UPGK is usually run by the village women's movement (PKK) and always relies on village volunteers called *kaders*. Usually four or five *kaders* per village organize monthly *pos yandu* (integrated health services including weighing) for children under five years of age. At these sessions, *kaders* assess each child's weight gain as adequate or not adequate for his or her age and, based on that determination, advise the family on appropriate care and attend to any observed illness. Other preventive health services are often offered, too.

UPGK has focused on improving household practices related to child care through nutrition education activities, recognizing that achieving and sustaining an increase of 200–300 calories per day in food intake makes a difference for many children in their growth and ultimately in the risk of illness and death (BASICS et al., 1995). Therefore, UPGK was one of the first programs to develop specific messages about key practices that affect food intake, such as unsupplemented breastfeeding in the first months of life, feeding frequency, amount of food per meal, and nutrient density.

During the early years of UPGK, the government undertook several projects to demonstrate how to achieve impact in the different program components. The pilot Nutrition Communication and Behavior Change Project (NCBC), implemented between 1978 and 1982, was able to achieve and measure significant improvements in child feeding practices and nutritional status by designing messages to improve key practices and by strengthening the counseling skills of community workers and supporting them through the mass media (Griffiths, 1990; Manoff International, 1984). NCBC showed many ways in which UPGK could be strengthened and provided the first evidence that a well designed communications program on child feeding alone could significantly improve children's growth.

In the mid-1980s, the Nutrition Directorate of the Department of Health of Indonesia decided to implement in UPGK the lessons learned from the pilot project. At that time, the US Agency for International Development (USAID) wanted to support such efforts as part of its interest in advancing knowledge on how to improve maternal and infant diets. In 1985, the USAID-funded Weaning Project joined forces with the Ministry of Health's Nutrition Directorate to formulate, implement, and evaluate province-specific educational strategies on child feeding to improve the nutritional status of infants and young children, thereby furthering the government's goal of promoting small and prosperous families. This chapter describes work done from 1985 to 1989 (Griffiths, 1991) and illustrates how the Nutrition Directorate built on lessons from the past to begin a process of local adaptation within its national program.

Although the Nutrition Directorate took the lead, the Indonesian Weaning Project[1] emphasized decentralized decision making and built partnerships for project funding, design, implementation, and evaluation. At the national and provincial levels, decision-making groups for program development and implementation consisted of the representatives from the Ministry of Health's nutrition and health education programs (key implementors), USAID's Weaning Project (technical assistance), UNICEF (the main funder of UPGK), and the National Family Planning Board (another key implementor and funder). Representatives from the program districts and subdistricts joined the provincial teams.

Although ultimately the activities of the Indonesia Weaning Project had to be applicable nationally across a country with tremendous cultural diversity, a few provinces were selected to begin the work. From the outset there was a recognition that the UPGK-strengthening process would require adapting a generic approach to specific cultural situations to learn what program activities and content could remain the same and what needed to change. Cultural adaptation did not mean just altering drawings and language, but also refocusing rationales and modifying the practices that could most impact child nutrition. With this in mind, the provinces that would test the methodology were chosen to provide wide cultural and program diversity. East Java and Nusa Tengarra Barat (NTB) provinces were selected.

East Java has the high population density (652 persons per square kilometer) characteristic of the wetland rice-producing regions of Java. There are highly urbanized areas with light industry. Although East Java had benefited from many programs, indicators such as female literacy (52% in 1983) were below the national average. In 1986, moderate and severe malnutrition was 12%, just below the national average (13%). NTB's population density is about half of East Java's.

There are no urban centers comparable to East Java's, and much of the population is rural. Female literacy was 43% in 1983. In 1986, moderate and severe malnutrition was 21%, well above the national average (Newcomer et al., 1986).

The main ethnic groups in East Java province are the Javanese and immigrants from the island of Madura off the north coast of Java. While the Madurese share many cultural traditions with the Javanese, they often remain apart and maintain their own traditions. Madurese are particularly devout Muslims, and Islamic religious leaders are more influential among them than the mostly Javanese government officials. The Madurese are outside of traditional Javanese class hierarchy and are viewed by the Javanese as having less self-control, being less disciplined. For example, they practice blood revenge for wrongs done to their family.

Javanese culture is stratified by social class and by level of adherence to Islam. However, many Javanese also have traditional religio-magical beliefs, believing that life is preordained and that they have little control over events. Traditional Javanese culture does not emphasize material wealth, but places importance on position. There is respect for those who contribute to the general village welfare over personal gain. And the spirit of *gotong royong*, or volunteerism, is promoted as a cultural value. Within social strata, differentiation is made between the person with *halus*, or refined manners, and the one who is *kasar*, or has rough manners. Kinship is bilateral, that is, determined by the ancestry of both parents. The most important unit is the nuclear family. For children, love is given unconditionally, but value is placed on the instructional role of the family, including grandparents. A child is acculturated to use self-control and to know appropriate manners (Bunge, 1983).

The main ethnic groups in NTB province are the immigrants from the island of Bali and the indigenous Sasak. Although their linguistic roots are similar and both groups maintain a caste system, many other beliefs and practices are different, including religion. The majority of the Balinese are Hindu and live primarily in the cities on the island of Lombok. The Balinese caste system is open, that is, it is possible to change castes. The Balinese, once rulers of Lombok with the Sasak as their servants, keep to themselves. Their Hindu faith means they place little value on wealth, except for its use in obtaining religious offerings. Balinese society is patrilineal, with group membership determined by one's father's ancestry. The extended family predominates, particularly for religious celebrations. Although the Sasak practice Islam, some maintain Sasak traditions more than others, who adhere solely to Islamic traditions. Sasak society can be divided into three classes, defined by behavioral norms and place of residence (neighborhood). Also, in spite of strong Islamic traditions limiting the role of women, Sasak women frequently manage household money and are active in family affairs (Bunge, 1983).

The UPGK programs in each province in 1985 were at different levels of maturity. UPGK was implemented early in East Java. The nutrition coordinator within the local Health Department understood program strengths and weaknesses. Attendance at monthly weighing sessions was high in the majority of villages, particularly among Javanese families. (The Madurese participated less than the Javanese, partly because they do not believe as strongly in the principle on which UPGK relies: self-help through community volunteerism. Furthermore, community women associated with the program tended to be of high status, to have husbands in government jobs, and to be Javanese; this often deterred Madurese women from enthusiastic participation.) In East Java there was also a very strong family planning program that provided an additional community outreach mechanism.

In NTB the program was newer and the infrastructure much less developed than in Java. Participation in monthly weighing sessions was lower than in Java, again in part because there was not such a high level of community volunteer spirit and because the communities were not as cohesive as in East Java. Also, people seemed less willing to accept new ideas from outside their traditional frame of reference. Program management was not as strong as in East Java because of less stability in program staff and because connections between the central program in Jakarta (the capital) and the provincial implementation team suffered from a feeling that the realities of NTB were not well understood in Jakarta.

During the four years of funding from September 1985 to December 1989, the program development and implementation plan was carried out in both provinces. The program included five phases:

- Assessment, November 1985–October 1986.
- Strategy formulation, materials design, and production, November 1986–February 1988.
- Implementation, March 1988–December 1989.
- Evaluation: baseline and follow-up surveys, July/August 1987–February 1989.
- Expansion, October 1988–December 1989, and 1990 onward.

Assessment Phase

Methods

The objective of the assessment phase was to gain an in-depth understanding, in the household and community context, of existing feeding practices and the reasons for them. It was also intended to identify the major resistances to changing those practices and the best motivations to encourage change. The assessment also explored the ways in which information in general, and health and nutrition information specifically, were communicated. The assessment studies were not intended to measure the prevalence of feeding practices, but rather to describe them in detail. The research was qualitative and involved a small sample from semiurban and rural locations in selected districts of each province.

The assessment of weaning practices had four main steps, each building on the findings of the preceding one (Griffiths, 1992). A local market research firm was hired to train Health Department staff and to supervise focus group discussions. Professional anthropologists and a nutritionist worked with the local research team to conduct in-depth interviews, observations, and trials of new feeding practices. The research team consisted of local health workers and social science or nutrition students who were willing to stay in the villages and who spoke the local languages. Staff from the provincial and national offices of the Health Department assisted the local teams. In addition to families, religious leaders, *kaders* (local nutrition volunteers), store owners, midwives, and village leaders were interviewed.

The first step in the assessment was to identify problems related to adequate dietary intake. This step entailed focus group discussions and in-depth household interviews and observations. Focus groups were held to determine general attitudes and perceptions about children, child rearing and feeding, and advice-seeking. In-depth household interviews and observations were then conducted in one semiurban and two rural villages in East Java and in two semiurban communities (one Balinese and one Sasak) and one rural village in NTB.

Researchers selected villages that were expected to show the range of differences in child feeding practices. Fifteen households with well- and undernourished children (determined from the child's growth chart), representing a cross section of ages under 24 months, were selected in each of the six villages. During three visits to each household, interviewers talked with mothers about their work; the availability, preparation, and consumption of food; health, morbidity, and mortality in the family; and information sources. Household conditions and possessions were observed to ascertain socioeconomic status and to understand information sources and feeding practices. A pre-coded 24-hour dietary recall was used to record each child's food intake. It allowed for analysis of calorie, protein, and vitamin A intakes.

The second step, problem analysis and concept formulation, was done at the provincial level by comparing real with ideal nutritional practices for each age group and then determining the beneficial and harmful practices contributing to children's nutritional status. Next, recommendations were drafted for changes in practices that could be adopted to narrow the gap between real and ideal practices.

This is usually where assessments stop. The recommendations from the in-depth interviews become the guidance for the program. However, learning from the earlier NCBC project, a key activity was the inclusion of a third assessment step: trials of improved practices (TIPs) (Dickin et al., 1997; Griffiths, 1992). TIPs involved taking the recommendations and concepts back to the mothers.

The TIPs were conducted with the same families that had participated in the in-depth interviews and observations. Since rapport had been established with these families, it was possible to talk with them about the feeding problems observed in their households and then to offer relevant recommendations on how to resolve these problems. With the interviewer, mothers decided on one or two new practices to improve the nutrient intake of their children, which they would try for one week. After a week the interviewer returned to the home to discuss the mother's experience, whom she had consulted, if she liked the new practice(s), if she felt she was successful, how her child had reacted, what she had changed, and if she would recommend the practice(s) to a friend or neighbor.

At the end of the TIPs, the field team knew which recommendations had been successful. In the fourth step of the assessment, researchers used focus groups to elicit the opinions of people who had not participated in the investigation of the new, recommended behaviors and to examine reasons that might persuade mothers to try the new practices.

Findings

The findings from the assessment research are reported in four areas important for programming: key child care concepts, current feeding practices, potential dietary improvements, and information sources.

Concepts Important because of Their Influence on Child Feeding. The following seven concepts were found to be significant.

Mothers' strong concern for pleasing their children and their family and their lack of confidence in their ability to improve their child's diet. Mothers wanted to be sure that their children were "satisfied." For example, mothers would not force an anorexic child to eat, because it would displease the child. This concern (particularly strong among the Javanese), often coupled with a mother's lack of self-confidence, limited the amounts children ate. The project needed to establish the link between a mother's ability to please her family, her knowledge of child care concepts, and having the confidence to do what is correct.

Parents' aspirations for their children. The higher aspirations expressed by mothers of well-nourished children compared with those of undernourished children indicated that offering some vision of the future could be an important motivator for improving feeding practices. However, aspirations needed to be tailored to each province: for parents in East Java, the meaningful appeal would be for a prosperous future; for those in NTB, it would be for increased happiness or a reduced burden in the near future—a response reflective of the lower socioeconomic status and lower level of ongoing development in NTB.

The desirable balance between the child's physical and psychological development. The effort to achieve this balance influenced the quantity and types of foods offered to a child, especially in Java, where parents did not want "fat" children or children who were accustomed to "good" foods and who might therefore become greedy. The child's psychological development sometimes motivated fathers' involvement. In NTB, fathers were responsible for character development.

Mothers' concerns for the cost of new practices, in terms of money and time. Appeals for changes in practices needed to address these two constraints honestly and directly, regardless of ethnic affiliation or the level of urbanity.

Mix of traditional and modern concepts about child care and use of health services. The positive aspects of traditional practices and customs for the mother should be transferred to the "new" or modified practices intended to improve nutritional status. For example, incorporate the feeding of colostrum (the fluid that flows for one to three days before breast milk) into the welcoming ritual for the newborn; train the traditional birth attendant to add a breastfeeding check to her usual postpartum visit; link the Javanese desire for a "refined," well-behaved child, to eating sufficiently and to alertness and brightness.

Lack of clear understanding of the relationship between adequate food intake and health and growth. Even mothers with more "modern" health ideas and those participating in government programs could not discuss these concepts clearly. Mothers feared "large" quantities of food and blamed them for making their children sick, even though sickness might be the result of food contamination, not the quantity of food. Few mothers could recall how much food their children had eaten, and they had no concept of how much a child should eat. When told about adequate quantities, they denied that their children could eat that much. By restricting food quantity, they felt they were keeping their child within realistic expectations, since some days there was less food than others. Restriction also was part of managing demand and teaching children about good manners. In Java it is culturally desirable to be thin, refined, and light, all of which are associated with low food consumption.

General contentment with life. Although parents saw benefits from other lifestyles and clearly recognized that their own lifestyle could and should be improved, in general they were happy with their lives. Surprisingly, differences in feeding practices and outlook on life were more pronounced between semiurban and rural populations than between provinces or even ethnic groups, except perhaps for differences between the Sasak and Balinese in NTB (although even here it is difficult to attribute all of the difference to ethnicity, since most of the Balinese are urban dwellers).

The Actual Practices Relating to Child Feeding and Child Care. Detailed descriptions of the diet and feeding of children under 24 months highlighted common practices across the provinces and local differences that merited attention. For example, practices in the first month of life were similar in all ethnic groups and locations. Prelacteal feeding with sugar water, honey, or teas, for one to three days, was used to mark the newborn's freedom from the womb and to satisfy the infant until the breast milk flowed. Generally, but not universally, colostrum was discarded because it was thought to be dirty and harmful. Prelacteal feeds, which were encouraged by traditional midwives, replaced colostrum. By 48 hours after birth, almost all mothers had begun to breastfeed and continued to breastfeed confidently and properly during this first month. However, few infants were exclusively breastfed, since they continued to receive small tastes of food, particularly from family members other than the mother, "to keep them quiet."

During months two to four, breastfeeding was continued on demand but generally was not done exclusively. There was predominant use of the left breast for feeding, due in part to the way mothers carried babies and breastfed while working. By the third month, many infants, especially in semiurban areas, received rice porridge in addition to tastes of other foods. In NTB, pre-chewed and fermented rice was given. Very small amounts of food were given at one time to prevent harming the child. This fear was especially prevalent among mothers with undernourished children.

From month five to eight, nutrient intake began to be inadequate: about 66% of infants' calorie requirement and 50% of their protein requirement were met. This situation was aggravated by a sharp increase in diarrhea and respiratory infections. Breastfeeding continued as in the month two to four period—on demand and primarily from the left breast. By the fifth month, infants in semiurban areas received a variety of starchy, "soft" foods. Mothers often prepared a "special" porridge for the child because they believed the child's food must be much softer than adult food. When teeth began to come in, the rice porridge became thicker. Green vegetables were often added to the rice porridge in East Java. In rural NTB, throughout this period, infants got only breast milk and rice.

By six months, many infants received some protein foods (tahu, or tempe, from soybeans) or eggs. Especially in semiurban areas, children began to receive snacks such as biscuits. However, food variety was kept at a minimum so "the child will not develop expensive habits." Diets were extremely low in fat. Semisolids were often given three times a day to well-nourished children and less often to undernourished children. Food quantities were not measured. Children were fed while the caretaker walked with the child, and the child was fed until "satisfied," usually based on cues from the child. Because they were often out of the house, mothers in semiurban areas were likely to entrust child feeding to other members of the family.

During months 9–18, dietary intake met only half of the caloric and protein requirements, and illnesses increased. On any given day, approximately one-third of these children had some symptom of an illness. Breastfeeding continued for most children, but frequency declined in the semiurban areas and some mothers in these areas weaned their children at this age. This was a time of transition to an adult diet. At about 10 months, children began to receive foods from the family pot, and at 18 months they received a full family diet. Food variety increased and was greater for the better nourished children, the semiurban children, and the Javanese and Balinese children. Fish, commonly available, was not given to children because it was thought to cause worms and accustom children to foods that are too expensive. Feeding frequency remained at three meals per day, although many children were given snacks to quiet them. Mothers tended to stop feeding when the child lost interest, not when the child had consumed a particular amount; consequently, many children ate very little. Frequently, mothers reported that the child "does not want to eat."

In the latter half of the second year of life, nutrient intake seemed to improve, but rates of malnutrition remained high because of illness. Children's diets did not change much during this period, although over half of the semiurban children were weaned at this age because they were thought to be "big enough" not to receive breast milk. In rural areas, weaning often occurred later. Feeding frequency continued to be three times per day. Mothers were likely to allow children to eat without adult supervision, to give them many snacks (often purchased), and to remain unaware of the amounts of food children ate.

Mothers continued breastfeeding during and after a child's illness. Breastfeeding was thought to help cure a sick child. Although mothers said they tried not to vary the feeding of their ill child, they fed less of other foods because they thought children were less hungry and feared that food might make the illness worse. Mothers fed sick children very cautiously and spent extra time with them. After the illness, mothers were willing to give more food only if the child would accept it.

Whether or not mothers worked for wages or were outside the home for many consecutive hours made no difference in children's nutritional status, caloric adequacy, or frequency of eating. Cessation of breastfeeding during the child's first year of life was not dramatically different among working and "nonworking" mothers, although mothers who worked tended to wean earlier. The difference was found in mothers who were paid for work at home or who worked a half-day or less outside the home. These mothers tended to have children who were fed less frequently and who had lower weight-for-age than mothers who worked long hours outside the home. The latter tended to entrust the care of their child to someone else, while women working at home or for shorter times outside the home had a minimal need for help with child care, trying to do everything themselves.

Dietary Improvement. In the trials of improved practices, or TIPs, almost every mother who tried to improve her child's feeding practices could do so. Low family income and a scarcity of resources were seldom reasons for not trying to do something, although the purchase of special foods was a problem in rural NTB. All mothers with children over one year old did at least one thing to improve the child's diet. Mothers who made limited changes in their practices had young children who were sick and would not eat, or who just refused additional food. The trials tested various improved practices and found certain ones to be feasible and key to nutrition improvement.

- Stimulate fuller lactation in initial months.
  Begin breastfeeding immediately at birth to welcome the child, and give colostrum rather than continuing to use honey or sugar water beyond the ritual feed.
  Breastfeed more frequently and use both breasts to satisfy the child.
  Decrease small "tastes" of food.
- Give "special" calorie- and nutrient-dense baby food made from family foods: Introduce the child to soft food during the fifth month. This food should not be watery but just soft/smooth.
  For a child 6–9 months old, offer a "special" soft mixed food (rice, *tahu/tempe*, green leaves) cooked with a source of fat (oil or coconut milk).
  After the child reaches 10 months, give adult foods to provide a complete meal. (Fruit was not stressed: all mothers gave fruit when it was available; if it had to be purchased, it was generally too expensive.)
- Increase the quantity of food consumed by young children (stressing frequency for younger children and amount per meal for older children):
  Feed children 6–9 months old four to six times per day, plus breast milk.
  Feed children 10–24 months old five times per day, combining meals and snacks in addition to breast milk.
  Give children 10–24 months old a larger portion of food than usual (increasing frequency was not favored by mothers of these children) and try to increase the variety of foods in their diet (add one food not usually given to the child).
- Feeding during and after illness:
  For sick children at least 4 months old, give a soft food in addition to breast milk.
  Increase portion size and feeding frequency by one additional feeding per day for the child recovering from illness.

Information Sources. Health information was not reaching the majority of families. About half the mothers in both provinces listened to radio and watched television (although not necessarily their own). Cassette recorders for popular music were available in many houses in semiurban areas. Print materials were seldom seen in the houses. Women rarely attended performances of traditional entertainment, but half attended various community meetings. In Muslim areas, attendance of *pengajian*, reading of the Qur'an, was high. Attendance at monthly village child- weighing sessions varied from 5% (rural NTB) to 65% (rural East Java).

The nutrition *kaders* were not recognized or sought out as people who could counsel about child care and feeding. *Dukun bayi*, traditional midwives, were sources of advice at birth and during the first months of a baby's life, but usually not after that.

Religious leaders were consulted on a variety of topics, although usually not child care, and their advice was highly esteemed.

Grandparents were frequent sources of advice. Only in NTB were fathers considered to take an active role in day-to-day child care decisions; therefore, their advice was sought on child care.

Warung, small stores or food stalls, were ubiquitous. Many families visited them every day, and others did so several times a week. The advice of the shopkeeper, if a woman, was solicited for problems a mother might be having in feeding her child.

The Communication Project

Strategy Development

After the assessment was completed, a three-day workshop was held to discuss the results and to formulate a project strategy and province-specific plans. For the first time since the project began, this workshop brought together members of the provincial and national teams, the advisory group, and representatives of the Ministries of Planning, Religion, and Agriculture who were active in UPGK, the National Family Planning Board, universities, private institutions, UNICEF, and USAID. Broad participation was desired to expose as many people as possible to the health and nutrition issues of the young child and to solicit ideas from many perspectives.

The national team presented the assessment findings. Provincial representatives critiqued the findings, which were then discussed by all workshop participants. Provincial specificity was appreciated and plans were made for undertaking similar work in other provinces. In small groups, participants discussed ideas for strategies and project activities that could be carried out at the UPGK monthly weighing sessions; within the UPGK multisectoral activities with Religion, Agriculture, and Family Planning; and by the private sector (mainly local and national nongovernmental organizations [NGOs]). Finally, the participants divided into two groups to examine work plans and budgets for East Java and NTB.

Key outcomes of this strategy formulation workshop were:

- The Weaning Project would limit itself to communication and training activities. Participants felt that other interventions, for example, production of a food or improved food distribution by market women, would overwhelm available staff and financial resources.
- The communication and training activities would have two foci: the UPGK monthly weighing sessions and other community programs such as family planning.
- Emphasis should be placed on strengthening the *kaders'* role as educators.

Following the workshop, the national team wrote a detailed communication and training strategy. A local company, P.T. Intervista, the pioneer of advertising in Indonesia with a history of public service work, was contracted by the Nutrition Directorate to add detail to the strategy, develop and test creative prototype materials, finalize them, and oversee their reproduction.

The objectives of the strategy that resulted from a process of continuous consultation between the agency and project groups at the national and provincial levels were to:

- Introduce an improved "product," good weaning practices (specific feeding behaviors) that would fulfill the needs of parents and improve children's nutrient intake.
- Create consumer acceptance for "good weaning practices" by promoting them through credible media and spokespeople with good coverage and frequent contact. This included better training of *kaders* to enhance their credibility as the "sales force" for good weaning practices.
- "Outsell" the competition—that is, old attitudes and practices related to infant and child feeding (and some "new" attitudes)—by improving knowledge and self-confidence of mothers in their ability to change and better nourish their children.

A second lesson from the NCBC project brought to this project was to segment (divide by common characteristic) the principal audience, mothers, in order to offer more precise advice (Griffiths, 1993). Mothers were assigned to segments according to the factor that most distinguished their feeding practices: the age of their child, then the child's state of health, and finally how busy the mother was. There were eight segments of the primary audience: pregnant women (preparation for child feeding); mothers with infants 0–3 months; those with infants 4–5 months; 6–9 months; 10–18 months; 19–24 months; mothers with children ill or recuperating from illness; and working mothers (inside and outside the home). Fathers, especially in NTB, and other caretakers of young children (under 24 months) were also important audiences.

The final strategy emphasized the unifying concepts or elements of the materials. For example, they promoted:

- *Ibu Gizi* (*Mrs. Nutrition*): She was the fictional spokesperson for the project, credible and authoritative because she was seen to be mature enough to know Indonesian ways, but young enough to know "modern" practices. She was the voice of all of the advice offered by *kaders* and others, who often lacked credibility. All print materials carried her picture, and she was the leading protagonist in the dialogues on radio and cassette.
- *The Concept of Good Weaning Practices:* This was the foundation of the strategy because it summarized the "product" the project was trying to sell. The assessment showed that mothers did not have a complete understanding of appropriate feeding practices and that they wanted a schedule or plan. They did not recognize what constituted a nutritious food for their babies or know adequate feeding frequencies or quantities. Emphasis was placed on conveying the idea that feeding changes as the child grows.
- *The Concept of Breastfeeding from Both Breasts at Each Feeding:* This concept was reinforced because it seemed to be the key to full breastfeeding (a key concept also in the NCBC project) and might be the key to mothers satisfying their baby with breast milk and eliminating or decreasing the early, small feedings of other foods.
- *The Concept of Nasi Tim Bayi* (soft, mixed rice for baby): The promotion of a "special," homemade, mixed (a combination of ingredients), soft food was critical to achieving project goals (and was a successful element of the NCBC project). *Nasi* (rice) is chosen to indicate that it is the family rice and not the usual rice flour porridge. *Tim* (steamed) is chosen to show that the food is soft. *Bayi* (baby) is part of the name to convey that it is a baby's food and special, different from the regular *nasi tim* because it is made from several ingredients (a carbohydrate, a protein, a vitamin-rich vegetable) and, in particular, a source of fat.
- *The Concept of Baby Weighing:* Weighing was emphasized because monitoring change in weight was key to the mother's understanding of whether she fed her child appropriately. Also, a mother's attendance at the weighing session ensured that she had an opportunity for intensive counseling on feeding.

The media plan was developed to ensure that communication would reach mothers and other family members through the UPGK program as well as through other channels, such as stores, and directly in their homes via radio. The principal media were *kaders*, traditional midwives, and other health personnel; community leaders, religious leaders, heads of women's groups, and others; store owners; radio; and print materials (e.g., posters) that carried the message in pictures and words.

A plan was developed so that various materials could be used by multiple media. For example, the dialogues would be used by the radio and put on audio cassettes for the *kaders* and store owners to use. Leaflets would be used by anyone responsible for talking about good weaning practices. The counseling cards and child feeding schedule would be for community and health center personnel or volunteers. Following is a description of the materials.

Audio cassette sets for tape players found in villages and for radio stations. One side of the cassette had the project jingle and popular songs interspersed with dialogues with *Ibu Gizi*. The other side had the dialogues alone. The dialogues addressed, in direct fashion, the questions and reservations expressed by the mothers in the assessment of particular practices. The side with the music could be used to attract people to a gathering or to a store, and the side with the dialogues used to counsel a mother during a home visit or at the weighing session. One set consisted of eight cassettes. Each cassette addressed a particular audience segment, for example, mothers with children six to nine months old. The messages on these cassettes were the same as those on the counseling cards.

Three posters with the major Weaning Project messages for stores, the village weighing posts, and health centers. One stressed immediate, exclusive breastfeeding after birth with colostrum and also continued full breastfeeding (use of both breasts). Another stressed that food does not need to be started until 4 months, that by 6–9 months the child should be eating *Nasi Tim Bayi,* and by 10 months the child should begin regular family foods. The third poster "advertised" *nasi tim bayi.* All of the posters featured *Ibu Gizi* and carried the reminder to consult the *kader*, village weighing post, or health center for more information.

The leaflet designed to be used by the kader or "teacher" when teaching the mother how to make Nasi Tim Bayi. It was kept by the mothers to assist them in their home preparation. Two recipe variations specified by mothers during the TIPs were presented, one using raw ingredients and another using already cooked foods.

A feeding schedule developed in response to the mothers' desire to have an overall plan for feeding. It was designed to fit into the national child health card and to be taken home by the mothers. It illustrated the age at which children should be introduced to specific foods and the frequency of feeding for children at each month from 0 to 24 months. Each box on the schedule corresponded to one feeding. Feeding included breastfeedings, first foods, *Nasi Tim Bayi,* family foods, and snacks. The schedule also reminded mothers to feed more and to breastfeed and/or give more food to a child recovering from an illness.

Counseling cards. These were divided by audience segment and used to assist the *kaders* in talking to a mother about exactly how she should feed her child. The nine cards emphasized the key behaviors feasible for mothers.

Implementation

Implementation began in December 1987. Trainers from all project areas were taught child feeding concepts as well as skills such as using the materials for counseling. In February 1988, approximately 1,000 *kaders*, two from each village health or weighing post, were trained for two days at their local health centers. Between January and April 1988, one-day orientations were held for intersectoral UPGK teams representing the Ministries of Religion, Agriculture, and Family Planning from the district and provincial levels; community leaders, including religious and neighborhood leaders and women's groups; midwives; and a few owners of small shops from each community.

The training and orientation sessions reviewed the project and its purposes, discussed the materials and the major messages, and finally provided practice (through role playing) on how to use and handle the materials. *Kaders* received longer training because of their critical job of counseling, including the correct use of the counseling cards. Immediate supervision of the distribution and use of the materials provided a follow-up to the training.

After the project was formally launched in March 1988, the national team monitored activities every other month. They developed a standardized form for reporting specific indicators of implementation, such as the presence of all materials with the appropriate people, how each educational agent was performing the required tasks, and how much mothers had contact with the project and recalled messages. Villages were picked at random for these visits. In addition, provincial representatives visited each district once a month, and district representatives monitored health centers twice a month. A health center representative was responsible for supervising each weighing post in the project villages once every three months.

After six months of project implementation, a team composed of representatives from the Department of Health, the advertising agency, and the technical assistance group carried out a detailed midcourse review, primarily of activities at the subdistrict and village levels, to begin planning for project strengthening and expansion. In general the project was working well, particularly in East Java. Many people reported on the project enthusiastically, saying that specific child feeding messages had been a missing element. The review showed that training had been implemented, the materials were well distributed and employed, and there was good recognition of project concepts and specific practices among both providers and families. Following are highlights of the findings and recommendations for project improvement.

- Implementation was very dependent on the strength of the ongoing integrated health delivery program offered at the village health post (*pos yandu*). Where the *pos yandu* was strong—that is, open regularly, well staffed and organized, and with good child weighing—the child feeding education was well implemented. Where the *pos yandu* program was weak (especially in rural NTB), the child feeding education was also poor. This is logical, because the project activities aim only to strengthen UPGK's educational component, not the infrastructure as a whole. The team recommended expanding the project educational activities only in areas with strong *pos yandu*.
- Community-wide activities needed to be strengthened, for example, by participation of more stores and community groups as providers of project messages. The team recommended that someone be hired to supervise these private sector activities, particularly to visit and distribute materials at the small shops.
- Some materials needed to be simplified. For example, the graphics on the *Nasi Tim Bayi* leaflet needed to be sequential; the set of posters needed to be reduced in number, and the messages they carried needed to be clearer; and the set of cassettes also needed to be reduced in number, one having songs and a few general messages and the others having specific dialogues.
- *Kaders* needed to be retrained after one year in communications skills, with special care taken to train only active *kaders*.
- Women's organizations, especially the PKK, needed to be encouraged to become active participants in the project advisory group and to make an institutional commitment to the project's educational activities. When they were involved, more education occurred at the village level.
- The provincial-level teams needed to have closer contact with the local radio stations to get them to play the dialogues during the time allotted for health programming.
- The supervision scheme and forms required simplification. Supervision (helping the providers improve their activities) needed to be stressed over monitoring (quantitative accounting).

Evaluation

Methods

The evaluation of this project was designed as two cross-sectional surveys (a pre/posttest design) among project and comparison groups of mothers and *kaders*. An additional feature was a cohort study in which a subsample of children under nine months of age at the time of the baseline was revisited during the postintervention survey. Comparison districts were matched demographically and socioeconomically with project districts. Both the comparison and project villages, or subvillage units in NTB, were randomly selected. Within these villages, all children were registered and households were selected randomly just prior to interviewing. A total of 780 mothers with children 0–2 years of age were interviewed. Of these, 143 were in the cohort sample. Two hundred forty *kaders* participated in an evaluation of their performance. After slightly less than a year of project implementation and before the majority of the recommendations from the midterm review were implemented, a repeat survey of the baseline was done to measure the impact of the project quantitatively.

During analysis each indicator was examined separately. In addition, for particular variable domains, composite scores were constructed to simplify comparison. For example, a composite socioeconomic score combining eight variables was compiled for each area. Families were also given a community participation score, comprising 11 variables. Composite project exposure, knowledge, and practice scores were also constructed. Highlights of evaluation results are summarized below.

Results

Briefly, this evaluation (Yayasan Indonesia Sejahtera, 1989) found that the Indonesia Weaning Project had improved mothers' and *kaders'* knowledge of child feeding practices, particularly knowledge of breastfeeding practices and introduction of complementary foods and appropriate mixed weaning foods (Table 9.1). Moreover, through this project, which brought educational inputs only, a significant impact was observed (relative to comparison sites) in children's calorie intake, the nutritional status of children, and in mothers' child feeding practices (especially those in the same areas where knowledge increased). The Weaning Project messages had a strong impact despite the fact that contact with the project was not universal and implementation of certain messages was not optimal.

Sociodemographic Characteristics. Project and comparison groups did not differ on a composite socioeconomic status (SES) score although there were some site-specific differences. Javanese, Balinese, and mixed ethnic areas had a higher SES score than Madurese and Sasak areas. Urban dwellers had a higher SES score than rural dwellers. Women's access and participation in community activities showed no significant difference between project and comparison groups. Significant differences in the age of children were not found between sites. Likewise, the percentage of children experiencing some illness the day before the interview (33%) was the same between project and comparison groups as was the rate of morbidity in the last month.

Project Exposure. At the time of the evaluation, within the project areas 80% of the mothers recalled seeing or hearing some project message, and 53% of project mothers correctly recalled the contents of at least one of the Weaning Project materials. Both mass media and *kaders* played important roles in disseminating messages. More mothers in the project areas (than in comparison areas) reported receiving information from their *kaders* both in general and at the last weighing session. In project areas, the mothers' perception of *kaders* as an important source of information on child feeding was higher as well. *Kaders* in project areas also reported giving information about child feeding and health to mothers at the weighing sessions significantly more often than their comparison counterparts (76.3% vs. 39.5%).

Knowledge. Mothers' knowledge about the Weaning Project messages for infants up to nine months of age was significantly higher in the project areas than in the comparison areas regarding the introduction of complementary foods, frequency of feeding, and ingredients of weaning foods, as well as the importance of giving only breast milk in the first four months of life. Maternal knowledge of feeding practices for older children was not as good as for the younger children. (The project placed less emphasis on those messages.) On the composite knowledge score, differences were significant between project and comparison groups (see Table 9.1). Project mothers' knowledge increased significantly between the baseline and final evaluation survey. The mother's residence in a project area as well as the number of project materials she could correctly recall were significantly linked to higher knowledge scores. Other determinants of knowledge were contact with the *kader* and attendance at the *pos yandu.*

Practices. Mothers' child feeding practices were influenced by exposure to the project (see Table 9.1). Mothers who had a correct recall of project materials (those mothers whose exposure to the project was verified) showed significant behavior changes compared with those mothers not exposed to the project, particularly on certain subtopics where their knowledge gains were high: giving colostrum, introducing foods later, preparing a special food for their child, and correctly preparing and giving the "special" mixed weaning food, *Nasi Tim Bayi.* (This last practice was corroborated by observation when possible.) The only significant change in practice noted for older children was that those in the project area received a greater variety of foods than did their counterparts in comparison areas.

Diet. The percentages of young children achieving recommended calorie and protein intakes in the project and comparison groups were analyzed. In the aggregate, no significant difference was seen. Significant differences were seen, however, for babies 6–9 months old (89.3% in the project area vs. 80.8% in the comparison area had adequate caloric intake) and in the numbers of children

Table 9.1 Summary of Project Results

	PROJECT GROUP	COMPARISON GROUP	p VALUE
Project exposure			
Mother ever seen or heard project message	80%	16.5%	≤ .01
Mother received advice at last weighing session	36.6%	24.1%	≤ .01
Mother received advice from community group	40%	14%	≤ .01
Mothers view *kaders* as source of information on feeding	33%	14.7%	≤ .01
Kaders report giving advice on child feeding at weighing sessions	76.3%	39.5%	≤ .01
Kaders report giving advice at community meetings	83.6%	38.6%	≤ .01
Knowledge			
Mothers knowledge score (% correct answers)			
Baseline	46.4%	45.4%	NS*
Endline	63.0%	55.5%	≤ .01
Kaders knowledge score			
Baseline	51.3%	51.1%	NS
Endline	81.1%	64.0%	≤ .01
Practices after one year			
Gave colostrum	50.1%	37.7%	≤ .01
Later introduction of foods	37.1%	28.2%	≤ .01
Correct preparation of *Nasi Tim Bayi*	23.1%	8.0%	≤ .01
Feeding more frequently (times/day)	4.4	4.3	NS
Feeding greater variety of foods (total types = 6)	4.2 types	3.7 types	≤ .0001
Diet after one year			
6–9 months old meeting caloric adequacy	89.3%	80.8%	≤ .02
10–24 months old meeting caloric adequacy	71.9%	71.9%	NS
25–28 months old meeting protein adequacy	75.2%	50.1%	≤ .005
Cohort sample—total caloric adequacy	79.5%	69.6%	≤ .02
Nutrition status after one year			
Weight-for-age (z score), controlling for age	–1.4	–1.6	≤ .015
Height-for-age (z score), controlling for age	–1.5	–1.6	≤ .02

*NS = not statistically significant.

25–28 months old meeting their protein requirement (75.2% vs. 50.1%). Mean percentages of requirements were also calculated. In the cohort sample (the subsample followed longitudinally), the percentage of children receiving their requirement was significantly different in the aggregate (79.5% vs. 69.6%). No significant differences were seen in intake at baseline. Higher weaning knowledge scores and contact with the Weaning Project were highly correlated with a higher percentage of recommended calorie intake.

Nutrition Status. The impact on growth was not expected to be large, given the relatively short implementation period. Analysis of the weight and height data, however, showed that the Weaning Project did have a statistically significant impact on the nutritional status (both weight-for-age and height-for-age) of children (Table 9.1). However, this impact was small and did not delay the alarming faltering of children's growth beginning around five or six months of age. Significant differences in nutritional status (weight-for-age) were noted at all five aggregates of monthly growth below 26 months. In addition to the age of the child, caloric adequacy (in itself positively correlated to knowledge and exposure to the project), socioeconomic status, ethnic group, and exposure of the mother to the project had a determining impact on the child's weight. Similarly, exposure to the project was found to influence height-for-age after controlling for age and socioeconomic status.

Kaders. A composite educator score showed that project *kaders* had a greater propensity to educate mothers and had better information with which to do this. For example, in addition to their offering advice significantly more often at weighing sessions, 83.6% of project *kaders* versus 38.6% of comparison *kaders* said they offered nutrition education at community meetings; this was confirmed. Higher levels of supervision were associated with increasing time spent teaching mothers. On a composite knowledge score, the two *kader* groups scored similarly on the baseline survey (51% vs. 53% correct responses, for project and comparison groups, respectively). At the time of the follow-up survey, both groups showed improvement, but the project group did significantly better (81.1% vs. 64% correct responses). Thus not only were the project *kaders* giving significantly more advice to mothers, but the advice they were giving was of better quality.

Besides these "impact" findings, the evaluation is replete with information on the extent and success of communication through various media. For example, the influence of the *kaders* is clear, although the reinforcement of several media was very important. A very provocative finding is the positive impact of the education on mothers merely living in the project area, but not necessarily participating in many project activities. Improvements in knowledge, attitude, and practices were seen even in project mothers who claimed not to recall exposure to project messages. This could be an indication of the "socialization" of new practices through daily observation and conversation which all health education programs seek. For example, significantly more project mothers reported giving advice on child health and nutrition to other mothers than did comparison mothers (20% vs. 7.5%). This confirmed the soundness of the project planning that aimed to get the messages into daily village life through shops and local leaders, not just through the health system, which, in places like NTB, often lacks credibility.

Overall, the hypotheses of the project were confirmed. The education project appears to have improved mothers' knowledge about infant feeding, positively changed practices, contributed to better diets being offered and consumed by young children, particularly in the first year of life, and led to slightly improved nutritional status.

Implications

Lessons from Education and Training

The Indonesia Weaning Project was the second time a pilot project in Indonesia demonstrated, through rigorous evaluation, that an enhanced nutrition education component adapted to meet local conditions could substantially improve the impact of the national nutrition program, UPGK. Several important lessons from the Weaning Project may be of use to planners of similar projects.

First, the communications did not just transfer nutrition information, but responded to the major problems mothers were experiencing in their feeding practices. Although extensive formative research has now been undertaken in five Indonesian provinces (South Sumatra, Central Java, D.I. Yogyakarta, East Java, and NTB), with similar key messages resulting, there have been important adaptations made for some province-specific details. Therefore, as the educational component is expanded, research should be done on a province-by-province basis, so that subtle differences in beliefs and practices can be noted, and responses to them can be formulated. At a minimum, from a set of key message themes, there needs to be adaptation of language, specific foods or preparation methods, and some of the rationales for undertaking certain practices.

During the Weaning Project, a rigorous protocol was tested for examining and better understanding families' child feeding practices. The national team learned the process and managed it. Building on past experience, it would be possible to streamline the assessment. For example, focus group discussions could be eliminated as the first step and used only at the end of the process. The initial household interview could be drastically reduced, relying more on what proved indispensable, the TIPs. With these changes, staff within the Nutrition Directorate could implement a provincial assessment in no more than four months.

The second lesson is that the messages that had the most impact were precisely stated and had a name or a product associated with them: *Susu Pelindung* (protective milk/colostrum) and *Nasi Tim Bayi*. These "products" were both new and appealing to the mothers. From this project, and NCBC, there is ample and adequate experience to move forward with province-specific adaptation of messages to improve critical breastfeeding practices and to introduce a homemade weaning food for children in the transition period prior to eating an "adult" meal.

However, the concepts such as frequency and quantity per meal were not captured effectively in the materials and, although stated precisely, were not disseminated well. To improve the impact of Weaning Project messages and materials, the following recommendations are made:

- The message about breastfeeding immediately should receive more emphasis. The poster about breastfeeding practices had a title of *"Susu Pelindung,"* or protective milk (colostrum), which stressed the feeding of colostrum rather than the need to begin breastfeeding immediately. The idea of selling "protective milk" was innovative and exciting, and the concept of a protective milk appeared to have changed perceptions of colostrum. However, the success of this concept was not coupled with the success of the accompanying message to breastfeed immediately.
- The concept of adult food and food quantities should be clarified. The messages for children over nine months old were difficult to evaluate because the "adult foods" were not defined precisely enough in each setting. Likewise, the amount fed per meal, although recognized as a problem at the time of assessment, was not communicated clearly enough for most mothers to act on. The expression of these concepts requires more cultural precision.
- The number of counseling cards should be reduced. One of the reasons that the messages for older children, sick children, and children cared for by working mothers were less successful was that *kaders* tended to learn and use only the first few counseling cards in the set (those for the younger children). The counseling cards were reduced in number from 16 to 9 to respond to this problem, and they were completely redesigned, with all major messages represented graphically on the front of the card, helping the *kader* quickly recall key messages.
- Use of the feeding schedule should be continued. This material, introduced only a few months before the evaluation, seemed to be essential in reinforcing messages (which are complex and difficult to understand) about transition ages and frequency of feeding. The feeding schedule also offered the mothers a reminder of what they should do and the *kaders* a way to follow up on their advice.

The third lesson from the Weaning Project is that in giving a precise message to a person precisely when it is needed, the important role of interpersonal communication, particularly via the *kaders*, cannot be underestimated. Giving *kaders* this specific information and training them in counseling seemed to increase both their confidence in giving advice and the mothers' receptivity, as the advice was more relevant and better presented than before. More emphasis should be placed on training *kaders* in communication skills, because they are the "sales force" for new concepts and products. In this same context, it is critical to remember that the *kader* and the entire educational system are only as strong as the basic program infrastructure. Thus enhanced educational components should first be incorporated into provinces where the basic program is functioning well.

Fourth, supervision of *kaders* emerged as an important determinant of their work as educators; in particular, the amount of time spent in educational activities had a significant impact for the project.

Fifth, the total package of educational materials and the mix of media seem to have been appropriate to the cultural context in the different provinces, since even those mothers who did not recall direct contact with the project were influenced by it. Clearly, some influence comes from word-of-mouth contact with other mothers, but some unconscious message reception occurs when the message becomes part of the environment, as happens when prompted by shopkeepers, religious leaders, women's organizations, and village leaders. For example, cassettes played during community work parties or at social gatherings may reach those who are not interested in regular health or government programs. It is important not to limit the project to health channels only, but to make it community-wide. In this context, the recommendation from the midterm evaluation to expand the use of store owners should be implemented.

Lessons from Project Organization and Management

In addition to these lessons from the education and training experience, there are lessons to be learned from the organization and management of this project.

First, from the outset, there was a commitment to building sustainable activities. The initial step in this process was the creation of a partnership between the technical assistance team and the in-country implementors, where each group had a voice in technical decisions and in the management of the project funds. The funding obtained for local expenses was administered and managed by Nutrition Directorate personnel, which meant that they developed a relationship with an outside funding agency (in this case, USAID/Jakarta). Sharing responsibility for project resources meant that decisions were mutually agreed upon and that all parties were ultimately accountable.

The second lesson is that decentralized decision making is also part of building a sustainable project. Creating the provincial project teams was a step toward this end, although involvement of the project implementors at the province level should have been much more consistent in overall project decisions.

Third, the advisory group proved invaluable as a mechanism for informing and receiving comments from leading nutrition programmers, the donor community, and other key individuals over the life of the project. However, even with the advisory board, more work should perhaps have been done with UNICEF and national-level UPGK program personnel to ensure that the results and products resulting from the Weaning Project would be adopted by

UPGK where funded by UNICEF. Expansion of project lessons and materials seems most likely by the NGO community, on a small scale, and through efforts carried out by the Center for Community Health Education (which has replicated the child feeding schedule nationally).

The fourth lesson is that the partnerships that were forged in-country among the Nutrition Directorate and a market research group, an ad agency, and an evaluation group strengthened the project and helped make collaboration with the private sector, both commercial and noncommercial, less formidable and more sustainable.

Fifth, the institutionalization of the project process calling for province-specific planning and cultural awareness seems to have taken place within the Nutrition Directorate, particularly among this project's personnel. The delineation of a manageable process for this adaptation and having advocates for it at the provincial level would help in its continuation.

Note

1. USAID Contract No. DAN-1010-C-00-4102-00, implemented by Manoff International, Inc., and its subcontractors.

References

BASICS (Basic Support for Institutionalizing Child Survival Project), the Nutrition Communications Project (NCP), and the Health and Human Resources Analysis for Africa Project (HHRAA/SARA) (1995) Malnutrition and Child Mortality: Program Implications of New Evidence. Washington, DC: BASICS, NCP, and HHRAA/SARA.

Bunge FM, ed. (1983) Indonesia. A Country Study. Washington, DC: US Government Printing Office.

Dickin K, Griffiths M, Piwoz E (1997) Designing by Dialogue. A Program Planners' Guide to Consultative Research for Improving Young Child Feeding. Washington, DC: USAID.

Griffiths M (1990) "Using Anthropological Techniques in Program Design: Successful Nutrition Education in Indonesia." In: Anthropology and Primary Health Care. J Coreil, JD Mull, eds. Boulder, Colo: Westview Press, pp. 154–169.

Griffiths M (1991) Improving Young Child Feeding Practices in Indonesia. Project Overview. Jakarta, Indonesia: Ministry of Health and The Manoff Group.

Griffiths M (1992) "Understanding Infant Feeding Practices: Qualitative Research Methodologies Used in The Weaning Project." In: RAP. Rapid Assessment Procedures. Qualitative Methodologies for Planning and Evaluation of Health Related Programmes. NS Scrimshaw, GR Gleason, eds. Boston: International Nutrition Foundation for Developing Countries.

Griffiths M (1993). "Defining Concepts and Strategies for Improving Young Child Feeding Practices: The Experience of The Weaning Project." In: Communication Strategies to Support Infant and Young Child Nutrition. P Koniz-Booher, ed. Cornell

International Nutrition Monograph Series, Nos. 24 and 25. Ithaca, NY: Cornell University.

Manoff International (1984) Report to the Indonesian Government. Nutrition Communication and Behavior Change Component of the Indonesian Nutrition Development Program, vols. I–IV. Washington, DC: Manoff International.

Newcomer W, Piwoz E, Griffiths M (1986) Literature Review. Indonesia Weaning Project. Jakarta, Indonesia: Ministry of Health and Manoff International.

Pelletier DL, Frongillo EA, Habicht JP (1993) Epidemiological evidence for a potentiating effect of malnutrition on child mortality. *American Journal of Public Health* 83:1130–1133.

Soekirman, Tarwotjo I, et al. (1992) Economic Growth, Equity and Nutritional Improvement in Indonesia. Jakarta, Indonesia: UNICEF.

UNICEF (1992) Food, Health and Care. The UNICEF Vision and Strategy for a World Free from Hunger and Malnutrition. New York: UNICEF.

Yayasan Indonesia Sejahtera (1989) Evaluation of the Indonesia Weaning Project. Jakarta, Indonesia: Yayasan Indonesia Sejahtera.

IV

INJURY AND OCCUPATIONAL HEALTH

10

Road Warriors: Driving Behaviors on a Polynesian Island

JUDITH C. BARKER

Ethnographic fieldnotes recorded on Niue Island (pronounced nee-oo-ā) in the southwestern Pacific late in 1982 document the circumstances surrounding the road traffic deaths of three men between 18 and 30 years of age. The loss of three young men in their prime is a tremendous blow to both family and society. With only 322 males aged 15 to 29 years on the island, such deaths have severe and long-lasting consequences.

The youngest had been employed by the Department of Public Works for only a few months. He was one of a crew of five men transferring a piece of heavy machinery to the wharf where it was to be shipped off the island for repair. The machine was packed in a large rectangular wooden crate which partly rested on one of the side rails as it was too large to lie flat on the truck bed. The crate was not secured in any way. Two of the crew sat in the cab of the truck next to the driver while another crewman sat on the tailgate. The victim, however, chose to stand on top of the precariously perched crate, just over a meter above the truck bed and about four meters above the roadway. He simply leaned on the truck's cab, making little attempt to hold on. During the drive to the wharf, the truck hit a pothole at moderate speed, causing the crate to bounce upwards suddenly and unexpectedly. This movement threw the youth sideways onto the road, directly under the rear wheels of the truck.

Two other youths died in a single road traffic crash as the result of impetuous, alcohol-impelled, jealous rages against one another; both were attempting to seduce the same young woman. The events were reconstructed thus. Both youths had spent the evening with friends, steadily consuming large quantities of alcohol. Both owned motorcycles. There was a long history of acrimonious encounters, fights, and intense and bitter rivalry between these protagonists. Around midnight on this particular Saturday night, one young man visited a dance on the east side of the island trying to locate the woman of his desires, while at the same time his rival was visiting a dance on the west side of the island for the same reason. In each locale, rumor placed the woman—with the rival, of course—at the other dance. Extremely jealous, drunk, enraged, and egged on by a youthful audience titillated by the possibility of a public display of aggressive, status-setting behavior, each man jumped on his motorcycle and raced toward the other dance. They met halfway—head on. Suggestions were made later that they deliberately rode directly at one another, each trying to be the most daring and to force the other to swerve away first in this last fatal game of "chicken." Caught in a web of social expectations and cultural values that supported such behavior, befuddled by alcohol, enveloped by overwhelming emotions, and riding powerful machines at high speed with no lights on unpaved roads in the middle of the night, neither had much chance of avoiding the tragic and fatal outcome.

To some degree, each of these fatal events involved the deliberate and conscious taking of risks, and, to some degree, lack of awareness and lack of availability of alternative, safer strategies. In part these deaths occurred because youths engaged in risk-taking behavior that was societally expected and approved. In part these deaths occurred because motor transport in this developing nation is inherently more risky than in the developed world, where there are better roadways, a greater variety of appropriate vehicles, stricter laws, greater enforcement of regulations, and public campaigns to heighten knowledge of and educate about road traffic issues (Forjuoh and Li, 1996; Soderlund and Zwi, 1995).

This chapter presents a case study of the causes of road traffic crashes (RTCs) in a Polynesian nation, Niue Island. Using anthropological methods, the island's road environment, transportation infrastructure, vehicle availability, road user behaviors, and their consequences are analyzed within the context of Niuean cultural values and social organization.

Roads, Traffic, and Crashes in Oceania

The island nations of Oceania are generally small in size, rarely rising above 200,000 and often being below 20,000 in total population. In these countries, the societal and financial costs of premature death can be severe and long-lasting, and not merely personal or familial.

Oceanic societies are experiencing the epidemiologic transition away from infectious disease as a leading cause of mortality or morbidity (Taylor et al., 1989, 1991). In most Pacific states now, unintentional injury is a leading cause of hospital admission and among the four leading causes of mortality, frequently accounting for more than 10% of deaths in any one year. A significant proportion of both fatal and nonfatal unintentional injury in Pacific societies is due to road traffic crashes (Baker and Crews, 1986; Barker, 1993; Taylor, 1985; Taylor et al., 1991).

In general, little detailed or accurate information is available about RTCs in Oceania. Both the quantity and quality of epidemiological data vary widely from nation to nation, but generally data are poor and outdated (Taylor et al., 1989). Traffic-related events and trauma are often poorly recorded, with little standardization of terminology, definition, or recording (Barker, 1993). Where documentation does exist, a fairly uniform and grim picture emerges.

The literature is dominated by reference to Papua New Guinea, where for several decades RTCs have been identified as a major public health problem (Jayasuriya, 1991). In the Pacific, mortality rates due to RTCs are several times higher than in industrialized countries. On Niue in 1979 and in Western Samoa between 1980 and 1986, for example, some 20% of all deaths due to unintentional injury were RTC-related. RTC mortality accounted for 60% of all traumatic deaths in Papua New Guinea between 1976 and 1985, and on Nauru between 1976 and 1981 (Barker, 1993).

In both developed and developing nations, young men between the ages of 16 and 30 are at greatest risk of injury or death from an RTC (Nelson, 1988; Smith and Barss, 1991; Soderlund and Zwi, 1995). This age–sex group, which so often contains the best educated and skilled youth who are being groomed for leadership, is also at greatest risk in Pacific nations (Barker, 1993). For example, Nauru is one of the smallest Pacific nations, with only 20 kilometers of sealed roadway, and a total population of around 4,000; the loss over a 5-year period of 21 males aged 15 to 34 years has had a major impact (Taylor and Thoma, 1985).

The type of vehicle using the roads is of major importance in determining outcome. Not only are open-backed trucks carrying passengers and overloaded light utility vehicles common on Pacific roads, but roll-over crashes frequently cause deaths or injuries (Nelson, 1988; Nelson and Streuber, 1991). Passengers and motorcyclists have very high fatality and injury rates, in large part because of head injuries. In the 1980s in Indonesia, where two-wheeled vehicles predominate, motorcycles were involved in 64% of all RTCs (Conrad et al., 1996). There were three times as many other motor vehicles as two-wheelers in Singapore in 1986, yet motorcycles were involved in 42% of RTCs resulting in injury (Wong et al., 1990).

In developing countries, the severity of injury in RTCs is often extreme (Smith and Barss, 1991; Soderlund and Zwi, 1995). Up to one-fourth of crash victims are admitted to the hospital following involvement in a motor vehicle collision on Pacific roads (Barker, 1993), "approximately double the proportion who would be admitted . . . in the UK or Australia" (Lourie and Sinha, 1983:188). Most deaths occur at the crash site, and most trauma involves severe head or chest injuries (Barker, 1993). Trauma care on these islands is limited in scope (Wyatt, 1980). Long-term morbidity or permanent disability as a consequence of RTCs has generally not been documented for developing nations, including the Pacific. Fitzgerald (M. Fitzgerald, personal communication, 1992), however, notes that many (young male) Micronesians need rehabilitation services because of trauma arising from motor vehicle collisions.

Levels of Motorization

Economic growth can lead not just to population growth but also to a rapid increase in the number of vehicles on a nation's roads (Jayasuriya, 1991; Soderlund and Zwi, 1995). Developing nations differ significantly with respect to the outcome of RTCs, depending on population size and number of vehicles, that is, on the level of motorization.

Most Pacific countries (e.g., Solomon Islands, Papua New Guinea, Western Samoa) exhibit RTC fatality rates consonant with low motorization; that is, the death rate from RTCs is low with respect to the total population but high with respect to the total number of vehicles in the country (Barker, 1993; Soderlund and Zwi, 1995). Figures for Papua New Guinea for 1976–1985 illustrate this: the fatality rate due to RTCs was only 1.5 per 100,000 population, but 67 per 10,000 vehicles (Sengupta et al., 1989). For countries with low motorization, the impact of RTC deaths on population structure or life expectancy is not yet great, but the chance of suffering fatal injury as a consequence of traveling in a vehicle is large.

A handful of Pacific nations (e.g., American Samoa, Nauru, New Caledonia), however, display an RTC fatality profile associated with highly motorized societies. Figures for New Caledonia in 1972, which demonstrate this, contrast markedly with those for Papua New Guinea presented above: New Caledonia's fatality rate was 46.2 per 100,000 population, but only 9 per 10,000 vehicles (Loison et al., 1974). In highly motorized countries, premature deaths due to RTCs have a significant effect on population structure and on health indicators, such as life expectancy and mortality rates (Taylor, 1985). By these measures, Niue is a Pacific nation with a high level of motorization and considerable societal costs from RTCs.

Methods

This account of driving behaviors on Niue comes from a systematic compilation and analysis of data collected in the course of other sociomedical research

(Barker, 1985). Transportation and RTCs were not initially a focus of interest, but after a few months I realized that they featured prominently in my field notes and in people's lives, so I began to pay them more focused attention and to collect data systematically.

Among the variety of methods used was historical research on government documents and archives, which uncovered factors affecting the development of Niue's transport system. Niue's hospital records were also examined to investigate the epidemiology of RTCs on the island. This case study would have been strengthened by other data, such as police and court records on the incidence and outcome of RTCs, specific investigation of the role of alcohol, assessment of public officials' awareness of RTCs and their policy responses, and a greater exploration of the meaning and impact of RTCs on individual Niueans and their families. Because my research was focused on a quite distinct topic, however, I did not have sufficient time or resources to gather these data or for this level of follow-through. Despite these shortcomings, the ethnographic approach, with its emphasis on understanding sociocultural context and on recording the minutiae of everyday life, enabled completion of this report.

The major method of gathering data was ethnography—the sustained observation of and participation in the daily life of ordinary Niuean people—over a 12-month period in 1982–1983. The island's population is bilingual, using primarily English to conduct business and Niuean for sacred occasions and for everyday life. I learned the native language and saw central Niuean values and concepts in action as I observed and participated in Niuean life. Along with many of the younger nurses, I lived at the hospital's staff quarters. In addition to yielding round-the-clock information about what was happening there, this also led to many conversations about the daily activities and thoughts of young Niueans, their families, and village communities. I attended a variety of social events, such as weddings, birthday parties, funerals, dances, and barbecues. I participated in church ceremonies; I helped weed gardens. I met a diverse group of people socially, interacting regularly with all manner of hospital staff, from cooks, janitors, laundry workers, and drivers, through clerks and accountants, to dentists, nurses, physicians, and ancillary professional staff.

I kept detailed field notes about the entire range of events, meetings, conversations, and issues discussed, while working in the villages, accompanying the clinical staff, or simply staying at home chatting. Field notes included extensive commentary on road and traffic matters—about my own and other people's transportation problems and their resolution; about who was involved in RTCs; about when, where, and how RTCs happened, and their consequences.

Firsthand experience of the island's transportation problems came about in several ways. During the first several months I had no vehicle and so relied on others to get around. Later, when I was able to rent a car, I drove people to events and transported goods for them. Accompanying the health department staff on their regular work assignments was also very revealing of the transport issues facing this tiny nation.

Niue in the 1980s

Although the situation on Niue has changed somewhat in the intervening years, issues arising in 1982–1983 are still all too pertinent today. Despite a devastating hurricane, occasional droughts, political change as older leaders died, and continued migration—all of which threatened economic stability and growth—life on Niue is very similar now to a decade ago. Niue continues to face major transportation problems and to experience consequences therefrom.

Over the past three decades, massive out-migration has occurred, especially by young adults, most of whom go to join family in New Zealand. Spurred in part by several destructive hurricanes, nearly one-fourth the total population has migrated off-island since the early 1970s. Despite this, Niue's total population is fairly stable, around 2,500 (Barker, 1985).

Niue is a single, isolated island in the western South Pacific Ocean, with a language, social organization, and pattern of daily life similar to but also somewhat different from other western Polynesian societies, such as Samoa or Tonga (Loeb, 1926; Smith, 1983). Compared with other Polynesian societies, distinctive features of Niuean society are a rudimentary and very flexible social hierarchy with no hereditary chiefs, intense egalitarian ideals, an emphasis on individuality and individual achievement, and a strong work ethic (Pollock, 1979; Ryan, 1977). These sociocultural features foster and reinforce the intense rivalry and aggressive behaviors of young adult men, or *fuata* as they are called. *Fuata* are engaged in establishing themselves as charismatic, fearless, assertive leaders who are physically strong, socially knowledgeable, politically savvy, and sexually successful—exactly the attributes and behaviors that in former times were associated with young men who were renowned warriors. The rival youths who died in the head-on RTC were *fuata*, young men engaged in high-stakes, risky status-setting behavior. Formal leadership devolves to *patu*, married men. Young adult men who marry and raise a family after establishing reputations as daring and fearless youth, and who are successful businessmen, administrators, or planters, become centrally concerned with village and island politics.

Niue has a high standard of living, in part because more than 80% of the workforce is employed in the service sector or the government (Connell, 1983). Although arduous because of the very rugged terrain and the lack of a protecting reef, slash-and-burn planting, hunting-gathering, and fishing are still important subsistence pursuits on this drought-prone island. Subsistence activity, as well as cash-cropping of copra, passion fruit, and limes, supplement wage income. Cash permits the purchase of durable consumer goods such as refrigerators, washing machines, and, especially, motorcycles (Pollock, 1979). In 1976, the average annual per capita income for employed persons on Niue was about US$400, and 25% of the population had annual incomes in excess of US$2,500 (Connell, 1983). Thus purchase of a motorcycle was a realistic and attainable goal (Pollock, 1979). The majority of these vehicles were Japanese-manufactured motorcycles which could be bought for around US$1,500. Motor vehicles were the third most frequent category of imports into Niue in 1983 (Development, 1983:17).

Motor Traffic on Niue

Motorized transport was introduced to Niue Island in the 1920s by the New Zealand Administration. Initially, motor transport was confined to a few vehicles for government use. At that time, too, prison labor was used to widen and level the 130 kilometers of tracks, navigable on foot or horseback, that connected the 13 coastal villages to accommodate motor traffic.

Throughout the 1950s and 1960s, ownership of a bicycle both accomplished the task of transportation and, at the same time, signaled high socioeconomic status. Private ownership of motor cars or trucks by individuals or families was limited to the small expatriate and merchant community and to only a few politically influential, wealthy Niueans. Since the mid-1970s, however, owner-ship of a motor vehicle has been a principal marker of social status, especially upward social mobility.

Road Environment

Major roads connecting the villages are flat with occasional undulations and gentle curves around large rocks, trees, or caverns. Several short sections of road, each about a kilometer long, traverse the steep rise that connects villages on the western side of the island with the large flat plateau in the center of the island and the eastern villages. Major roads are two lanes wide so that vehicles travel-ing in opposite directions can pass each other at any point without hindrance. Narrower, twistier, and bumpier minor roads or bush tracks have relatively little traffic, being used mainly by families with land in the area to reach their gar-dens. Often these roads or tracks are accessible only by two-wheeled vehicles or by foot.

The road surface itself constitutes a significant hazard, particularly for mo-torcycle traffic. The principal roads are well maintained, although the pounded coral road surface readily forms potholes and gets extremely slick when wet or overlaid by drifts of finely pulverized coral, resulting from the passage of traffic. In 1982, only in Alofi, the capital, was the roadway paved.

Vehicle Type

Public sector services operated a small fleet of cars, vans, and heavy-goods trucks. Private citizens owned a variety of types of vehicle, many of which were of quite ancient vintage, representing a broad array of manufacturers. While many larger, wealthier families owned cars or utility trucks, most privately owned vehicles on Niue were two-wheelers.

Young adults—both men and women—coveted motorcycles. Not only are they relatively inexpensive to purchase and cheap to operate or repair, but they have other desirable features. Motorcycles are mechanically reliable; have a limited ability to carry passengers and therefore offer to youth a welcome degree of independence and freedom from familial and societal scrutiny; can be driven fast; can be used for stunts; and, depending on the rider's desires, can be either quiet or conspicuously noisy. Machines with modest 50cc or smaller engines, essentially motorized bicycles, imported in small numbers during the 1970s, were no longer glamorous in 1982. They had been displaced in the prestige stakes by bigger, glossier, more powerful machines, with engines of at least 250cc or, preferably, larger capacity, made by Kawasaki, Suzuki, and Honda.

In 1982, I conservatively estimated that one in every three Niuean households had some type of motorcycle; thus there were approximately 250 to 300 motorcycles on the island, the majority less than five years old. Privately owned utility trucks, vans, or cars were far fewer, probably not more than 100 in total.

Societal Infrastructure

Drivers. In 1982, virtually all adult males between 15 and 60 years of age (i.e., about 850 men) and approximately one-half of women aged between 15 and 45 years (i.e., about 325 women) could drive a motorcycle. Few people over 60 years of age knew how to ride a motorcycle, however, and virtually all who did were male. About one-third of the people who could drive a motorcycle could also drive a car or truck. Again, young adult males far outnumbered females with respect to this skill.

"Driver" was a major category within the hierarchy of government jobs. Because it was a secure job and reasonably well paid, it was a prized occupation, reserved for men, especially young men with few other job skills but with families to raise.

Though any family member who could drive could request access to a motor vehicle for a particular purpose or occasion, the owner of the vehicle (i.e., the primary person who arranged for its importation and payment) was said to have priority. In cases of conflict, in keeping with the general dominance of males and of older people in Polynesian societies, men are usually more successful than women in arguing for and winning access to a machine. Older men especially were able to commandeer vehicles for their use, including vehicles belonging to their sons. A female motorcycle owner could be forced to succumb to the wishes of a brother if he demanded use of her vehicle, especially if he claimed it was for transporting produce from bush garden to village home or for attending to business that affected the entire family.

Licensing and Law Enforcement. Driving licenses were not issued until a person reached 16 years of age, but all boys and many girls knew how to—and frequently did—drive a motorcycle well before then. Driving licenses were renewed annually, and were very inexpensive, around one dollar. When in 1982 I applied for a license to drive on Niue, I was not asked to take any test of vision, knowledge of traffic laws, or driving ability.

No doubt there are official traffic laws on Niue, but few were ever mentioned by the people I interacted with daily. Traffic regulation was generally presented as being mostly a matter of common sense.

Enforcement of traffic rules was socially difficult, largely because in this very small-scale society the village policeman and his past and present personal and family circumstances were well known to everyone, and these factors would be brought into play in any encounter. Police had to balance carefully: on the one hand, they had do their job but not too zealously; on the other hand, they had to do their job while upholding or acquiescing to basic Niuean cultural values. For example, police often had to contend with an offender's claims of family connectedness and expectation of kin loyalty, as well as with the offender's memories of youthful pranks by the now-grown policeman, and knowledge of less than meritorious activities by the policeman's kin.

Transportation System. As on many Pacific islands, transportation is a major issue, in part because government services and private businesses are highly centralized. The hospital, sawmill, high school, coconut cream factory, bakery, government services such as the post office, mercantile businesses, and garages, for example, were all in or near Alofi. This meant that most employees or customers had to commute daily to and from their home villages, to work, to shop, and to engage in business. Adequate and reliable access to motor transport, then, was essential for economic activity. Even though most people on Niue owned or could get access to motor vehicles, not everyone could do so.

If requested, the owners of the two privately operated garages on the island would arrange the rental of a car or van, usually their own or a family member's vehicle. Such transactions, however, were very expensive, around US$20 per day in 1982. Renting a car was undertaken almost exclusively by expatriates on the island for relatively short periods of time.

Niue had no private bus service, although one or two men with vans occasionally hired themselves out. This service was most consistently available on

Friday mornings when a round trip was made between outlying villages and Alofi. This coincided with the major shopping event of the week, which drew people from all over the island—an informal market for the exchange of produce. Using this bus/taxi service was not cheap, however, costing about two dollars for the round trip.

Many people preferred alternative means of transport. Older people especially were indignant about the need to pay for bus service. They vocally contrasted it to the long-established local custom that at any time, day or night, any car, truck, or van driver would stop and pick up someone who was walking on the road. Hitchhikers would be delivered as close as possible to their destination for free. Indeed, it was very bad manners for a driver to pass someone on the road and not stop to offer a lift or to help if a vehicle had broken down. Only drivers of motorcycles with very small engines were exempt from this informal rule about providing rides. People rarely refused a lift when offered it, unless they were very close to their destination.

The Niuean government recognized transportation as one of its central problems and dealt with it in two ways: first, by taking services out to the villages, and second, by bringing to Alofi people who required specialized services. The Health Department, for example, operated a mobile outpatient clinic four days a week. Known as Island Round, this included a van, carrying a doctor and nurse, which visited every village. People needing attention hung a flag outside their houses to signal the van to stop. Similarly, once a month, the Post Office would send a van to each village to disburse pension monies. In another form of transport, available on weekday mornings, women from a particular region of the island who were attending the antenatal clinic or people scheduled to get treatment at the dental clinic would be gathered up by a Health Department van and brought to Alofi. After treatment, they would be returned to their village, again by a Health Department van. The next day, people from a different region of the island would be taken to and returned home from various clinics. Outside regular working hours, on evenings or weekends, the ambulance would be dispatched to transport patients needing urgent attention to and from the main clinic.

Similarly, heavy-goods vehicles (10 ton trucks), operated by the Public Works Department, provided transport to and from work for people in all government departments. Several trucks were in daily use, with the drivers resident in the furthermost villages. When necessary, the truck picked up or let off employees at other villages en route. During the drive, some 15 to 20 passengers sat on the flat bed of the open-backed vehicles.

Vehicle Maintenance. Vehicle maintenance and repair on Niue was performed by two garages near Alofi, which serviced privately owned vehicles, and by the Public Works Department, which maintained the government's fleet of motor vehicles. While everyone strove to keep vehicles functioning mechanically as income permitted, there were few evident standards governing vehicle maintenance.

Whether private or government owned, vehicles were often in a very poor state of repair. Four-wheeled vehicles seemed to be in worse repair than motorcycles. Constant problems bedeviled vehicle maintenance on the island: first, combating the effects of a harsh environment; second, obtaining the equipment and parts needed for repair in a timely fashion; and third, keeping as many vehicles as possible functioning mechanically, so that transportation services on the island did not grind to a complete halt.

The hot, humid, wet tropical climate quickly causes rust. Although the rust was often merely cosmetic, it was also a major factor in the creation of structurally unsafe vehicles. Cracked windows, missing or malfunctioning door handles, dents and scratches, even holes in the side panels of vans, were far from ideal, but they were not as potentially dangerous as large rust holes in the floor, wobbling seats attached only by partly rusted bolts, doors that no longer closed, or windshield wipers that had fallen off—all seen with equal frequency. At the time of the study, bald tires, worn so extensively that the canvas or steel webbing was visible, were common on private more than on government vehicles.

Both private and government repair facilities had to order supplies and parts from overseas and then simply wait an unknown length of time, often several months, for them to arrive. Large or heavy parts had to come via the once-a-month cargo steamer serving the island. Private vehicle owners coped with these contingencies on an individual basis, usually being forced simply to wait until supplies or parts arrived. Perhaps because of these obstacles, not to mention the expense of undertaking repairs on Niue, many people postponed maintenance as long as possible. Vehicles awaiting repair were usually still in use, sometimes with severe consequences. One young man, for example, spent three months in the hospital because parts did not arrive before his motorcycle's brakes failed one morning as he descended a hill on his way to work. Despite his nickname, "Rapido," earned because of his usual rather reckless driving style, he had not been speeding at the time or the outcome might have been fatal. The compound fractures of his arm and legs, and his other wounds, healed, he learned to walk again, and eventually he returned to work—but he neither walked as well nor progressed as fast as he would have had this RTC happened in a country where support services such as physiotherapy were available.

The Niue Government had slightly more flexible options with respect to vehicle repair than did the private citizen. Mindful of the deleterious impact of the climatic conditions and of the vagaries of purchasing and shipping parts, the government purchased identical vehicles by the fleet. When the need arose, the mechanics "cannibalized" the vehicle in the worst state of repair, moving working or salvageable parts to the other vehicles in order to keep as many as possible on the road. Even so, there were occasions when so many of the Health Department's vans were in for repair at the same time that some regular preventive services, such as the Public Health Mosquito Control Team or the Child Welfare Well-Baby/Vaccination Clinic, had to be curtailed or postponed so that clinical services, such as Island Round, could be maintained. There were even times when transport for clinical services came about only because some other government department put its regular activities on hold temporarily. So, for example, for a two-week period in March 1983, Island Round was undertaken first using a van lent by the Education Department and later a van belonging to the Customs Department.

Driver Behavior

Factors such as climate, road surface, vehicle type, laws, enforcement, and vehicle maintenance created an environment conducive to RTCs. Much more opportunity for misadventure, however, was due directly, even solely, to driver behaviors. Discussion here focuses intently but not exclusively on motorcycles and their drivers because of their prominence on Niue.

Passenger Transport. Frequently, motorcycles were used to transport more than a single person, especially for short distances, such as from house to bush garden, or from one end of the village to the other. Adults and children older than about five years generally sat behind the driver and hung on. If the passenger was seated properly on the motorcycle, this practice was reasonably safe.

Toddlers, even infants on rare occasions, were usually placed behind the driver and tied on by a length of cloth that encompassed both driver (mother, usually) and child. Transporting infants on motorcycles was roundly discouraged, but Niueans recognized that sometimes it was difficult to avoid this situation. Occasionally a young child was simply perched in front, between the driver's legs. If the child was tall enough, he or she hung on to the handle bars; nothing else secured the child. This was recognized as a dangerous practice and, if seen, was likely to draw censure from others.

On utility trucks, overcrowding was common. Passengers sat in the open bed or on the side rails, often with arms or legs protruding over the side. People were mindful of the danger to some passengers, however, as infants and toddlers were usually placed in the cab. Out of respect, the oldest passengers would also get preferential seating in the cab where they would care for children too small to ride in the back. School-age children and teenagers were routinely assigned to the open bed, with younger children placed in the center, the older children on the outside.

Transport of Goods. Utility trucks and vans often hauled loads far exceeding their capacity, resulting in considerable wear and tear, especially on brakes and tires. I heard accounts of several RTCs involving vans and pickup trucks that were attributed to mechanical failure.

More commonly, however, large or heavy loads, such as 30-kilogram sacks of taro, were perched on the front or back of motorcycles. Many RTCs—both major and minor—resulted from the unexpected shifting of these precariously balanced loads. A road fatality in 1979 occurred as a 60-year-old planter was transporting his harvest home. Apparently unable to see the road because of the sacks of taro balanced on the handlebars, the driver hit a pothole, losing control. Motorcycle, driver, and load fell in such a way that the heavy sacks and the vehicle landed on top of the driver, with the handlebars piercing his chest. Severely injured, he died in the hospital later that evening. He was not discovered for several hours after the event because this RTC took place on a Sunday morning, a time when most people were in church and there was little inter-village traffic. Unlike the vast majority of Niueans who consider Sunday the Sabbath and a day on which any kind of work, including harvesting food, is forbidden, this man was a Seventh-Day Adventist.

Vehicle Headlights. A very common habit was that of riding at night without using headlights. When (or, more often, if) oncoming traffic or an obstacle on the road was observed, lights were switched on; as soon as the hazard was passed, the headlights were switched off again. While this habit prevents easy identification of the driver, who may well be a youth on his way to an assignation (an occasion on which he will not be riding fast or noisily), it also creates numerous RTCs because potholes are not avoided, and pedestrians or wandering animals are struck.

In August 1982, for example, an elderly man walking between houses in his village about 8:30 P.M. was struck by a motorcycle being driven without lights by a young man who had his mother as a passenger. The old man was badly shaken but not seriously hurt, and he was released to go home after receiving attention at the hospital for cuts and severe bruising. This incident, however, nearly precipitated an inter-village feud. Apparently the woman and her son were well known locally as troublemakers. At the scene, the woman, who was inebriated, was overheard to say that the old man was a longtime enemy of hers and she wished her son had caused him more physical damage. These remarks did not sit well with the witnesses who had arrived to investigate the commotion, especially with the injured man's sons, who had to be physically restrained from beating the driver and his mother and from going to attack their kin in the neighboring village. It was several weeks before inter-village animosity and tensions diminished. The elderly man's family was not mollified until months later when the driver was convicted of criminal negligence and heavily fined.

Livestock. Dogs were typically unchained, but livestock was supposed to be penned at all times. At night, however, pigs were often allowed to roam free to forage for food. Thus pigs and dogs comprised significant hazards when they wandered onto the roadway in search of a warm place to sleep.

About 10 o'clock one night, I heard that a nurse and her three-year-old daughter had been injured earlier that evening in an RTC. During her break, the nurse had ridden her motorcycle to her boyfriend's home, where his mother had been caring for the little girl. The nurse was driving the child home, where the nurse's mother would care for her. Because the headlights were off, the motorcycle struck a pig lying unseen in the middle of the road, and both mother and child fell off. The nurse suffered relatively minor injuries to her elbow, but the child was hospitalized because she suffered a concussion when she hit her head on the road and sustained a deep burn on her leg from the motorcycle's muffler.

Physical Protection. Even when it existed, protective gear was rarely used. If cars, vans, or trucks had seat belts, these were not used. Similarly, protective gear, such as crash helmets, was rarely used by motorcycle riders, largely because such equipment makes riding very uncomfortable in a hot, humid, tropical climate. Absent, too, were shirts or pants long enough to cover the motorcycle rider's arms or legs. Even feet, highly vulnerable to damage from misadventure on a motorcycle, were typically not well protected: riding barefoot was not quite as common as wearing floppy, thonged sandals, but use of more substantial footwear was rare. The few individuals who routinely used helmets and other protective devices were well-educated young women, all nurses (Barker, 1993).

Spiritual Dangers. Like many Polynesian peoples, Niueans are somewhat fatalistic and tend to accept life's misfortunes stoically. On Niue, as in many Pacific societies, there is a feeling that "accidents" are not random in timing or target (Feinberg, 1979; Hooper, 1985). Misfortune, "accidents," and sudden, severe, or long-lasting ill health are regarded as forms of supernatural justice, of retribution for past misdeeds committed by either the afflicted individual or his or her immediate kin.

An aspect of the road environment that has considerable influence on driver behavior on Niue is the association of specific locales with *aitu* and their activity. *Aitu* are ghosts of the dead who interfere in the affairs of mortal beings (Barker, 1985; Goodman, 1971; Shore, 1978). Such ancestral spirits are dangerous, powerful, and often malevolent. So-called accidents, especially those that occur at night and involve severe property damage, severe injury to people, or death, are usually attributed to *aitu*.

People who die suddenly and violently, as in RTCs, are said to have particularly resentful, vengeful spirits, or *aitu*. For a period after a fatal event, *aitu* lurk at the locality where the death occurred, hoping to capture someone else to share the spirit's journey into the next world. Sites of fatalities become places to avoid, places in which to behave in an exceptionally correct and circumspect manner lest one draw the attention of or trigger the wrath of the *aitu*. Sites of fatalities are made *tapu* (sacred and taboo) by placing a *fono* (supernatural edict restricting access) for a specified period of time. Thus for a month after the double fatality in 1982, few people would drive alone or on motorcycles past the spot at which the two youths died. Men who normally rode to work on motorcycles using this route joined others on the back of the Public Works truck, for there is safety in numbers.

Encounters at night with harbingers of misfortune, such as screech owls, thought to be a form of *aitu*, or nearly having a traffic "accident" at some haunted locale, will induce a person to abandon the journey. In these circumstances, it is simply not prudent to continue traveling, especially if one is alone. For example, in January 1983, one of the nurses telephoned the hospital about 10 P.M. to say she would not be coming in for night duty. The next afternoon she arrived for work six hours early, well before dark, and explained what happened the previous evening on her way to work. Driving past a place known to be haunted by a teenage brother and sister who had died in a dengue fever outbreak five years earlier, she heard and saw a screech owl, and then suddenly felt very faint. She stopped driving momentarily, starting again as soon as the dizziness passed. But she was worried because the screech owl now seemed to be accompanying her, always just ahead of her, almost leading the way, just like an *aitu* enticing a person into mortal danger. Then to her immense surprise she fearfully realized that she was driving not in the direction of work but of home. She had absolutely no recollection of turning her motorcycle around. Heeding these omens, however, she continued until she reached her home and stayed there.

Alcohol, Entertainment, and Sports. In keeping with the measured pace of life common in Polynesian societies, most drivers on Niue proceeded at a moderate speed in a quiet and unobtrusive manner; in contrast, young motorcycle riders developed a characteristic, personal style of driving, including speed, noise, and stunts. Young men tuned their motorcycles to produce a distinctive sound, by which they could be identified (if they wished). Riding style made the government-issued license plates redundant: no one needed to check a number to identify any vehicle or its young driver.

On an island with limited mass media and few entertainment outlets, riding motorcycles was nightly sport. There was no television station, no daily newspaper, a short and staid daily radio program, and movies or dances only once a week. Private clubs, the restaurant/bar, and the hotel, however, were open nightly and all weekend, providing venues for (primarily but not exclusively young) men to socialize with companions and consume alcohol.

Older men and women tended to be more circumspect about alcohol, generally drinking at home or at special events. And some Niueans abstained from consuming alcohol, including adherents of the Mormon faith, some pastors of other churches, older women, and women from poor families. Wherever and whenever people gathered socially, especially men or the young, beer and liquor were usually readily available. Weekends—when dances, feasts, boys' first haircutting rituals, and birthday celebrations were typically held—had a higher occurrence of RTCs than did weeknights.

Pumped up by their participation at social venues which invariably included drinking, young people gathered late at night on particular stretches of roadway to continue socializing and to compete in various ways. Although some competitions involved youths from different parts of the island, most such sport was limited to rival youths from the same or a nearby village.

Almost always undertaken just by moonlight, motorcycle sports took several forms. One sport was the race, with several participants speeding in the same direction, vying to reach a stated goal first. Another competition was more like jousting, where contestants rode as fast as possible directly toward each other, trying to see who "chickened out" and swerved away first. Stunts were added and especially enjoyable entertainment, both for the young men and for their girlfriends, who formed the requisite audience. Stunts, sometimes called "wheelies," included racing noisily and speedily along, then braking sharply to induce a curving skid that flung up thick sprays of coral dust; driving very fast while standing up and rocking the motorcycle from side to side as far as possible; and raising the front wheel of the motorcycle off the ground while driving as fast as possible. Not surprisingly, drivers often lost control during stunts and ended up injuring themselves or others, and even more frequently damaging their vehicles.

There were two badges of honor among the youth for prowess and participation in motorcycle sports. One hung on bedroom walls: calendars from manufacturing companies featuring photographs of scantily clad women draped over large and shiny motorcycles. The second badge of honor was on arms or legs, the scars or still-healing wounds from muffler burns or road abrasions caused by the fine coral sand. These almost ubiquitous scars were eloquent testimony to the prevalence of RTCs on Niue.

Teenagers and young adult men in the process of establishing reputations as *fuata* were road warriors, using motorcycles to engage each other in symbolic and real combat. Rivalries between young men often took the form of outrageous, foolhardy, or dangerous dares: who could seduce which woman; who could beat whom in a midnight motor vehicle race; who backed down first when playing "chicken"; who survived dangerous stunts. Mixed with large doses of sexual insecurity and jealousy, with real and imagined slights and insults between rivals, and with a great deal of alcohol, these competitive desires set the stage for explosive and tragic situations.

Without a *fuata* tradition to impel them, females generally drove less aggressively than their male counterparts. Not for them the stunts, races, and dares, although ordinary speeding was common, especially after alcohol was consumed. Consider, for instance, the story of two young women, cousins, from a west coast village. One time in 1980, they were attending a dance at an eastern village. In the course of the evening both consumed a number of alcoholic drinks. Around midnight, riding home in tandem on a single machine without using the head-light, they struck another unlit motorcycle going in the opposite direction. The young woman driver told me, "I'd always been hell on wheels. I rode my bike like a man—fast, with lots of noise. People used to tease me about that all the time. Now, I'm very quiet. After that month in hospital, I just putter along." Although she eventually recovered from her knee and facial injuries, she is still occasionally beset by severe pain, stiffness, and a limp.

On occasion, some Niueans, women especially, acknowledged regretfully the link between alcohol consumption and undesirable outcomes, such as lack of money for household essentials, inability to fulfill family obligations, or RTCs. Talk was resigned and pessimistic, however, doubtful that things would ever change for the better.

A float in the October 1982 Independence Day parade symbolized well this pessimism, rooted in the complex intertwining of the public/private and political-economic/policy arenas of this small-scale society. The owner of the snack-food restaurant-bar presented a float proudly advertising the source of his prosperity—and of many RTCs, not to mention marital discord and domestic violence. A huge plywood replica of a whiskey bottle was attached to the bed of a beat-up utility truck. Lolling on the truck bed were several young men, acting as if they were drunk, waving genuine, full whiskey bottles in the air, making ribald remarks and calling out loudly to onlookers, urging them to patronize the restaurant-bar and to participate in the fun. That the restaurant-bar owner happened also to be the government minister responsible for health services and health policy, and for regulating traffic and transport policy, was an irony that did not escape many in the audience. Women, middle-aged and older women especially, loudly and bitterly voiced their disapproval of this particular mixed message.

Road Traffic Crashes on Niue

Clearly, in the early 1980s there was plenty of opportunity for misadventure on Niue's roads. Road traffic crashes were, in fact, common and consequential events.

Several authors estimate the cost of RTCs to developing nations to be 1%–2% of gross domestic product (Jacobs and Sayer, 1983; Soderlund and Zwi, 1995). In 1977, Niue's gross domestic product was US$750,000; one percent was the average revenue earned by 36 people. With very limited options for developing a stable manufacturing sector (Development, 1983), road traffic crashes under-mined or severely delayed Niue's plans for, and ability to achieve, social and economic development.

Unintentional injury—a large proportion of which was the result of RTCs—was a leading cause of morbidity and mortality on Niue (Barker, 1985, 1988; Taylor et al., 1987; Taylor et al., 1989). My field notes record both directly ob-served RTC incidents and outcomes and reports of RTCs from others. My records also indicate that alcohol consumption played a dominant role in both minor and major RTCs. I estimate that close to half of all RTCs on Niue in 1982–1983 were alcohol-related. Although my notes document several instances of vehicles other than motorcycles being involved in an RTC, the vast majority of all RTCs on Niue, both minor and major, involved motorcycles and their rid-ers. RTCs resulting in minor injuries were many times more common than those resulting in hospital admission (Barker, 1993).

RTCs and Medical Care

For a Pacific nation, Niue spent a considerable amount on health care: around US$100 per capita in 1979. Approximately 100 times this per capita expendi-ture (or 3% of the total health budget) was spent on health-related travel and transport, mainly to ensure access to clinical services but also to provide public health and preventive and ambulance services (Niue Government, 1981). For the populace on Niue, health care services, including hospitalization, were free, accessible, and available 24 hours a day, 7 days a week.

For the period 1977–1982, the hospital's Ward Admissions Book documented a total of 96 people admitted because of RTCs, an annual incidence of 6.4 per 1,000 (Barker, 1993). Almost half (47%) the RTCs on Niue resulting in hospi-talization involved multiple admissions. Most (67%) multiple-admission crashes involved two people, but 16% resulted in four people being hospitalized at one time. This represented a significant and sudden increase in workload for the island's medical services: four people occupied one-quarter of the available hospital beds. Twice as many males as females were involved in multiple-admission RTCs, a significant difference (Fisher's exact $p < .05$).

In 1982, some 11.2% of all adult male hospital admissions were the result of RTCs, matching some of the highest RTC admission rates in the world (Barker, 1993). Note that these figures *exclude* RTC-related deaths that occurred before reaching the hospital, as well as less injurious RTC events. In contrast, female RTC victims comprised a more usual and more modest proportion of admis-sions, just 1.9% of all adult female admissions for other than obstetric reasons.

The exact ages of adult admissions were largely unknown; hospital staff routinely recorded specific age only for children under 16 years and for older people, those over about 60 years (Barker, 1985, 1988). Of those admitted to the hospital because of RTCs, 9% were children under the age of 16 years, and none was elderly. Field notes revealed that the majority of RTC events involved young adults between 18 and 30 years of age.

Medical services on Niue were limited. Standard care and routine surgery were available for the most commonly encountered acute and chronic illnesses or emergency situations, such as appendectomies or cesarean sections (Barker, 1985). Patients requiring a specialist's attention were sent overseas, mostly to New Zealand, as soon as practicable. Such patients were usually evacuated on the scheduled weekly flight, but for cases of extreme trauma a plane was specially chartered or diverted. One Sunday morning in November 1982, for example, a flight out of American Samoa on its way to Fiji was diverted to Niue to deliver special medications needed to treat a middle-aged man who had been badly injured in an RTC during the night. The combination of too much alcohol, not using lights, traveling downhill too fast, and riding a poorly maintained motorcycle resulted in the driver losing control and plunging into a deep drainage ditch at the side of the road. After being medically stabilized, this patient was sent for thoracic surgery and rehabilitation on the next scheduled flight to New Zealand two days later.

In 1979, nearly 1% of the total Niuean health budget of approximately US$350,000 (which included salaries) was used to send four patients overseas for specialist care, on regular commercial flights at rates heavily subsidized by the airline (Niue Government, 1981). Thus the treatment of RTC victims who needed evacuation was very costly.

Road Traffic Crashes in Developing Nations

Throughout the developing world, RTCs and their human and societal aftermath are becoming recognized as major public health concerns. Smith and Barss (1991:233) claim that "motor vehicle crashes are the largest single cause of death from unintentional injury in most developing countries for which data are available." Between 1968 and 1983, road traffic mortality increased by more than 200% in African countries, by 150% in Asian nations, and by 400% in Papua New Guinea, while over the same period in Europe it decreased by more than 20% (Jayasuriya, 1991; Soderlund and Zwi, 1995). In 1986, in several countries in the Americas, road traffic mortality accounted for more than 30% of all deaths by violence (Yunes, 1993). Nelson concluded that "in developing countries there is not an increased risk of [an RTC] but an increased risk of casualty once an [RTC] occurs" (Nelson, 1988:192), in part because of sparse trauma and medical services.

Misadventure on the roads has multiple and complex causes (Nelson, 1988). Cultural values and other important factors affecting traffic safety have been identified as:

- Road environment (e.g., road surface, climate, terrain)
- Vehicle characteristics (e.g., vehicle size and type, occupancy)
- Societal infrastructure (e.g., availability and adequacy of vehicle maintenance, presence of paratransit vehicles such as horse-drawn buggies or rickshaws, legal statutes and licensing controlling access to and operation of vehicles, enforcement of laws, population density)
- Road user characteristics (e.g., driver experience, driver behavior)

Of these, driver behavior has been identified as by far the most important factor in motor vehicle collisions, accounting for around 60% of road crashes in Europe and the United States (Evans, 1996; Hingson et al., 1996). In the developed world, road user behaviors have been amenable to some change, for example, through media campaigns against drunk driving, enactment and enforcement of speeding laws, and improved technology such as passive restraints. When deeply embedded within cultural values that uphold risk-taking and fatalism, and when societal infrastructure limits economic and policy options with respect to transport, as is often the case in the developing world, road users can be recalcitrant and reluctant to change their behavior.

Culture, Risk, and Intervention

Before the social and economic consequences of RTCs can be adequately assessed, however, developing nations need to document fully the circumstances surrounding motor vehicle collisions. Without examining the sociocultural norms and mores that sustain road behaviors and risk-taking, an understanding of the causes of injury will remain sketchy; efforts to design interventions will fail because they do not address the local sociocultural environment; and evaluation of the efficacy of intervention will remain elusive.

Attempting to inhibit motorization or hamper individual use of vehicles is counterproductive in developing nations with poor transport systems. To develop economically, nations need to be able to transport goods and people, but they need to do so safely. Concerted efforts need to be made to improve roads, to provide safer and more extensive public transportation, to increase safety standards, to foster better vehicle maintenance, to educate drivers, and to promote prevention in order to reduce the impact, both short-term and long-term, of road traffic crashes and motor vehicle–related injuries. Soderlund and Zwi (1995:181) note that efforts to reduce RTCs and their consequences in developing countries will work best with a "multi-sectorial involvement to promote healthy public policy rather than . . . focus on the transport sector alone." An example is Nelson and Streuber's (1991) suggestion that developing nations offer tax incentives to encourage the purchase of enclosed vans that would reduce reliance on overcrowded, open-backed vehicles for transporting passengers.

Better engineering and the enactment and enforcement of laws regulating road traffic are interventions that have reduced crash involvement and injury in the wealthier nations (Forjuoh and Li, 1996; Soderlund and Zwi, 1995). Examples of effective interventions are improvements in the design, construction, and maintenance of roads and/or vehicles; use of passive restraints such as seat belts, of reflective clothing, or of protective devices such as helmets; enhancement of the visibility of vehicles, for example, through the use of daytime running lights; and provision of safe public transport. Despite the success of these types of intervention, "the key to avoiding crashes is changing the behavior of road users" (Evans, 1996:785). Behavior change is usually undertaken through educational interventions, often centered around issues such as speeding and alcohol. Educational interventions, however, are difficult to implement and sustain, especially when situated in a sociocultural context that encourages or accepts certain types of risk.

In developing societies, the young, educated elite—those being groomed for leadership roles—are at greatest risk for premature death and injury from RTCs (Nelson, 1988). Young adult males are overrepresented in RTC statistics not just because of their greater access to and use of vehicles but also because societal perception and acceptance of risk is enacted through culturally encouraged behaviors.

On Niue, these are *fuata* behaviors, warrior behaviors. On Niue, youth are road warriors. Roads and motorcycles are a readily available means for Niuean youth to engage each other competitively, to become men, just as they did in the past by preparing for warfare against rival factions or invading strangers. *Fuata* behaviors are not new. Nor are they created by overseas education or travel, but they are exacerbated by this experience of the outside world. Visits to neighboring metropolitan countries induce new rivalries and foster desires for ownership and mastery of a key symbol of contemporary adulthood on Niue—the motorcycle.

Considering the Pacific region as a whole, *fuata*-like behaviors are not confined to Niue. When compared with other New Zealand drivers, Maoris, the indigenous Polynesian inhabitants, are also overrepresented in RTC statistics (Langley and McLoughlin, 1989). Marshall's (1979) discussion of "weekend warriors," drunken Micronesian youth in Truk, who are given to outbursts of rage and violence, and Freeman's (1983) discourse on male aggression and violence in Western Samoa, point to similar roots and social-psychological functions. In these societies, aggressive competitiveness and exaggerated, socially approved, glorified risk-taking are expected and valued aspects of individual (male) maturation. Noninjurious, culturally appropriate alternatives for competition, for display of maturity and demonstration of sociocultural competence, need to be developed. Educational endeavors will fail, however, if they are mere importations from outside, based on very different understandings of and tolerance for particular risks.

Cultural theory conceives of risk deriving as much from the sociocultural context in which people live as from their individual thoughts and actions. This differs from other dominant theories of risk in three assertions:

1. Individuals actively perceive, construct, and resist risk, and are not merely passive recipients of information.
2. Cultural, social, and institutional imperatives and values that operate in the recognition and selection of risks must be attended to.
3. Societal management consists not just of highlighting and attending to certain risks, but also of tolerating other risks and actively suppressing from recognition yet other risks (Douglas and Wildavsky, 1982; Rayner, 1992).

Thus far, however, few studies of roads, traffic, or driver behaviors have looked at sociocultural factors that influence risk acceptance or risk avoidance. This case study does just that. It situates human behavior in its sociocultural context and argues that successful intervention to reduce traffic-related injury must take into account not just the material environment of roads, equipment, or technology, but also the human environment constituted by and through particular behaviors, social relations, and cultural perceptions.

References

Baker PT, Crews DE (1986) "Mortality Patterns and Some Biological Predictors." In: The Changing Samoans. Behavior and Health in Transition. PT Baker, JM Hanna, TS Baker, eds. New York: Oxford University Press, pp. 93–122.

Barker JC (1985) Social Organization of Health Services for Preschool Children on Niue Island, Western Polynesia. PhD dissertation. San Francisco and Berkeley: Medical Anthropology Program, University of California.

Barker JC (1988) Admission of geriatric patients to hospital on Niue Island, 1977–1982. New Zealand Medical Journal 101:638–640.

Barker JC (1993) On the road to health? Road traffic accidents in Pacific societies: the case of Niue Island, Western Polynesia. American Journal of Human Biology 5:61–73.

Connell JC (1983) Migration, Employment and Development in the South Pacific. Country Report Number 11—Niue. Noumea, New Caledonia: South Pacific Commission.

Conrad P, Bradshaw YS, Lamsudin R, Kasniyah Y, Costello C (1996) Helmets, injuries and cultural definitions: motorcycle injury in urban Indonesia. Accident Analysis and Prevention 28:193–200.

Development (1983) Small island states. Development 6 (1), March. External Aid Division, Ministry of Foreign Affairs, New Zealand.

Douglas M, Wildavsky A (1982) Risk and Culture. An Essay on the Selection of Technological and Environmental Dangers. Berkeley: University of California Press.

Evans L (1996) Comment: The dominant role of driver behavior in traffic safety. American Journal of Public Health 86:784–786.

Feinberg R (1979) Anutan Concepts of Disease. A Polynesian Study. Laie, Hawaii: Institute for Polynesian Studies, Monograph Series, No. 3.

Forjuoh SN, Li G (1996) A review of successful transport and home injury interventions to guide developing countries. *Social Science and Medicine* 43:1551–1560.

Freeman D (1983) Margaret Mead. The Making and Unmaking of an Anthropological Myth. New York: Cambridge University Press.

Goodman R (1971) Some *aitu* beliefs of modern Samoans. *Journal of the Polynesian Society* 80:463–479.

Hingson R, McGovern T, Howland J, Heeren T, Winter M, Zakocs R (1996) Reducing alcohol impaired driving in Massachusetts: the Saving Lives Program. *American Journal of Public Health* 86:791–797.

Hooper A (1985) "Tahitian Healing." In: Healing Practices in the South Pacific. CDF Parsons, ed. Honolulu: Institute for Polynesian Studies/University of Hawaii Press, pp. 158–198.

Jacobs JD, Sayer I (1983) Road accidents in developing countries. *Accident Analysis and Prevention* 15:337–353.

Jayasuriya R (1991) Trends in the epidemiology of injuries due to road traffic accidents in Papua New Guinea. *Asia-Pacific Journal of Public Health* 5:41–48.

Langley JD, McLoughlin E (1989) Injury mortality and morbidity in New Zealand. *Accident Analysis and Prevention* 21:243–254.

Loeb EM (1926) History and Traditions of Niue. Honolulu: Bernice P. Bishop Museum. Bulletin No. 32. [Millwood, NY: Kraus Reprint Co., 1978]

Loison G, Bourre AL, Nalo C, Tamson R (1974) The health implications of urbanization in the South Pacific. *Journal de la Société des Océanistes* 30:79–104.

Lourie J, Sinha S (1983) Port Moresby road traffic accident survey. *Papua New Guinea Medical Journal* 26:186–189.

Marshall M (1979) Weekend Warriors. Alcohol in a Micronesian Culture. Palo Alto, Calif: Mayfield.

Nelson DC (1988) Growth in Vehicle Populations and Motor Vehicle Related Fatality Rates in Developing Countries. PhD dissertation. Berkeley: Department of Civil Engineering, University of California.

Nelson DC, Streuber JV (1991) The effect of open-back vehicles on casualty rates: the case of Papua New Guinea. *Accident Analysis and Prevention* 23:109–117.

Niue Government (1981) Annual Report of the Niue Health Department for 1979. Alofi: Niue Government.

Pollock NJ (1979) Work, wages and shifting cultivation on Niue. *Pacific Studies* 2: 132–143.

Rayner S (1992) "Cultural theory and risk analysis." In: Social Theories of Risk. S Krimsky, D Golding, eds. Westport, Conn: Praeger, pp. 83–116.

Ryan TF (1977) Prehistoric Niue. An Egalitarian Polynesian Society. Master's thesis. Auckland, New Zealand: Department of Anthropology, University of Auckland.

Sengupta SK, Patil NG, Law G (1989) Seat-belt message and the law? *Papua New Guinea Medical Journal* 32:199–202.

Shore B (1978) Ghosts and government: a structural analysis of alternative institutions for conflict management in Samoa. *Man* 13:175–199.

Smith GS, Barss P (1991) Unintentional injuries in developing countries: the epidemiology of a neglected problem. *Epidemiologic Reviews* 13:228–266.

Smith SP (1983) Niue: The Island and Its People. Suva, Fiji: Institute for Pacific Studies, University of the South Pacific. [Reprinted from *Journal of the Polynesian Society* 11 and 12, 1902 and 1903]

Soderlund N, Zwi AB (1995) Traffic related mortality in industrialized and less developed countries. *Bulletin of the World Health Organization* 73:175–182.

Taylor RH (1985) Health in the Pacific Islands. Honolulu: Pacific Islands Development Program, East–West Center. [Mimeo]

Taylor RH, Lewis ND, Levy S (1989) Societies in transition: mortality patterns in Pacific island populations. *International Journal of Epidemiology* 18:634–646.

Taylor RH, Lewis ND, Sladden T (1991) Mortality in Pacific island countries around 1980: geopolitical, socioeconomic, demographic and health service factors. *Australian Journal of Public Health* 15:207–221.

Taylor RH, Nemaia HT, Connell JC (1987) Mortality in Niue, 1978–1982. *New Zealand Medical Journal* 100:477–481.

Taylor RH, Thoma K (1985) Mortality patterns in the modernized Pacific Island nation of Nauru. *American Journal of Public Health* 75:149–155.

Wong TW, Phoon WO, Lee J, Yiu IPC, Fung KP, Smith G (1990) Motorcyclist traffic accidents and risk factors: a Singapore study. *Asia-Pacific Journal of Public Health* 4:34–38.

Wyatt GB (1980) The epidemiology of road accidents in Papua New Guinea. *Papua New Guinea Medical Journal* 23:60–65.

Yunes J (1993) Mortality from violent causes in the Americas. *Bulletin of the Pan-American Health Organization* 27:154–167.

11

Balancing Risks and Resources:
Applying Pesticides without Using Protective
Equipment in Southern Mexico

LINDA M. HUNT,
ROLANDO TINOCO OJANGUREN,
NORAH SCHWARTZ, AND
DAVID HALPERIN

The "green revolution" has resulted in immense increases in agricultural productivity throughout the world over the past half-century. An important part of the technological innovations accompanying this revolution is the introduction of a variety of chemicals generically known as "pesticides," which have been developed and widely marketed for the control or destruction of unwanted species of plants or animals that interfere with agricultural production. In recent years, pesticide use has reached massive proportions worldwide with about 2.5 million tons being applied each year (Pimentel et al., 1992), reflecting a dramatic increase in the use of these chemicals since the early 1970s. The total annual cost worldwide was estimated at US$7.7 billion in 1972, rising to over $25 billion in 1990 (1985 US dollars)(Tolba and El-Kholy, 1992). The most rapid growth has occurred in developing countries, which now account for about 20%–25% of pesticide use (Forget, 1991; McConnell and Hruska, 1993; Pimentel et al., 1992).

   Although these chemicals clearly improve farm productivity, they pose serious health dangers for the people who apply them, both in short-term toxicity and in long-term biological effects. There are currently more than 15,000 individual pesticide compounds being used worldwide, most of which have been demonstrated to be acutely toxic to human beings (Davies, 1987; Ecobichon et al., 1990). The negative health impact of exposure to these chemicals, both through direct physical contact during application and through ingestion of residues in produce and water supplies, has been widely reported in the public health literature (Ecobichon et al., 1990; Levine, 1986; Loevinsohn, 1987; Pimentel et al., 1992; Ragsdale and Menzer, 1989; WHO, 1990; Wilkinson and Baker, 1990). The acute effects of pesticide exposure can be fatal; they may include symptoms such as skin and eye burns, headache, nausea, blurred vision, muscle cramping, vomiting, and difficulty breathing. Information on the chronic health effects of pesticide exposure is not conclusive, but there is increasing evidence that many pesticides are carcinogenic (WHO, 1990), may produce immune dysfunctions (Fiore et al., 1986; Thomas and House, 1989), and may cause permanent neurological damage (Ecobichon et al. 1990; Lotti, 1984).

Every year there are an estimated 3 million severe, acute pesticide poisonings worldwide and approximately 220,000 deaths associated with pesticide exposure (McConnell and Hruska, 1993). Although developing countries account for only about a quarter of the pesticides used globally, they account for more than 50% of the poisonings and up to 99% of the deaths (Jeyaratnam, 1990; Pimentel et al., 1992; WHO, 1993). The excessive health burden in developing countries may be caused by the wide availability of pesticides banned in other countries due to known health hazards; generally inadequate safety standards and poor enforcement; low education levels resulting in limited knowledge of the health risks and needed precautions; and inadequate availability and use of protective clothing and washing facilities (Forget, 1991; Pimentel et al., 1992; World Resources, 1986).

Although the use of appropriate protective measures can significantly reduce excessive exposure and the associated health effects (FAO, 1985; ILO, 1977; Nigg et al., 1986; WHO, 1985), it is often observed that agricultural workers fail to take proper precautions when applying pesticides (see, for example, Avory and Coggon, 1994; Bwititi et al., 1987; Jeyaratnam, 1985; London, 1993). On the assumption that this is primarily due to lack of information, knowledge, and awareness (WHO, 1990), major public health efforts throughout the world have been undertaken to teach agricultural workers the dangers, proper handling, and protective measures for use of these chemicals. However, only limited success in changing behavior has been reported (Avory and Coggon, 1994; London, 1993).[1]

Does this indicate that ignorance persists in spite of educational efforts? Have instruction programs failed to communicate adequately the facts about the dangers and recommended precautions in pesticide use? Have the farmers failed to learn basic information repeatedly presented to them? Or could other factors explain this phenomenon?

In research with *campesinos* (peasant farmers) in the border region of southern Mexico we have observed an anomalous situation that has led us to reexamine the assumption that ignorance underlies the failure of people to use proper precautions in handling pesticides. For the *campesinos* we studied, failure to use protective measures was not associated with lack of knowledge and understanding of the toxicity of pesticides or of the recommended protective practices. Instead, cultural, practical, and perceptual factors seem to underlie their pesticide use behavior.

Background

Pesticides in Mexico and Chiapas

Mexico provides a good example of some of the problems associated with the expanding use of pesticides in the developing world. The market for pesticides in Mexico has grown dramatically in the past two decades: in 1960, some 14,000 tons were sold; in 1972, sales reached 22,000 tons; in 1983, around 34,000 tons; and in 1986 sales reached 60,000 tons (Ortega-Ceseña et al., 1994). It is estimated that, in Mexico, 11.5% of toxic exposures to pesticides are fatal (WHO, 1993). Although legislation regulating pesticide availability (but not procedures for application) exists in Mexico, modeled after US regulations, no procedures for ensuring compliance have yet been implemented. For the most part, enforcement is pursued only in response to crisis situations (Ortega-Ceseña et al., 1994). Research about the health effects of pesticides in Mexico is scarce and concentrates almost exclusively on the central and northern parts of the country, with almost no studies reported for the south of Mexico, where agriculture is the primary means of subsistence (Ortega et al., 1993).

Chiapas, where our study was conducted, is the southernmost state of Mexico, with 58% of the population devoted to agricultural work (INEGI, 1990). Corn and beans are the primary crops. Our study concentrated on the Guatemalan border region of Chiapas, a predominantly rural area of high-altitude valleys and tropical jungles. Economically and in terms of its general health infrastructure, it is one of the poorest regions in Mexico (Hunt, 1996). The majority of the inhabitants are mestizo, (i.e., of mixed European and indigenous ancestry) but there is also a notable indigenous presence in the region, with about 25% of the population being ethnically Mayan and maintaining Mayan traditions.

The border region is a subtropical zone where a wide variety of unwanted plants and insects present serious threats to modern crops. In Chiapas, reliance on pesticides is particularly pronounced. According to a 1988 survey, 72% of the *ejidal*[2] farms and communities in the border region have incorporated pesticides into their production, 20% more than the national average rate of pesticide use (INEGI, 1988a, 1988b).

The intensive use of agrochemicals in this area began in the mid-1970s with a development program of the Mexican Federal Government, run by an agency known as SARH (Secretaria de Agricultura y Recursos Hidráulicos). In cooperation with several banks, SARH embarked on an intensive campaign promoting the use of agrochemicals, offering farmers throughout Mexico technical assistance and bank loans for purchase of the chemicals. The program included sending agricultural technicians to rural areas to promote the use of the chemicals and teach the proper handling, storage, and protective techniques. A few local farmers from each community were also trained as technicians and were meant then to advise and oversee the use of the chemicals in their local communities. As part of the Mexican government's efforts to economize in response to the economic crisis of 1982, the program has since been suspended, but agrochemicals continue to be widely used in southern Chiapas, as they are throughout Mexico. Currently there are still a few agricultural agents assigned to the region, but they are responsible for covering huge areas. We are told by local residents that, on arriving in a community, these agents have time for little else than getting the local authorities to stamp their work-log books, proving they visited the community, and then moving on to the next community.

Although pesticides are used extensively in the border region, the available information about their health effects there is minimal. A few studies indicate that toxic exposure to pesticides is a serious health problem, in spite of nearly two decades of technical training and instruction in the use of agrochemicals. These studies show that serious levels of pesticide exposure among agricultural workers in this area are not uncommon. For example, a 1987 study of 150 agricultural workers in Tapachula, Chiapas, measured the enzyme cholinesterase levels (an indicator of exposure to organophosphates, a common class of toxic pesticides), and found that 22% had enzyme levels equivalent to severe intoxication (Herrera and Rodas, 1987). Similarly, a study of 199 farmers in the border region compared their enzyme levels before and after they applied pesticides in their usual manner and found statistically significant increases following use; the differences were more pronounced among farmers from poorer communities (Tinoco and Halperin, 1998). Another study found that 57% of farmers in one community of the region reported that, while working, they had experienced symptoms compatible with organophosphate intoxication (Tinoco and Halperin, 1992).

Protective Equipment for Pesticide Application

The health risks associated with pesticide use can be reduced by implementing appropriate safety precautions, such as proper storage and the use of protective clothing and equipment (Forget, 1991; ILO, 1991; London, 1993). Although this is common knowledge in southern Mexico, a general lack of public concern for the safe handling of pesticides is evident as one travels through the region. In the border region, it is commonplace to see people, sometimes children, applying pesticides using backpack sprayers, with no protective equipment of any kind. They are often wearing only a tee shirt, slacks, and sandals as they walk through thick foliage that is wet with chemicals.

The Study

To explore the factors that might underlie these practices, we have combined data collected by both survey and ethnographic techniques. The research was conducted between 1990 and 1993. We developed a questionnaire, based in part on the Hispanic Health and Nutritional Examination Survey (HHANES), which included questions about characteristics of work, exposure, and symptoms related to pesticide use, actions taken in the case of exposure, and knowledge and practices in the preparation and handling of pesticides (NCHS, 1984). One hundred and nineteen men from Tziscao who had worked as farmers in the past two years answered the questionnaire. This was a self-selected sample: the researcher (RTO) described the project to the general assembly of the town, and the men in attendance agreed to cooperate with the study. Subjects were drawn from consecutive men coming to a public health clinic in the town during the research period.

In addition, 18 men were interviewed (by LMH) using open-ended, ethnographic interview techniques. Subjects were selected for this phase of the study from families of men who had been diagnosed with cancer (leukemia or lymphoma) in the Comitan General Hospital within six months prior to the interview. This selection method was chosen to maximize the likelihood that the subjects would have heightened concern and awareness about the health hazards of pesticides. These interviews followed a loosely structured series of questions, focusing on the history of their use of pesticides both at home and in the fields, understandings and perceptions of the dangers they present, experience and interpretation of symptoms associated with exposure, what they do if exposed, and their concepts and practices for taking protective measures. The interviews were tape recorded and transcribed.

Thirteen women from the same community were also interviewed (by NS) using similar ethnographic techniques. This was a "snowball sample," which began with the daughter of the municipal president, who suggested for interviews other women who used pesticides either in their garden or home for insect and pest control. These women were interviewed, and in turn suggested other women for the study. Because women's use of pesticides is distinct from men's, the women will be discussed separately.

Early in the data collection period, a series of provisional categories and a filing and retrieval system were established for the ethnographic data. All field notes and transcripts were indexed by topic. A method for standardizing interview data and displaying data was developed (Miles and Huberman, 1994), and content analysis was conducted (Bernard, 1990). This analysis took place in several steps. First, initial matrixes were built of blocks of text (quotations and summations) for each subject, with cells displaying, for example, reported pesticide handling behaviors, symptoms experienced, and subjects' evaluations of the health impact of pesticide use. These initial matrixes were reviewed for trends and patterns across subjects. Patterns identified in these reviews were the basis of further classification of the data, which were then summarized into higher level matrixes grouping subjects, for example, by types of behavioral precautions taken, and by their expected outcome.

Observation in the community of actual behavior in mixing, applying, and storing the chemicals was also part of the ethnographic data collection. This occurred on an informal basis, both in the fields and in the homes of subjects, in the course of visiting the community to conduct interviews.

Knowledge and Behavior

Knowledge of Handling Recommendations

Of the 119 men answering the survey, 90% reported having used pesticides within the past year. The most commonly used pesticides were parathion and paraquat, an insecticide and a herbicide, respectively, both highly toxic. Many of those we spoke with in the ethnographic interviews said they had first learned about pesticide use through agricultural extension agents from programs of SARH or similar agencies. They said they get their current information for choosing and handling chemicals from reading product labels, advice from clerks in grain and feed stores, and advice from other farmers. All those who said they relied on friends and family for such information also mentioned technicians or labels as an information source.

Generally, people in this study displayed a thorough understanding of the recommended use and handling of the pesticides they employ. The survey group was asked the purposes for which they used specific pesticides, and how they prepared them. The agricultural engineer who conducted these surveys (RTO) found that 70% of the responses indicated the chemicals were being used appropriately, and a surprising 99% of the respondents described correct mixing procedures in preparation for application. These findings indicate that basic practice in preparation and use of these chemicals is consistent with what they have been taught.

Our data also indicate that these *campesinos* well understand that pesticides can be highly toxic. All of those we spoke with in the ethnographic interviews told us that the chemicals were dangerous to humans and could prove fatal to anyone exposed to large quantities. Many told stories of fatal or near-fatal poisonings they had heard about within their community, but they emphasized that these events were due to some physical weakness (such as aging or infirmity) or error on the part of the person affected. For example, a common view of why some people get sick from pesticide exposure is expressed in the following quote:

> There are people who suffered from this. One fellow, who lives over there [pointing to the next farm] was spraying insecticides and he was dying, he got poisoned. . . . But that's rare around here—I don't know if he was using too high a dose or what. I think that must be why.

It is interesting to note that a 1990 study found that 56% of paraquat poisoning deaths in southern Chiapas were the result of deliberate ingestion of the chemical with suicidal intent (Tinoco et al., 1993). Clearly, where pesticides are a preferred method of suicide, their toxicity must be well known by the community.

Nearly everyone we spoke with in the ethnographic interviews also knew the recommended procedures for protecting oneself from toxic exposure while applying the chemicals. They were able to describe a full array of precautionary measures for using pesticides, including washing hands after use, bathing following exposure, keeping the pesticide in its original container, destroying empty containers, keeping pesticides out of reach of children, keeping children and pregnant women from being exposed, and using protective equipment while applying pesticides. Everyone was able to list all recommended protective gear: boots, gloves, overalls, and face mask. All were aware that the chemicals could enter the body of a person spraying them in the fields. Most thought that toxic exposure occurred through the nose and mouth and some thought that exposure occurred through the skin as well.

Although in ethnographic interviews people commonly reported that they kept their young children from touching or using the chemicals and avoided exposing pregnant women, we found virtually no one who regularly took any precautions to protect themselves from exposure, beyond simply washing their hands or bathing after use. It should also be noted that such bathing often took place in irrigation ditches of fields treated with pesticides, which probably increased exposure to the pesticides. When asked what one should do to protect oneself, most said that it would be best to use protective equipment. However, none owned or had ever used any of this equipment. As one farmer explained:

> The best thing would be to buy protective equipment, and fumigate like that, with everything, the mask, boots, gloves, overalls. . . . But nobody uses it, not one person from here. It would be just me if I would have bought it [laughs].

Consistent with the ethnographic interviews, the questionnaire survey group also showed very little use of protective equipment. Ninety-three percent said they had never used protective equipment of any kind, and only six people (7%) said they had occasionally covered their mouths with a scarf or worn boots while spraying, but none reported doing this on a regular basis. When asked how regularly they used protective equipment, 98% said "never."

Thus we come to an anomalous finding: although nearly everyone in this study showed a good understanding of the toxicity of pesticides, and of how they ought to be handling the chemicals, and took steps to protect others, no one reported taking precautionary measures on a regular basis to protect his own health. To understand this paradox, let us examine the personal experiences and perceptions of risk discussed by our subjects and consider how these perceptions interact with socioeconomic and cultural factors to affect pesticide handling practices.

Personal Experience and Precautionary Measures

The usual way of applying pesticides in southern Mexico is from a backpack sprayer: the pesticide is sprayed from a hose attached to a metal or plastic tank carried on the applier's back. Many in our study were using sprayers they had purchased 10 or 15 years earlier, which often leaked or spilled pesticides onto the user. Indeed, 89% of the men in the survey sample said they had experienced spills while applying pesticides.

Although firsthand experience with high levels of exposure to pesticides was clearly common, this seems rarely to have translated into an increased sense of personal danger. In fact, those who had experienced spills were not more likely to use protective equipment than those who did not. Using Fisher's Exact Test (2-tail),[3] we performed a test of covariance between use of protective equipment and experience of spills and found no significant association between these two variables ($p = 1.000$). We also found that the number of spills people had experienced did not increase their likelihood of using protective equipment: there was no significant difference in average number of spills and use of protective equipment ($p = .90$).

It may seem curious that having experienced spills was insufficient to instill a sense of personal risk in most of our survey group. However, the failure of people to take protective action, in spite of frequent spills, is less surprising when one considers that the associated symptoms, most commonly nausea or headache, were not considered serious. Furthermore, 30% of those experiencing spills reported no symptoms at all. It seems that when a spill is perceived to have no noteworthy adverse effect, the individual may feel that protection is not really necessary.

More than half (59%) of the survey sample said that they had, at one time or another, gotten sick while using pesticides. The symptoms most frequently mentioned included headache, dizziness, cough, and conjunctivitis, as well as stomach pain, burning eyes, and skin irritation. In the ethnographic interviews men expressed a rather casual attitude about these symptoms. For the most part they were viewed as temporary, minor inconveniences that a healthy person could easily endure. Work in the fields is hard, our subjects reasoned, and challenges the body in many ways. The headache and nausea that often come with pesticide exposure were viewed as one more thing a farmer must bear. People discount the importance of symptoms when they find that simply washing the exposed area relieves the burning, or that the headache goes away within a few hours, causing no serious inconvenience. Despite this lack of expressed concern, we did find a statistically significant relationship between the use of protective equipment and the experience of symptoms (Fisher's exact p = .030), indicating that many who reported using protective clothing had also previously experienced symptoms.

Experience and Perceived Risk

Thus the anomalous situation of knowing pesticides are toxic, but seldom taking protective action, may be explained, at least in part, by the experience that no serious harm seems to accompany exposure. While exposure to pesticide spills was common, and minor transient symptoms were also fairly common, those we interviewed had never experienced serious health effects firsthand. Furthermore, while most said they had heard of people who had become very ill from pesticide exposure, none in our study had personally witnessed anyone in such a state. The lesson learned from personal experience was that pesticide spills were of no real consequence; they were something one could easily endure, producing essentially only short-term superficial symptoms. As one *campesino* observed, "The headache only lasts a couple of hours, and we're young, we can tolerate it."

In reviewing the literature on differences in responses to health risks among ethnic minorities, Vaughan (1993) points out that the frequency of exposure to a hazardous agent and the immediacy of the onset of negative outcomes are important factors in the assessment of risk. Discounting of future consequences or evaluating one's present state to indicate future vulnerability may become important in making decisions about taking risks, especially when situational indicators of risk are not obvious. Vaughan argues that the sense of risk is reduced when the risk is familiar, negative effects are not immediate, and consequences are viewed as common and relatively mild.

In peasant communities such as this, people often rely on an empirical process to assess the value or danger in many things they encounter (Castañeda, n.d.). Individuals make judgments about risks in the world around them based on previous experiences, both their own and what they hear about from the people around them (Ramos et al., 1995). Past experience can affect risk perception in two distinct ways. On the one hand, when people observe serious consequences of a behavior, they may perceive it as dangerous and avoid it. Castañeda, for example, found farmers in central Mexico avoided pesticides altogether after they had become very ill using them. On the other hand, when someone's experience has been that exposure leads to only fleeting and superficial consequences, the perception that there is no real need for special precautionary measures is reinforced. As Douglas and Calvez observed, "If a person . . . takes great risks in the name of their own experience or knowledge, the evidence of this person is stronger than anything else" (1990:41).

The Familiar and Unavoidable

The criteria by which people assess risk, and decisions about risk reduction behaviors, are patterned by the cultural and practical context in which they find themselves (Douglas and Calvez, 1990). People tend to minimize possible dangers in familiar activities (Douglas, 1985). This may partially explain the sense of subjective immunity these *campesinos* had in using pesticides: because of leaching of the soil and changes in the pest population, the men felt it was no longer possible to farm productively in the area without using the chemicals. The following comments by four individuals express this common perception:

> Well, if you didn't fumigate there wouldn't be any *milpa* (corn crop) at all, because it would get destroyed. That's why you've got to be fumigating forcefully. This time I sprayed six times, and the bug is still winning.

> When we first began to use these products, we felt it helped a whole lot, because the harvests came out much better and much more easily. But today, the harvests have been less and less, because the earth is getting burned-out, the nutrients are being destroyed, because of the application of these products. . . . But you can't avoid using them. They are very basic to our work.

> This year there were a few people who didn't have enough money to buy chemicals, and their *milpa* isn't growing well, they don't have anything. . . . You used to be able to grow without chemicals, but now the earth is used up.

> Our production is double with the chemicals, but the problem is that they heat up the earth. When you use these chemicals the land erodes. . . . The land gets sterile. . . . It takes two or three years for it to recuperate.

The farmers often spoke of pesticides with resignation. Although the chemicals had improved production, at the same time they had caused a dependence which was expensive and unhealthy, and was harming the land in the long run. Many farmers were very frustrated by the situation, but they felt there was nothing to be done about it. They felt they *had* to use pesticides, regardless of the ecological and health dangers.

The Cultural and Practical Context

Thus we found that these *campesinos* understand that pesticides are dangerous and know the recommended handling precautions, but they rarely follow procedures for protecting themselves from exposure in the fields. While they perceive the use of pesticides to be a necessity, the use of protective equipment is uncommon, and is viewed as something of an extravagance. How, then, do local cultural concepts of vulnerability, the local physical environment, and economic context contribute to this situation?

Culture and Perception of Vulnerability

Previous studies often reported that people commonly hold an optimistic bias, or the belief that they are not personally susceptible to given health risks (e.g., Timko and Janoff-Bulman, 1985; Weinstein et al., 1991). This tendency has been shown to be particularly pronounced among Latino populations (Perry and Mushkatel, 1986; Turner and Kiecolt, 1984; Vaughan, 1993). Individuals' perceptions of their personal vulnerability may reflect cultural notions of weakness and strength. Studies among Mexicans and Mexican Americans report many people believe only the weak and infirm are vulnerable to health risks from pesticide exposure (Castañeda, n.d.; Lantz et al., 1994). Castañeda, for example, found the farmers in central Mexico understood individual vulnerability to be a function of the "nature" of a person. She describes men who view themselves as so strong and healthy that they can even taste the pesticide they are mixing to judge its concentration, without risk of ill effect.

Consistent with these previous studies, we found that the cultural expectation that healthy males are strong and able to sustain a certain degree of hardship was a factor in the perception of personal risk. In discussing their perceptions of personal vulnerability to pesticides, several people mentioned that those who can't tolerate pesticide exposure are the very old, the very young, and pregnant women. The instructions they had received for precautions in pesticide use had emphasized that children and pregnant women should not use the products. This, coupled with the observation that men who got sick while applying the chemicals would feel better in a few hours, led many to believe that to admit susceptibility to toxic exposure was to appear weak and unmanly. A strong man, a *macho*, wouldn't be bothered by the symptoms. The following quotations illustrate how the experience of toxic symptoms is associated with weakness:

[Whether the pesticides affect you] depends on aging. The body gets contaminated and weakened, even though it gets used to using [pesticides], but each time the body is less resistant, for whatever changes aging has caused, everything is changing.

Here we don't cover anything, we just go like this. If there are boots we put on boots, and when there's not, we don't, But really, it hasn't affected us. Some people do get sick, they get things like headaches. That may be because their body is run-down, or who knows, maybe it's their blood. That's probably it, because it affects very old people and very young about the same.

The reluctance of the men of this region to use the protective equipment could be rooted, at least in part, in this cultural concept. A man who covers up to apply pesticides is a fearful man, or he is a weak man who can't tolerate a minor physical challenge.

Practical Concerns

When asked directly why they didn't use protective equipment, people consistently cited two practical considerations: expense and discomfort.

Previous studies among Mexican and Mexican-American farm workers report that economic considerations, such as the cost of the equipment or the fear of job loss in retaliation for asking employers for equipment, are important in the infrequent use of protective equipment (e.g., Lantz et al., 1994; Vaughan, 1993). Likewise, in our ethnographic interviews, nearly everyone said the recommended equipment was expensive and they simply couldn't afford it. They said they could barely afford the pesticides themselves, and the equipment was something they couldn't ever imagine being able to buy.[4] Framed in economic terms, the decision to forgo protective equipment begins to seem a rather reasonable choice. When faced with several independent risks, individuals must make choices about how to allocate resources to reduce those risks (see, for example, Elliot and McKee, 1995). When allocating very limited financial resources to farm production, the purchase of agrochemicals, which ensure an increased crop yield, clearly must take precedence over the purchase of protective equipment, whose very necessity is viewed skeptically for all of the reasons cited above.

Another frequently mentioned factor discouraging use of protective gear is the heat and fatigue they cause. The standard protective gear (rubber boots and gloves, heavy overalls, goggles, and face mask) was designed for use in nontropical regions and is very heavy and hot. Like previous studies (e.g., Chester et al., 1990), we found that workers consider such clothing unacceptable: in the intense heat and humidity of the fields of southern Chiapas, the physical discomfort makes it impossible to work very long while wearing such covering. As one man explained, it is very impractical, since stopping to take rests to cool off and catch your breath results in so much lost work time that it's very costly to production.

Special Issues for Women and Children

Women are estimated to perform 50% or more of agricultural labor in developing countries worldwide (Charlton, 1984; FAO, 1994). Studies in Latin America have reported similarly high rates of involvement of women in agriculture (Arizpe and Botey, 1989; Ashby, 1985; Nash, 1982). Still, studies of pesticide use among female farmers and farm workers are rare (McDuffie, 1994). Indeed, the primary focus in our research project has been on male farmers. However, preliminary data indicate that the use of pesticides by women and children for household purposes may merit special consideration. One of us (NS) conducted community observations and exploratory interviews with 13 women from the Tziscao region. The women, all of whom were mothers, were asked open-ended questions about their use of pesticides. Their practices in handling and storing the materials in and around the home were also observed in the course of the interview visit. The women were asked about the types of chemicals used, reasons for using pesticides, manner and location of use, storage methods, perceived risks to themselves and their families, and precautions taken.

The women reported frequent use of pesticides in the home for purposes ranging from killing ants in the kitchen to preventing pests from destroying crops in their communal gardens (*hortalizas*). They reported using backpack sprayers once every other week to fumigate the garden. When asked about the risk they perceived in using these chemicals, their answers ranged from "there are no risks" to "we can die." Many reported experiencing symptoms they associated with pesticide use, including headaches, colds, and eye pain. The measures they said they took to protect themselves were similar to those reported by the men: not storing chemicals in the house, avoiding direct contact with the chemicals, washing hands after use. A few also mentioned covering the mouth with a scarf, but like the few men who reported doing this, none said they did this on a regular basis. Also, as with the men's interviews, pregnant women, children, and the elderly were seen to be at greatest risk and were subject to more stringent restrictions on their handling of the chemicals, such as avoiding work in the garden or field at the time of spraying.

Some unexpected behaviors indicate that there may be a serious gap between the cognitive awareness of the dangers of pesticide use and everyday practices among the women. It was not uncommon for women to say that they used pesticides as a treatment for head lice. Five of the mothers described applying various insecticides to the heads of their children. One mother applied the chemical for three minutes to her child's hair before washing it, while another let it stay in overnight and repeated the application on the following night. Although all of these women indicated they knew pesticides were dangerous and discussed preventing their children from having contact with pesticides, they nevertheless applied them directly to their children's bodies.

Another anomaly was apparent in the storage of the chemicals. All the women interviewed discussed the importance of storing chemicals out of the reach of children, yet in at least two households, bags of pesticides were observed to be within easy reach of children (on a tabletop or under a bed).

Overall, although the women seemed to understand the danger of pesticides and the appropriate precautions, they shared the men's generally casual attitude about day-to-day exposure to these chemicals. It seems that the women also minimize the dangers of pesticide exposure in daily practice, perhaps because, like the men, they observe no immediate adverse effects. However, these preliminary interviews are not sufficiently detailed to draw any clear comparisons and contrasts between the women and the men.

Conclusion

Pesticides present serious health risks to any population that uses them, but in developing countries, where distribution and use of pesticides is not well regulated, these health risks are particularly pronounced. Unsafe handling practices, such as those we observed in Chiapas, are common and have not been remedied by repeated educational campaigns.

In this study we combined survey methods with ethnographic techniques to examine the basis of infrequent use of protective equipment when applying pesticides in this region. By drawing on these complementary methods, we have been better able to understand how people think about pesticides and why they handle them the way they do in this setting. Analysis of the survey of men resulted in the seemingly anomalous finding that high levels of knowledge were not predictive of use of protective gear. This finding contradicts the basic assumption underlying many interventions for promoting protective behaviors: that people fail to comply with safety recommendations because of lack of knowledge. Through the use of the anthropological methods of open-ended interviews and observations and their associated data analysis techniques, we were able to shed considerable light on the apparent paradox. Combining these methods has indicated several considerations which should be recognized in developing strategies for promoting the adoption of protective practices in handling pesticides.

We identified a number of important interacting factors associated with the infrequent use of protective equipment among our study population. Most of the people we interviewed had personal experiences with high levels of pesticide exposure and perceived that resulting symptoms were infrequent, transitory, short-lived, and did not result in any observable serious health effects. Experience tells them that health risks of exposure may be unpleasant but are of no real consequence. Furthermore, pesticides are viewed as a necessity for agricultural production. The unavoidability of pesticide use leads to a process of normalizing and minimizing the sense of related danger. These combined factors result in a general sense that protective measures are not of great urgency.

The local cultural and practical contexts further contribute to the situation. The common concept that only the weak and infirm are susceptible to marginal health risks is reinforced by the formal instructions that emphasize that children and pregnant women are particularly vulnerable. To use protective equipment would require a sense of personal vulnerability that men may not experience or not wish to display. Finally, but perhaps most important, the cost and discomfort associated with the equipment present important practical barriers to its use in this setting.

We conclude that the marginal sense of personal risk perceived by the *campesinos*, combined with the practical and social costs of using protective equipment, results in the decision to forgo the use of protection, in spite of awareness of the toxicity of the pesticides. In a world where there are many present dangers and many physical hardships, the risks encountered in pesticide use are but one factor. Decisions about how to apply and respond to the knowledge of pesticide toxicity occur within a framework of cultural concepts of gender and risk as well as pragmatic considerations; therefore, they can best be understood through the use of research techniques capable of considering the broader social and cultural context of local life. By thus framing our analysis, what at first appeared as contradictory phenomena became more comprehensible. We began to see noncompliant behavior not as an indication of simple ignorance or lack of understanding, but instead reflecting an interplay between risk assessment and resource allocation on the part of the *campesinos*. They were involved in a process of balancing the perceived personal danger encountered in unprotected use of pesticides against the practical, social, and economic costs they would incur in taking the precautions.

Recommendations

The standard protective equipment recommended for pesticide application is both too expensive and too cumbersome to be widely used in developing countries and tropical regions. Efforts to develop gear that is more affordable and appropriate for this climate are essential (see, for example, Chester et al., 1990) but, if left to market forces, will not be forthcoming. Incentive programs would be needed to encourage its development and distribution. Controlling the cost of the equipment, perhaps through government subsidies to farmers for its purchase, would also be likely to increase its use.

Given the many barriers to the regular use of protective equipment, high exposure to pesticides is likely to continue. It is essential that developing countries and the international community better regulate the distribution and use of agrochemicals. For example, it is not uncommon for pesticides which are illegal in the United States to continue to be sold in countries that have more lenient regulations (Simonian, 1988). Given the likelihood that people in these countries will come into direct contact with these chemicals, careful regulation is of great importance.

Most studies of pesticide use fail to examine the role of women. Our preliminary work with the women of this region indicates that they may be important users of pesticides as well as sources of pesticide exposure for children. It would seem important, therefore, that women not be excluded from future studies of pesticide use or from future intervention development efforts (Boserup and Lijencrate, 1982; Sims et al., 1985).

By combining survey methods with anthropological research techniques, this study has opened new insights into the conceptual and practical basis of behaviors that are a great public health concern. This has enabled us to move away from the usual assumptions about the relationship between information and action, and to better understand how and why specific knowledge translates into practical actions in this local setting. Use of these complementary methods has great potential for helping to move international public health efforts away from the frustrating dead end of repeatedly providing information that the target population cannot or does not apply. Instead, such research can lead to a productive appreciation of the cultural and practical factors which underlie failure to comply with health recommendations.

Notes

1. For example, Avory and Coggon (1994) report that farmers in Hampshire, England, regularly read pesticide labels and use appropriate mixing techniques, yet they rarely comply with recommendations for using protective equipment, even when they have completed training in pesticide handling.

2. The *ejido* is a form of land tenure common in Mexico wherein the state grants a group of individuals ownership of a tract of land, which they then divide into separate plots for use by individual families. Originally, in this system, the land could change hands only as inheritance given to one's children; it could not be sold. The system was intended to ensure that families retained their subsistence base, in spite of fluctuating economic pressures. However, in 1993 the federal law was changed, and these lands can now be bought and sold. This decision, which provoked much debate and social protest, was a central issue put forth by the Zapatista movement of 1994. About 20% of the farms in the border region are *ejidal* (Secretaria de Programación y Presupuesto, 1990).

3. This statistic was chosen because it is useful for testing probabilities in small samples with small expected values (Fisher and van Belle, 1993).

4. The full recommended protective gear, including boots, gloves, overalls, and face mask, currently costs about US$150 in Comitan, the central market city of the area. The average yearly cash income in Tziscao currently ranges from about US$800 to $1,500. Moreover, due to the lack of demand, the gear is not readily available for purchase in the region.

Acknowledgments

This research was supported in part by a research grant from the Fundación México en Harvard, A.C., and by the Tinker Foundation Graduate Student Research Travel Grant though the Center for Latin American Studies at the University of California at Berkeley. An earlier version of this chapter was presented at the National Meetings of the American Public Health Association, San Francisco, 1993.

References

Arizpe L, Botey C (1989) "Las políticas de desarrollo agrario y su impacto sobre la mujer campesina en México." In: La Mujer en el Desarrollo de México y América Latina. L Arizpe, ed. Mexico City, Mexico: UNAM/CIM, pp. 83–107.

Ashby J (1985) "Women and Agricultural Technology in Latin America and the Caribbean". In: Women, Agriculture, and Rural Development in Latin America. J Ashby and S Gómez, eds. Italy: CIAT/IFDC.

Avory G, Coggon D (1994) Determinants of safe behaviour in farmers when working with pesticides. *Occupational Medicine* 44:236–238.

Bernard HR (1990) Research Methods in Cultural Anthropology. Newbury Park, Calif: Sage Publications.

Boserup E, Lijencrate C (1982) "La integración de la mujer al desarrollo, ¿como? ¿cuando? y ¿porque?" In: Secretaria de Programación y Presupuesto (SPP) Serie Lecturas III: Estudios sobre la mujer. 1. Empleo y la mujer. Bases metodológicas y evidencia empírica. Mexico, DF: SPP, pp. 99–113.

Bwititi T, Chikuni O, Loewenson R, Murambiwa W, Nhachi C, Nyazema N (1987) Health hazards in organophosphate use among farm workers in the large-scale farming sector. *Central African Journal of Medicine* 33:120–126.

Castañeda X (n.d.) The Social Construction of Risk Perception in Rural Adolescents of Mexico. Cuernavaca, Mexico: National Institute of Public Health. [Unpublished document]

Charlton S (1984) Women in Third World Development. Boulder, Colo: Westview Press.

Chester G, Adam AV, Inkmann Koch A, Litchfield MH, Tuinman CP (1990) Field evaluation of protective equipment for pesticide operators in a tropical climate. *Medicina del Lavoro* 81:480–488.

Davies JE (1987) Changing profile of pesticide poisoning. *New England Journal of Medicine* 316:807–808.

Douglas M (1985) Risk Acceptability According to the Social Sciences. New York: Russell Sage Foundation.

Douglas M, Calvez M (1990) The self as risk taker: a cultural theory of contagion in relation to AIDS. *Sociological Review* 38:445–464.

Ecobichon DJ, Davies JE, Doull J, Ehrich M, Joy R, McMillan D, MacPhail R, Reiter LW, Slikker W, Tilson H (1990) "Neurotoxic Effects of Pesticides." In: The Effect of Pesticides on Human Health. R Wilkinson, SR Baker, eds. Princeton, NJ: Princeton Scientific Publishing Co., pp. 131–199.

Elliott S, McKee M (1995) Collective risk decisions in the presence of many risks. *Kyklos* 48:541–554.

FAO (Food and Agriculture Organization of the United Nations) (1985) Guidelines on Good Labeling Practice for Pesticides. Rome: United Nations.

FAO (Food and Agriculture Organization of the United Nations) (1994) A Rural Social Agenda. The FAO Perspective. Document submitted to the United Nations Preparatory Committee for the World Summit for Social Development.

Fiore MC, Anderson HA, Hong R, Golubjatnikov R, Seiser JE, Nordstrom D, Hanrahan L, Belluck D (1986) Chronic exposure to aldicarb-contaminated groundwater and human immune function. *Environmental Research* 41:633–645.

Fisher LD, van Belle G (1993) Biostatistics: A Methodology for the Health Sciences. New York: John Wiley & Sons.

Forget G (1991) Pesticides and the Third World. *Journal of Toxicology and Environmental Health*. 32:11–31.

Herrera C, Rodas M (1987) Intoxicación por Plaguicidas: Determinación de la Actividad de Colinesterasa en Personas Expuestas a Insecticidas Organofosforados en el Municipio de Tapachula, Chiapas, México. Tesis de Licenciatura de Químico Farmacobiologo Chiapas, México: Universidad Autónoma de Chiapas.

Hunt LM (1996) "Inequalities in the Mexican National Health Care System: Problems in Managing Cancer in Southern Mexico." In: Society, Health, and Disease: Transcultural Perspectives. J Subedi, E Gallagher, eds. Upper Saddle River, NJ: Prentice Hall, pp. 130–147.

ILO (1977) Safe Use of Pesticides. Occupational Safety and Health Series Report No. 38. Geneva: International Labor Office.

ILO (1991) Safety and Health in the Use of Agrochemicals. A Guide. Geneva: International Labor Office.

INEGI (1988a) Encuesta Nacional Agropecuaria Ejidal 1988, vol. II. Ejidos y Comunidades Agrícolas. Mexico, DF: Instituto General de Geografía e Informática.

INEGI (1988b) Encuesta Nacional Agropecuaria Ejidal 1988, vol. III. Unidades De Producción Con Tierras Ejidal y Comunal. Mexico, DF: Instituto General de Geografía e Informática.

INEGI (1990) Chiapas, X Censo General de Población y Vivienda 1990, vol. 1. Resultados Definitivos. Mexico, DF: Instituto General de Geografía e Informática.

Jeyaratnam J (1985) Health problems of pesticide usage in the Third World. *British Journal of Industrial Medicine* 42:505–506.

Jeyaratnam J (1990) Acute pesticide poisoning: a major global health problem. *World Health Statistics Quarterly* 43:139–144.

Lantz PM, Dupuis L, Reding D, Krauska M, Lappe K (1994) Peer discussions of cancer among Hispanic migrant farm workers. *Public Health Reports* 109:512–520.

Levine RS (1986) Assessment of mortality and morbidity due to unintentional pesticide poisonings. Unpublished World Health Organization (WHO) document. WHO/VBC/86.929.

Loevinsohn ME (1987) Insecticide use and increased mortality in rural central Luzon, Philippines. *Lancet* 1:1359–1362.

London L (1993) Agrichemical safety practices on farms in the Western Cape. *South African Medical Journal* 84:273–278.

Lotti M (1984) "The Delayed Polyneuropathy Caused by Some Organophosphorus Esters." In: Recent Advances in Nervous System Toxicology. CL Galli, L Manzo, PS Spencer, eds. New York: Plenum, pp. 247–257.

McConnell R, Hruska AJ (1993) An epidemic of pesticide poisoning in Nicaragua: implications for prevention in developing countries. *American Journal of Public Health* 83:1559–1562.

McDuffie HH (1994) Women at work: agriculture and pesticides. *Journal of Occupational Medicine* 36:1240–1246.

Miles M, Huberman AM (1994) Qualitative Data Analysis. An Expanded Source Book, 2nd ed. Thousand Oaks, Calif: Sage Publications.

Nash J (1982) "Algunos aspectos de la integración de la mujer en el proceso de desarrollo: un punto de vista." In: Secretaria de Programación y Presupuesto (SPP) Serie Lecturas III: Estudios sobre la mujer. 1. Empleo y la mujer. Bases metodológicas y evidencia empírica. Mexico, DF: SPP, pp. 29–67.

NCHS (National Center for Health Statistics) (1985) Plan and Operation of the Hispanic Health and Nutrition Examination Survey 1982–84. Programs and Collection Procedures Series 1, No. 19. DHHS Pub. No. (PHS)85-1321. Hyattsville, Md: Dept. of Health and Human Services (DHHS).

Nigg HN, Stamper JH, Queen RM (1986) Dicofol exposure in Florida citrus applicators: effects of protective clothing. *Archives of Environmental Contamination and Toxicology* 15:121–134.

Ortega J, Carreón T, López L, Chávez R, Hernández M (1993) La investigación en México sobre el impacto en la salud por contaminantes ambientales. *Salud Pública de México* 35:585–591.

Ortega-Ceseña J, Espinosa-Torres F, López-Carillo L (1994) El control de los riesgos para la salud generados por los plaguicidas organofosforados en México: retos ante el Tratado de Libre Comercio. *Salud Pública de México* 36:624–632.

Perry RW, Mushkatel AH (1986) Minority Citizens in Disasters. Athens: University of Georgia Press.

Pimentel D, Acquay H, Biltonen M, Rice P, Silva M, Nelson J, Lipner V, Giordano S, Horowitz A, D'Amore M (1992) Environmental and economic costs of pesticide use. *Bioscience* 42:750–760.

Ragsdale NN, Menzer RE, eds. (1989) Carcinogenicity and Pesticides. Principles, Issues and Relationship. Washington, DC: American Chemical Society.

Ramos R, Shain R, Johnson L (1995) "Men I mess with don't have anything to do with AIDS": using ethno-theory to understand sexual risk perception. *Sociological Quarterly* 36:483–504.

Secretaria de Programación y Presupuesto (SPP) (1990) Agenda Estadística Chiapas, 1990. Mexico City, Mexico: SPP.

Simonian L (1988) Pesticide use in Mexico: decades of abuse. *Ecologist* 18:82–87.

Sims H, Poats SV, Cloud K, Nureme HR (1985) "Conceptual Framework for Gender Analysis in Framing Systems Research and Extension." In: Working Together. Gender Analysis in Agriculture, vol 1. Case Studies. H Sims, SV Poats, eds. West Harford, Conn: Kumarian Press.

Thomas PT, House RV (1989) "Pesticide-Induced Modulation of Immune System." In: Carcinogenicity and Pesticides. Principles, Issues and Relationship. NN Ragsdale, RE Menzer, eds. Washington, DC: American Chemical Society, pp. 94–106.

Timko C, Janoff-Bulman R (1985) Attributions, vulnerability, and psychological adjustment: the case of breast cancer. *Health Psychology* 4:521–544.

Tinoco R, Halperin D (1992) Pesticide use in Chiapas, Mexico. Paper presented at the Annual Meeting of the National Council for International Health, Washington, DC. June 23–25.

Tinoco R, Halperin D (1998) Poverty, production and health: inhibition of erythrocyte cholinesterase via occupational exposure to organophosphate insecticides in Chiapas. *Archives of Environmental Health* 53:29–35.

Tinoco R, Tinoco R, Parsonnet J, Halperin D (1993) Paraquat poisoning in southern Mexico: a report of 25 cases. *Archives of Environmental Health* 48:78–80.

Tolba MK, El-Kholy OA (1992) The World Environment, 1972–1992. London: Chapman and Hall.

Turner R, Kiecolt K (1984) Responses to uncertainty and risk: Mexican-American, Black, and Anglo beliefs about the manageability of the future. *Social Science Quarterly* 65:665–679.

Vaughan E (1993) Chronic exposure to an environmental hazard: risk perceptions and self-protective behavior. *Health Psychology* 12:74–85.

Weinstein ND, Sandman PM, Roberts NE (1991) Perceived susceptibility and self-protective behavior: a field experiment to encourage home radon testing. *Health Psychology* 10:25–33.

WHO (1985) Safe Use of Pesticides. 9th Report of the WHO Expert Committee on Vector Biology and Control. WHO Technical Report Series No. 720. Geneva: World Health Organization.

WHO (1990) Public Health Impact of Pesticides Used in Agriculture. Geneva: World Health Organization.

WHO (1993) Plaguicidas y Salud en Las Américas. Serie Ambiental No. 12. Washington, DC: World Health Organization.

Wilkinson R, Baker WR, eds. (1990) The Effect of Pesticides on Human Health. Princeton, NJ: Princeton Scientific Publishing Co.

World Resources (1986) A Report by the World Resources Institute and the International Institute for Environment and Development 1986. New York: Basic Books.

V

COMMUNITY HEALTH

12

Prospects for Family Planning in Côte d'Ivoire: Ethnographic Contributions to the Development of Culturally Appropriate Population Policy

RUTH P. WILSON,
CAROLYN F. SARGENT,
SHEGOU DARRET, AND
KALE KOUAME

Here we examine the results of the Policy Ethnography for Family Planning Study (PEFPS)[1] designed to collect information for the development of culturally appropriate population policy and family planning services in Côte d'Ivoire (Wilson, 1991). This study was requested by the Côte d'Ivoire Ministry of Health and Social Protection (MHSP) and the Regional Economic Development Support Office of the United States Agency for International Development (REDSO/ USAID) to complement quantitative studies conducted for planning purposes. Qualitative data on the importance of the extended family among urban Ivoirians and the role of various social segments in decision making for maternal and child health and birth spacing are discussed in the context of family planning program development. This study demonstrates the importance of the cultural context in addressing the full integration of family planning services in the health services of Côte d'Ivoire.

Background

Family planning affects maternal and infant mortality—two major health problems in African countries—and may thus be a preventive health measure (Fathalla, 1990; Singh and Ratnam, 1990). If African women were to have only

257

the number of children they wanted, it is estimated that the average number of births would be reduced by 17% (Maine et al., 1987). It is also anticipated that the high rates of Ivoirian maternal mortality (estimated at 597 deaths per 100,000 births for 1988–1994)(Sombo et al., 1995) would be reduced through elimination of certain high-risk births. Maternal deaths occur most often in women who have many or frequent pregnancies, or those who conceive very early or very late in their fertile years (Singh and Ratnam, 1990).

Infant mortality is also a serious problem in Côte d'Ivoire: the estimated infant mortality rate is 89 deaths per 1,000 live births (Sombo et al., 1995). Infant deaths are also associated with short birth intervals, extremes of maternal age, and large numbers of births (Centers for Disease Control, 1983). In developing countries, the lack of access to health personnel trained to identify and treat the complications of pregnancy magnifies the effects of these factors (WHO, 1991).

Côte d'Ivoire has a birth rate of 50 live births per 1,000 women of childbearing age (WHO, 1991) and a fertility rate estimated at 5.7 live births per woman (Sombo et al., 1995). Its annual population growth rate was estimated at 3.6% in 1985 (Futures Group, 1988) and 3.8% in 1992. As such, the population is expected to double in 20 years. Voluntary use of contraceptives is the strategy recommended to reduce fertility rates, curb population growth, and decrease maternal and young child deaths. However, Côte d'Ivoire has one of the lowest estimated rates of contraceptive use in western Africa (3%), with only 1% of women surveyed reporting use of modern methods (Population Reference Bureau, 1991).

There have been indications of an unmet demand for family planning services in Côte d'Ivoire. For example, although only 8% of the 5,000 women interviewed in 1984 in Abidjan (the commercial center and largest city) reported ever using modern contraceptives, 40% said they were interested in using them (USAID, 1991). In 1987–1988, another study of 1,207 Ivoirian women ages 15–49 near Bouaflé (a medium-sized Ivoirian town) found that 58% wished to limit family size, 47% wanted to space births, and 48% said they were ready to use modern contraceptive methods (Tafforeau and Timyan, 1987). And in 1990, three private clinics that provide family planning services in Abidjan recorded a surge in the number of users (Huntington, 1991).

During the past three decades, the Government of Côte d'Ivoire (GOCI) has encouraged rapid population growth. However, the 1986 collapse of coffee and cocoa prices plunged the Ivoirian economy into a recession from which it has yet to fully recover (US State Department, 1990). The combination of a declining economy and a rapidly growing population constrains efforts to improve the health status of the Ivoirian people. This has led to increased attention to population issues and the rethinking of population policy.

Before 1986, family planning services were provided in the offices of a few private practitioners and at Association Ivoirienne Pour le Bien-Etre Familial (AIBEF) clinics located in three university teaching hospitals, at government-sponsored maternal and child health clinics, and at freestanding clinics. Health care providers in the public sector referred clients to AIBEF, to private practitioners, or to Promotion de la Vie Familiale (PROVIFA), a group of nuns who provided counseling on natural birth spacing.

Indicators of change in the government's position on population issues include the following: (1) a proposal made by the government's Human Resources Development Policy Committee that a national population policy be formulated and a family planning program be implemented; (2) the creation in 1991 of a post for a National Family Planning Coordinator; (3) the reversal of the law forbidding pharmacies to sell condoms; (4) the convening of a National Seminar on Family Planning (Côte d'Ivoire Ministry of Health, 1991); and (5) the government's support for development of a joint GOCI–USAID family planning program (USAID, 1990).

As a part of this effort, the GOCI sought better understanding of the cultural context of population issues, as discussed by Ford and Arcury (1984) and Knodel and van de Walle (1979). The present study was commissioned in the early phases of policy and program development.

Research Setting

At the time of this study Côte d'Ivoire had an estimated population of 13 million (Reddy, 1994), including members of more than 60 ethnic groups. The research was focused in Abidjan, the commercial center of the country. Abidjan had an estimated population of 2.7 million residents, approximately one-fourth of whom were immigrants from neighboring countries. Family structures were varied: some were polygamous, others monogamous; some were extended, others were nuclear families; some groups traced their descent through maternal lines, others were patrilineal. Most health services were delivered at the university hospital clinics and at a network of 10 government-sponsored maternal and child health (MCH) clinics.

Methods

Focus group and individual interviews were the primary sources of data. Focus group interviews were conducted because previous experience had shown that this method of data collection can yield reliable behavioral and qualitative data on family planning issues (Haryono et al., 1981; Schearer, 1981; Stycos, 1981). Individual interviews were used when focus group discussions were not appropriate, that is, when interviewing senior government officials or supervisors of health personnel.

Semistructured interview guides were used to conduct the focus group and individual interviews with three types of respondents: (1) governmental and nongovernmental officials involved in developing the new population policy; (2) health care providers (including supervisors of health centers, physicians, nurses, nurse assistants, midwives, and social workers) in both public and private facilities; and (3) potential adolescent and adult users of family planning services (male and female adolescents and adults representing different age groups). Each semistructured interview guide contained a list of all of the key questions that interviewers were to ask during an interview.

Focus group and individual interview data were supplemented by discussions with key informants and field observations of Abidjan residents in their everyday activities, recorded in field notes by the ethnographer and one of the research assistants.

Site Selection

Sites were selected to represent the diversity of the city and the places where one might find the major stakeholders in family planning program development (government offices, health facilities, youth centers, etc.).

Policymakers were interviewed at their offices located in three Abidjan communes.

Health care provider interviews were conducted at health facilities where the staff had experience with family planning services. Interview sites were the three AIBEF clinics in Abidjan where family planning services were provided, one private clinic that offered maternal and child health (MCH) services, two private organizations that disseminated family planning advice, and four government-sponsored maternal and child health clinics and three university hospital clinics where family planning services were extended on an unofficial basis, in the absence of a formal government planning policy. These facilities were located in 6 of Abidjan's 13 communes.

Consumers of family planning services were interviewed at maternal and child health clinics, employment centers, youth centers, and outdoor restaurants.

Research Staff

The core research staff included an anthropologist/ethnographer (RPW), a physician from the National Family Planning Coordinator's Office (SD), a medical sociologist from the National Institute for Public Health (KK), and three research assistants. Four of the six core staff members were Ivoirians. Core staff, unlike other staff members, participated in all phases of the research process: research design, data collection, analysis of the data, and review of the final report written by the anthropologist.

Additionally, six Ivoirian interviewers who had the equivalent of at least two years of university education were trained to conduct and record the interviews. Two staff members were present at each individual interview; one posed the questions and took brief notes while the other recorded responses and took more extensive notes. Three staff members were used for each focus group; one posed the questions while two recorded responses.

Respondent Selection

Key Informants. Selection of key informants from the client and policymaker groups was based on their availability and willingness to speak frankly with the ethnographer and on their involvement in and understanding of some aspects of family planning policy or program development.

Policymakers. Policymakers were selected from a list, generated by five key informants and the core research staff, of officials in governmental and nongovernmental agencies who were involved in the development of population policy in Côte d'Ivoire. The five policy-level key informants were each asked to select 20 individuals from the list to be interviewed. The 20 most frequently selected individuals were interviewed.

Health Care Providers. The selected health care providers were health center staff who were experienced in maternal and child health or family planning services. At each selected health care provider site, the research team presented the chief of staff with a letter from the Ministry of Health explaining the research team's mission and the purpose of the study and proposing a date for group interviews. The team attempted to conduct interviews of at least two professional health workers delivering services to reproductive-aged women or their children. If the chief of staff provided services to reproductive-aged women (e.g., a chief of obstetrics and gynecology or a chief of the pediatric unit), he or she was interviewed individually.

The chief of staff selected focus group participants from staff members who were responsible for taking care of mothers who had recently given birth or women who were of reproductive age. Separate focus groups were conducted for nurses, physicians, and midwives.

Consumers. Adolescents and both married and unmarried adults were interviewed in focus groups. Directors of services at employment agencies, health clinics, and youth centers requested volunteers for the focus groups. At the outdoor restaurants, the research assistants asked volunteers to participate in the focus groups. Focus group participants were selected by age, marital status, and sex. Interviewed in 25 same-sex groups were the following: (*1*) male and female adolescents between the ages of 16 and 19 years; (2) unmarried men and women 20–30 years of age; (3) unmarried men and women over the age of 30; and (4) married men and women. No incentives were offered to study participants.

Interview Instruments

A draft interview guide was prepared that covered the main themes of the study: (1) the changing shape and roles of the modern Ivoirian family; (2) the role of government, society, and the family in maternal health and birth spacing; (3) the old population policy and the challenges and strategies in developing and implementing a new one; and (4) the challenges and strategies in integrating family planning into child survival activities. These themes, which were considered important by policymakers and program managers attending a USAID-sponsored child survival conference in Swaziland, had not been fully addressed by previous family planning surveys, such as Demographic and Health Surveys, KAP (knowledge, attitude, and practice) surveys, or situation analysis studies. Here we provide the results of responses to the first two themes, the only ones for which we collected data from all three groups of respondents.

The draft interview guide was prepared in English, then translated into French. The first draft included questions on each of the four themes. The French version of the draft interview guide was reviewed, translated back into English for verification, and revised by the core research group. The interview guide was then pretested on several policymakers, health care providers, and potential consumers. Based on the pretests, the research group determined which themes and open-ended questions should be included during interviews for each respondent group and interview format.

The interview guide for policymakers contained 35 questions which covered the four main themes of the study. Two interview guides were developed for health care providers; one for the individual interviews contained 36 questions, and one for the focus groups contained 13 questions. Policymaker and health care provider interviews also included questions that elicited information about respondents' professional training, vocation, and thoughts about the type of consumer information that might be useful for policy and program planning. Consumer focus groups were asked 18 questions related to two of the main themes, in addition to several questions about teenage pregnancy.

All interviews were conducted in French with two exceptions: one consumer focus group was conducted in Djoula (a local trade language), and one policymaker interview (of a USAID staff member) was conducted in English. Each focus group and individual interview took from 45 to 90 minutes. Most of the questions were open-ended, and participants were allowed multiple responses to open-ended questions. Interviews were conducted in June and July 1991.

Data Analysis

Analyses of the interviews were conducted in three stages: during the period of data collection in the field; immediately after the fieldwork (when the preliminary report was written); and prior to preparing the project report (Wilson, 1991). During the first stage of the analysis, the teams of interviewers expanded their interview notes from the individual interviews and focus group discussions, resulting in a more detailed version of the responses. A transcript of each interview was typed and entered into an individual data file. At weekly meetings, the core research staff reviewed the transcribed interviews and developed a consensus on how the data would be coded and interpreted.

During the second stage of the analysis, we used GOfer (Microlytics, 1989), a software program for text management, to regroup the data into separate files by question and type of respondent. Interviewers coded these regrouped data files by systematically interpreting and categorizing phrases and concepts that appeared in the transcripts. Frequency tables of the codes provided an indication of the relative importance of a certain idea or value and allowed comparisons by type of respondent.

At the third stage of the analysis, an independent recoding of the GOfer data files was done by a research assistant at the Centers for Disease Control and Prevention (Atlanta, Georgia) who was unfamiliar with the study results. The first author then compared the codings conducted at the second and third stages of the analyses and reviewed the coding categories and the relative frequency of each category. Final synthesis of the data results was based on information from all three stages of the analysis.

Results

Respondent Characteristics

Key Informants. Key informants included two staff members from the Côte d'Ivoire Ministry of Health and Social Protection (MHSP); three non-Ivoirian USAID senior staff members knowledgeable in maternal and child health/child survival programs and ongoing family planning policy activities; and two Ivoirian educators, one male social science professor at the university and one female instructor at a vocational training school. Also included as key informants were two Ivoirian women who were street food vendors (one in her twenties, the other over 50), and one seamstress in her early thirties.

Policymakers. The 20 policymakers included 16 Ivoirians and 4 non-Ivoirians who were senior administrative staff at the MHSP, USAID, AIBEF, UNICEF, the United Nations Fund for Population Activities, and several other nongovernmental organizations. Thirteen were men, seven were women.

Health Care Providers. Of 126 health care providers interviewed, 38 were interviewed individually and 88 were interviewed in focus groups. Individual interviews were conducted with 10 men and 28 women. Thirty individual respondents (79%) were married, and all but one had at least one child. Among the female respondents, the average number of children per woman was 3.4, with a range of 1–9. Nine male respondents had children; the mean number of offspring was 4.4, with a range of 1–9. Twenty individual respondents were midwives, thirteen were physicians, three were nurses, one was a nurse's aide, and one was a social worker.

The 14 health care provider focus groups had an average of 6 persons, with a range of 4–8. Seven groups were composed of midwives, three of physicians, two of nurses, one of nurses' aides, and one of health agents from PROVIFA. Interviewers recorded sex, age, and number of children for respondents in 10 of the 14 focus groups. The mean age of the 62 participants for whom age was recorded was 38 (range 26–54).

Most of the respondents in the individual (27/38) and focus group interviews (13/14) were from the public sector.

Consumers. Twenty-five focus group interviews were completed with 158 consumers. The average size of the groups was 6, with a range of 5 to 10 participants per group.

Perceptions of the Family in Abidjan

Translated statements from interviews demonstrate that respondents view the contemporary urban family structure as the extended family, in its varied forms:

POLICYMAKER: With the ethnic diversity in Côte d'Ivoire, the definition of a family differs from one ethnic group to another. There are those who follow the patrilineal system and those who follow the matrilineal system (*Akan* and *Senufo*). Attachment to the family is very extensive and the bonds are very strong between the family members. The children are important according to the groups concerned. The value of the family cannot be considered in a general sense. If a FP [family planning] program is constructed, it must not be a standardized program in every country, but must be looked at according to the regions.

HEALTH CARE PROVIDER: The Ivoirian family is the African family. It is a very broad family. Almost everyone is a part of it (cousins, nephews, even the aunts). We are Africans and we should remain so. It is the lack of financial means; otherwise we should have many children, because children are very important. There is also polygamy, which has tended to decrease.

Although respondents valued the extended family structure, they voiced concern and criticism about contemporary inequities related to sharing the burdens of extended family life:

HEALTH CARE PROVIDER: The Ivoirian families are very big. The people are unhappy. They live under bad conditions. When only one person works in the family, he/she has the responsibility for the whole family and even for the [other] relatives in the village. I myself take care of my relatives in the village. I have many charges. Almost all of my salary goes to my relatives. With each death, for example, grandiose funeral ceremonies are organized.

TEEN CONSUMER: In the Ivoirian family, the fathers are often absent. The children live with the mothers. In the European family, both parents live together. In the mixed family, it depends. In the village, the people live together, and the older relatives also live with the family.

ADULT CONSUMER: Life is difficult right now. Before, we had as many children as we wished. One could have 10 children. There were no problems because one cultivated [farmed] to nourish them. Now, it is otherwise. Life is expensive. It is necessary to have only a few children in order to be able to care for them.

Responses of study participants suggest that most urban Ivoirians prefer large families. The family was generally described as *la famille élargie* (the extended family), which included one's spouse, children, parents, siblings, and other relatives (living and dead). Although the extended family was recognized by most as the major family structure, respondents also indicated that family size was becoming smaller. Policymakers and health care providers mentioned the smaller, nuclear family more frequently than did consumers.

When asked about their own families, health care providers in individual interviews recognized the nuclear unit as the core family unit in urban Abidjan. The nuclear unit was described by respondents as comprising a man, a woman, and all their children, the last including the couple's biological offspring and/or any younger kin for whom they assumed responsibility.

All three groups of respondents volunteered statements about the problems associated with modern life. Among health care providers and consumers, discussions of family life often centered around the financial difficulties associated with providing housing and food for all family members in Abidjan, where the cost of living is high and housing is scarce. Among consumers, discussions about economic difficulties were often linked with concern about the need to limit the number of births.

Essential Elements of Family Life. The most consistently reported essential element of family life was "solidarity." When asked to explain the meaning of "solidarity," respondents used words and phrases such as "understanding," "tolerance," "fellowship in the large family," "cohesion," "hospitality," and "a sense of community within the family life."

Translated statements from participants in all three respondent groups suggest the term "solidarity" is used to express the strong bonds that link the individual to his or her lineage through the duties, obligations, rites, and privileges
of that group:

> CONSUMER: It is necessary to conduct a synthesis among two lives: modern life and
> traditional life. This allows us to develop and to better adapt ourselves to this course
> of life. We must not copy the Western way of life. It is necessary to keep the African
> bonds, cultures, and solidarity while improving them.

> CONSUMER: To live in solidarity, teamwork, fraternal and communal life.

> POLICYMAKER: Family solidarity, but adapt it so that each one takes his destiny by the
> hand without counting on someone with more means.

This sense of solidarity, or corporateness, was one of the values that Ivoirians in
this study said they wanted to maintain as the family structure changes.

Statements from respondents suggested that they saw no conflict between
family solidarity and limiting fertility levels:

> HEALTH CARE PROVIDER: Solidarity above all. Intervals between births are also
> important.

> HEALTH CARE PROVIDER: In the city where the people are emancipated, polygamy is
> less pronounced. The law will decide on its fate in the future. In any case, if it is not
> done openly, it is done in secret (mistresses). It is necessary to have fewer children
> and to live in a reduced family. It is necessary to plan the births in order to better
> care for the children.

Among policymakers, health care providers, and consumers, there was an
expressed desire to retain the importance of family life, traditional and civil
marriage, and education for the children (including both formal schooling and
proper upbringing). All respondent groups expressed a desire to limit births to
the number of children one can afford.

In Côte d'Ivoire, a woman's contraceptive practices may limit her births, but
this might not result in a smaller family size. The practice of child fosterage
(Bledsoe, 1990; Omari, 1989), which we observed in Abidjan, is another way
that African family structure can influence a woman's decision regarding childbearing. An Ivoirian woman may volunteer to adopt a relative's child into her
own household, or the decision may be thrust on her by her spouse or by other
kinsmen (Etienne, 1979). For example, parents can decrease their family size
and obtain inexpensive child care for young children by sending toddlers to live
with kinsmen in the rural areas, or they can increase family size by fostering
school-aged children of kinsmen from the rural areas. The foster children can
gain assistance such as educational opportunities not available in the rural area;
they also give assistance by assuming responsibility for some of the household

chores, including child care. Fosterage is perceived as an aspect of the practice of "solidarity," as discussed by one study respondent:

POLICYMAKER: The characteristic of social life here is the spirit of sharing with the family. This has ramifications on money. People with money are called upon to share resources and they support a great number of people. Those who care, have difficulty saving. They can't invest for the future. This is not a value judgment, but this is what I have observed.

The stability of contemporary couples and their unions (cohabiting without formal marriage, polygamy, and monogamy) was a concern of men and women in all respondent groups. Observations at the Office of the Magistrate where marriages are performed suggest reasons for this concern. In each district, the magistrate performs marriages on a specific day of the week. On the day that marriage procedures were observed, all of the newlyweds were in their mid- to late thirties and some of the men were older. When the anthropologist asked a key informant and other research team members why there were no young couples, she was informed that "young people cannot afford to be married." Ideally, a man must first have "a position" before he enters a civil marriage, and that takes a long time for many men in Abidjan. A couple might live together until the man finds a stable position. In another discussion, a male informant further explained why respondents were concerned about the institution of marriage: "In the context of a dwindling economy, there is stiff competition among women for employed men." He also explained that "Ivoirian men consider their home where their children are. And before a couple is formally married, whether by traditional or legal marriage, it is to a woman's advantage to have many children. A man is less likely to leave a woman with whom he has children."

In Abidjan, marriage is often the formal legitimation of an existing union, and respondents associated marriage with an increase in prestige in the community. Through marriage, a man publicly assumes the role of family "provider" and thus announces that he has obtained economic stability, during a period when attaining this goal has become increasingly difficult. On the other hand, a woman who may have already given birth to several of her mate's children solidifies her children's inheritance and formalizes their kinship links through marriage.

Aspects of Family Life That Need Improvement. Statements from all respondent groups indicated that the education of children and adults and the need to increase the amount and quality of the communication among family members were aspects of family life that could be improved. Some respondents also reported the need to limit births.

Of 20 policymakers, 16 referred to the education of adults or children as a way of improving family life. Most policymakers saw the state and the government ministries as the primary force responsible for improving family life, although the family responsibility was mentioned in five responses and the role of private associations was mentioned in four. Comparatively, statements from health care providers indicated that parents *and* the government were responsible for improving aspects of family life in Côte d'Ivoire. Health care providers also mentioned that responsibility for improving family life should be shared by the family, health care providers, society, the elite, religious chiefs, and youth. Consumers specifically mentioned the role of staff at the government-sponsored maternal and child health clinics (to educate and better care for women, and to inform the population about family planning) and of fathers (to be responsible for their children, honor legal marriage, and eliminate the practice of polygamy).

The Role of the Government, Health Care Providers, and the Lay Population in Maternal Health and Setting Reproductive Goals

Role of the Government. Policymakers saw the government's role in maternal health and family planning programs as (*1*) providing the infrastructure, equipment, and staff necessary to deliver basic health care services to the population; (*2*) conducting research on the needs of the population; (*3*) ensuring that health care providers have been technically trained to deliver family planning services; and (*4*) determining and developing policies.

Health care providers in public and private health centers identified the following five areas as the government's responsibility in maternal and child health: (*1*) providing material and financial resources; (*2*) training health personnel; (*3*) sensitizing and educating the population; (*4*) creating the substructures for delivering services; and (*5*) establishing standards of care and providing guidelines for service delivery.

Consumers said that they wanted the government to make all services and medications accessible by reducing or eliminating the cost and stocking the health centers with medicines. Focus group participants often expressed hostility and anxiety when discussing the possibility of additional fees for contraceptive services. The need for the government to inform the population about changes in fees and service delivery was also mentioned.

Role of Health Care Providers. Although respondents in each category indicated that health care providers were responsible for delivering services, health care providers themselves perceived their role also to include informing, advising, and educating consumers. Responses of health care providers in individual and focus group interviews were similar, regardless of their affiliation with a public or private health facility or type of facility. In the two independent codings of health care provider data, the order of the frequency of the coded responses was constant: highest ranked (as indicated by the greatest frequency of individual and focus group interviews in which mentioned) was the role of informing, advising, and educating the public; preventive and curative services were second.

In contrast to discussions among health care providers, focus group discussions among consumers indicated a basic concern with the conduct of the staff during the provider–client interaction. During the clinical encounter, consumers often perceived the health care providers' behavior and tone of voice as harsh. Of 45 statements on this topic by consumers in focus groups, 13 referred to the staff's need to receive and treat patients kindly. Spirited discussion of this topic occurred in every age group and type of consumer focus group. Eight groups referred to the need for health care providers to act in a more nurturing manner when treating patients.

Role of the Lay Population. Policymakers said that the public's responsibility included paying for care, using the health services, self-motivating through education, adhering to government guidelines, and being responsible for good health. In contrast, health care providers' statements regarding the people's responsibility could be categorized into two themes: understanding and following advice of health care providers; and sharing the cost of health services. Consumer respondents said that the people's role included assisting the family financially, sensitizing the population, observing proper hygiene, and helping the government to construct or equip the health facilities where family planning services could be delivered. Half of the statements that suggested providing financial assistance to families came from adolescents.

Responsibility for Birth Spacing. Respondents in all three categories viewed "the couple" as the unit responsible for spacing or limiting births. When asked about the meaning of "the couple," the respondents and the Ivoirian interviewers agreed that the term included the man and woman involved in a sexual union, as well as their kin who have some influence over the number of children a couple should have. Responses such as "the individual," "a man," or "a woman" were the least frequently cited by all respondent types.

In individual interviews of health care providers regarding responsibility for childbearing decisions, the second most frequently cited responses referred to "the government" or "the health care providers" (staff who deliver services) as having responsibility for birth spacing. In the 15 health care provider focus groups, consensus from about half indicated that "the couple" had this responsibility, and one-third placed the responsibility on the government.

The dominant response from the consumers interviewed was also "the couple," and statements from several consumer focus group participants suggested that this dominant response may be the norm, but that the modern urban family structure is in a state of flux. Traditional as well as modern norms may govern sexual and marital relationships. For example, one consumer focus group participant said, "It is better if the two can reach an agreement; if not, it is the woman who has to take charge." A few statements from consumers indicated that the individual woman or man may have some influence in determining family size. For example, this statement from another consumer focus group suggested the role that men may have in birth spacing: "Men need to be aware of the health risks [of pregnancy] for women and the alternatives, because men have a lot of influence." In this and other statements, respondents acknowledged male pressure on women to conceive and have children. Other statements from informants confirmed that the more children a woman has with her mate, the more likely their union will be established by either traditional or civil marriage.

Field Observations

During the course of the fieldwork, the research team visited many sites frequented by Abidjan residents: health centers, hospitals, churches, homes, marketplaces, grocery stores, nightclubs, beauty shops, employment sites, government social service offices, the university campus, and rural villages where some urban respondents go on weekends to visit their relatives. The integration of various aspects of different cultures was evident in the varied hairstyles and fashions, as well as in the diverse types and cost of durable goods sold in the central market in Treichville, one of Abidjan's oldest and most densely populated communes.

Urban residents were avid consumers of modern health services at all of the health facilities that we visited. Waiting rooms at the AIBEF clinics, the MCH clinics, and university hospitals were usually filled or overflowing with patients seeking care, and the pharmacists and drug sellers in the marketplaces had a steady stream of customers. The influence of modern medicine was apparent from the type of medicines displayed in stores and sold in small markets and vendor stands throughout the city and suburbs.

The extent to which many modern concepts and practices, including health-related practices, have diffused into modern, urban Abidjan culture is impressive, standing in stark contrast to the reported low usage rate of modern contraceptives.

Policy Implications

This chapter summarizes similarities and differences among study respondents on two research themes: perceptions of the family, and the role of various social segments in provision of maternal health services and in decisions about child spacing. Individual and group interviews, field observations, and key informant interviews were used to identify and describe cultural factors that could assist in the development of culturally appropriate population policy in Côte d'Ivoire.

Study findings should be considered valid for several reasons. First, each interview guide was translated into French, translated back into English, and pretested with subjects similar to our respondent population. Second, the focus groups represented a cross section of the health care provider and consumer populations. Third, the data from the health care provider focus groups were consonant with and complemented those from individual interviews. Fourth, four of six members of the core research team were Ivoirian researchers who were involved during all stages of data collection, interpretation, and analysis and who were familiar with the local languages and cultural practices.

The data from the two study themes reported here have implications for both policy and program development.

Implications of Theme 1: Perceptions of the Family

The large extended family was the valued form of family structure in contemporary Abidjan; respondents also recognized the need to limit births. African societies are stereotypically described as preferring large numbers of children (Frank, 1987). This might suggest that Africans have little interest in birth spacing or in limiting the number of births. However, the timing of births has traditionally been an important concern of African societies (Mabogunje, 1981; Omari, 1989) and has been suggested as the rationale for several fertility-inhibiting cultural practices, such as prolonged breastfeeding and postpartum sexual abstinence (Schoenmaeckers et al., 1981). Statements from our study respondents indicating an interest in birth spacing or limiting family size are supported by a surge in the number of new users of modern contraceptives (Huntington, 1991) and a growing interest in the use of modern contraceptive methods (Tafforeau and Timyan, 1987; Timyan, 1987).

Ivoirians' interest in limiting family size seems unfettered by their appreciation for strong, extended family linkages (Côte d'Ivoire Ministry of Health, 1991; Timyan, 1987). Solidarity reinforces social and biological ties and supports cultural practices such as fosterage. Through fosterage, an individual in an extended family may enjoy the benefits of a large family without giving birth to a lot of children. Respondents in our study suggested that when there are too many relatives and too few resources to share, the concept of solidarity can be weakened, as can extended family links.

There is a need to broaden the focus of family planning services from women of childbearing age to all adults in the extended family. If the target of family planning is not broadened, cultural practices may present obstacles to individual fertility regulation. In Abidjan and elsewhere in Africa, initial response to the acceptance of modern contraceptives was slow. This may have been influenced by a culturally inappropriate campaign that focused on individual women rather than on a more relevant network of persons who can influence long-term use of contraception. For example, early works by Fortes (1949, 1953) documented the corporate nature of societies that are organized in matrilineal or patrilineal descent groups. Whether matrilineal or patrilineal, men wield considerable power in African family decision making because ancestry and inheritance rights are reckoned through maternal or paternal male relatives. Men (in their roles as spouses) were found to have a critical role in a woman's decision to seek and use family planning services in the Ivorian Demographic Health Survey results of 1992 (Sombo et al., 1995), the Ivorian Abidjan PEFPS (Wilson, 1991), in Zimbabwe (Mbizvo and Donald, 1991), and in Tanzania (Omari, 1989).

Recently, a study of women using family planning services in Abidjan indicated that the objection to a pregnancy by a mate was the most frequently cited reason for having an abortion (35%) (Huntington et al., 1993). Demographic Health Study results concur with findings in our study on the decisive role of men: in Côte d'Ivoire, when spouses disagree on desired family size, women tended to want fewer children than men (Sombo et al., 1995). Taken together, these data suggest that program planners should target both men and women for family planning services and make a focused effort to target men.

Family planning messages in the media might identify birth spacing and birth limitation as a concern of all family members (youth, young adults, and the elderly) and the Ministry of Health should consider directing family planning information to members of the entire extended family in Côte d'Ivoire.

Instability in the economy seems to be influencing family structure as well as marital and childbearing strategies. Although Abidjan residents expressed appreciation for the concept of family solidarity, policymakers and health care providers interviewed individually felt that family solidarity is burdensome when only a few family members are employed and can earn money for the family. The statements of study respondents suggest that Abidjan residents recognized the constraints that the economy placed on family structure and sought solutions at the individual and social level. Consumers wanted fathers to exercise more responsibility for their children, and policymakers and health workers wanted families to limit their births to the number each couple could support. Respondents stated that marriage is an institution that Abidjan residents would like to preserve, but economic forces seemed to influence this institution too.

Respondent statements regarding the pressure on women to have children before marrying their mates (who may be financially unstable early in the relationship) are echoed by Bledsoe (1990): "A woman can press her economic demands on a particular man, whether or not they [the couple] call their relationship a marriage, with far greater leverage if she has a child by him." In this cultural context, it is advantageous for a woman, especially if she is uneducated or from a family of lower socioeconomic status, to have numerous children with her partner without limiting or spacing births. According to Bledsoe (1990), children can legitimize a woman's claim to her partner's resources and increase the probability that their relationship will be formalized by legal or traditional marriage. A sound population policy should focus on employment, education, and the provision of job skills, as well as the limitation of births.

Implications of Theme 2: Role of the Government, Health Care Providers, and the Lay Population in Maternal Health and Fertility Regulation

The government, health care providers, society, and extended family members were perceived to share responsibility for maternal and child health and birth spacing. In many Western societies, it is assumed that the individual (usually the woman in the case of family planning services) is responsible for health care decision making (Caldwell, 1993). Statements from study respondents suggest that residents in Abidjan may perceive the responsibilities for maternal and child health and child spacing to be distributed to a larger social unit, not just the individual mother. As such, it might be acceptable for the government to develop plans for population control that indicate the individual's role within the context of family health and community health, as well as the health of the nation.

Study findings regarding the influence of the couple and other family members in reproductive decision making suggest that plans for the distribution of contraceptive information and services should target women of childbearing age, their mates, and other relatives. According to Freeman (1987), "Small primary groups of relatives, friends, and neighbors are universally the people through whom most traditional and new behavior patterns are learned and validated." For program managers using this approach, the structure of Ivoirian families can be viewed as an enabling rather than an inhibiting factor. For example, family planning products could be marketed as commodities that can improve the quality of life for the extended family, a concept that supports the continuity of family solidarity and requires full support by all family members. If practiced by most adults (males and females), family planning may increase the number of employed adults in a family who can financially support unemployed extended family members.

Consumers are concerned about the costs of family planning services and access to contraceptive information. Differences in points of view expressed by health care providers and consumers regarding the financing of family planning services have historical sources. Before this study, consumers in Abidjan had enjoyed the benefits of 30 years of free service at the clinics and hospitals. Although the current trend in economic development may encourage a fee-for-service system for cost recovery (World Bank, 1987), consumers in Abidjan should be informed that the bulk of the cost is subsidized by the government and the fees consumers pay for services are a relatively small proportion of total costs.

Adolescents in Abidjan and elsewhere in Africa (Adetoro et al., 1991; Barker and Rich, 1992) have expressed interest in contraceptive services. Adolescent respondents in our study were especially concerned about the costs of family planning services. In the past, the youth were betrothed or married during their adolescent years, and the traditional social institutions, such as initiation schools, prepared them for their responsibilities in marriage and sexual relations. Westernization has brought the acceptance of extended adolescence, during which teenagers pursue highly valued formal education with the hopes of obtaining employment. At the same time, these traditional institutions for training youth are collapsing and have not been selected as the conduit of new contraceptive technology (Omari, 1989). For adolescent girls, an unplanned pregnancy usually means the termination of education or leads to an abortion (Boohene et al., 1991; Nichols et al., 1986). In Côte d'Ivoire, abortions are illegal, although key informants in our study noted the availability and routine use of abortion as a method of family planning in Abidjan (see also Huntington et al., 1993). In this regard, Abidjan adolescents may be similar to other African youth (Barker and Rich, 1992). A population policy that makes family planning services available and affordable for adolescents can shield them from unwanted pregnancies and the need to seek septic illicit abortions.

Health care providers and their clients had different attitudes toward the importance and quality of patient–provider relations. The family planning literature has suggested that patient education and interpersonal communication skills are often overlooked but can influence acceptance and continued use of contraceptives (Bruce, 1987). A Nigerian study of physician attitudes and practices provides a good example. Although physicians in the study reported having smaller family size than most Nigerians and were more likely to be practicing family planning, 40% believed family planning was foreign to their culture and that it promoted promiscuity (Covington et al., 1986). Attitudes such as this could have an important effect on service delivery. It is recommended that health worker training should emphasize the two key components of quality service delivery: technical competence and interpersonal skills.

Caldwell and Caldwell (1990) have suggested that unilineal (matrilineal or patrilineal) descent systems and African religious beliefs have encouraged high rates of childbearing and discouraged the use of modern contraception throughout sub-Saharan Africa. Perhaps one reason for the slow adoption of modern contraceptive technology in Abidjan and throughout Côte d'Ivoire is the absence of cultural approaches that address the complex of deep-rooted values on which Ivoirian society is based. The delayed diffusion of contraceptive technology (relative to the diffusion of other technological advancements) is also undoubtedly influenced by government policy related to the availability of contraceptives and family planning information. Statements on the two themes discussed in this chapter suggest that traditional values about gender roles and the structure and role of the family may have a strong influence over a woman's decision to seek out and use modern contraceptives.

Conclusions

Implications of the study data for Ivoirian population program and policy development include the following:

1. There is support for family planning among policymakers, health care providers, and consumers.
2. Family planning should be promoted as a means of increasing Ivoirian family solidarity.
3. The target population for family planning services should include women of childbearing age and their mates, influential members of their extended family, and youth.
4. Health care provider training in family planning services should emphasize interpersonal as well as technical skills.
5. The degree to which consumers will financially support a fee-based family planning service is uncertain and needs further assessment.

Côte d'Ivoire is responding to a growing demand for family planning services. The Ministry of Health has developed a draft plan for population policy that includes standards of care for public and private family planning services. The results of our study can help to ensure that these services will be delivered in a way that is acceptable to the health care providers and to consumers. In modifying policy and developing programs there is a need for usable data that reflect the understandings, values, and desires of the consumers. The challenge lies in the successful integration of these findings into policies and programs.

Note

1. Van Willigen and Dewalt (1985) refer to policy ethnography as a data collection technique. In this chapter the term "policy ethnography" refers to applied ethnographic research for policy development. Policy ethnography, like traditional ethnography, uses basic anthropological techniques: participant observation, key informant interviewing, and structured and semistructured interviews conducted individually and in groups. The data are used for policy formation and program evaluation.

Acknowledgments

Funding for this study was provided by the United States Agency for International Development (USAID) Africa Child Survival Initiative–Combating Childhood Communicable Diseases (ASCI-CCCD) Africa Regional Project (698-0421) and the Ministry of Health and Social Protection in Côte d'Ivoire. We thank Nanette Barkey (American Public Health Association intern), Constance Binde (Ivorian Center for Economic and Social Research, Abidjan, Côte d'Ivoire), and Yvonne Bosso (Ministry of Womens Affairs, Abidjan, Côte d'Ivoire), who served as research assistants for the project and members of the core research staff. Additionally, we thank Lynn Mohammed of REDSO/ USAID; Sylvia Acquah of the CCCD Project in Abidjan; James Herrington, the CCCD technical officer; Modupe Broderick, the CCCD project officer, Côte d'Ivoire; and Charles DeBose of USAID/REDSO. For technical and editorial reviews we are indebted to Maureen Birmingham, Emmanuel Joseph, Cathy Melvin, Melinda Moore, Kathleen Parker, George Stroh, Virginia Sturwold, and Andrew Vernon (Centers for Disease Control and Prevention), Chris Elias (the Population Council), Judith Timyan (Population Services International), and other peer reviewers.

References

Adetoro OO, Babarinsa AB, Sotiloye S (1991) Sociocultural factors in adolescent septic illicit abortions in Ilorin, Nigeria. *African Journal of Medicine and Medical Sciences* 20:141–153.

Barker GK, Rich S (1992) Influences on adolescent sexuality in Nigeria and Kenya: findings from recent focus-group discussions. *Studies in Family Planning* 23:199–210.

Bledsoe C (1990) Transformations in sub-Saharan African marriage and fertility. *Annals of the American Academy of Political and Social Science* 510:115–125.

Boohene E, Tsodzai J, Hardee-Cleaveland K, Weir S, Janowitz B (1991) Fertility and contraceptive use among young adults in Harare, Zimbabwe. *Studies in Family Planning* 22:264–271.

Bruce J (1987) Users' perspectives on contraceptive technology and delivery systems: highlighting some feminist issues. *Technology in Society* 9:359–383.

Caldwell JC (1993) Health transition: the cultural, social and behavioral determinants of health in the Third World. *Social Science and Medicine* 36:125–135.

Caldwell JC, Caldwell P (1990) High fertility in sub-Saharan Africa. *Scientific American* 262:118–125.

Centers for Disease Control (1983) Family Planning Methods and Practice. Africa. Atlanta: Centers for Disease Control, Center for Chronic Disease Prevention and Health Promotion and Division of Reproductive Health.

Côte d'Ivoire Ministry of Health (1991) Seminaire national sur la planification familiale en Côte d'Ivoire, Grand Bassam, Ivory Coast, April 1–6.

Covington DL, Otolorin EO, Janowitz B, Gates DS, Lamptey P, Ladipo OA (1986) Physician attitudes and family planning in Nigeria. *Studies in Family Planning* 17:172–180.

Etienne M (1979) The case for social maternity: adoption of children by urban Baule women. *Dialectical Anthropology* 4:237–242.

Fathalla MF (1990) "The Challenge of Safe Motherhood." In: Health Care of Women and Children in Developing Countries. HM Wallace, K Giri, eds. Oakland, Calif: Third Party Publishing Co., pp. 219–228.

Ford TR, Arcury TA (1984) Population and health in the developing world: research perspectives for medical anthropologists. *Social Science and Medicine* 18:855–859.

Fortes M (1949) The Web of Kinship among the Tallensi. London: Oxford University Press.

Fortes M (1953) The structure of unilineal descent groups. *American Anthropologist* 55:17–41.

Frank O (1987) The demand for fertility control in sub-Saharan Africa. *Studies in Family Planning* 18:181–201.

Freeman R (1987) The contribution of social science research to population policy and family planning program effectiveness. *Studies in Family Planning* 18:57–82.

Futures Group (1988) Côte d'Ivoire: Population et Developpement. Réssources pour l'Analyse de la Population et de son Impact sur le Développement (RAPID). Washington, DC: The Futures Group.

Haryono S, Piet N, Stirling F, Ross J (1981) Family planning attitudes in urban Indonesia: findings from focus group research. *Studies in Family Planning* 12:433–441.

Huntington D (1991) Trip Report—Côte d'Ivoire. New York: Population Council. Unpublished report.

Huntington D, Mensch B, Toubia N (1993) A new approach to eliciting information about induced abortion. *Studies in Family Planning* 24:120–124.

Knodel J, van de Walle E (1979) Lessons from the past: policy implications of historical fertility studies. *Population and Development Review* 5:217–246.

Mabogunje AL (1981) "The Policy Implications of Changes in Child-Spacing Practices in Tropical Africa." In: Child Spacing in Tropical Africa. Traditions and Change. HJ Page, R Lesthaeghe, eds. London: Academic Press, pp. 303–315.

Maine D, et al. (1987) Prevention of Maternal Deaths in Developing Countries. Program Options and Practical Considerations. World Bank paper prepared for the International Safe Motherhood Conference, Nairobi, February 10–13.

Mbizvo MT, Donald JA (1991) Family planning knowledge, attitudes, and practices of men in Zimbabwe. *Studies in Family Planning* 22:31–38.

Microlytics (1989) GOfer 2.0, MS-DOS Version. Pittsford, NY: Signum Microsystems.

Nichols D, Ladipo OA, Paxman JM, Otolorin EO (1986) Sexual behavior, contraceptive practice, and reproductive health among Nigerian adolescents. *Studies in Family Planning* 17:100–106.

Omari CK (1989) Socio-cultural Factors in Modern Family Planning Methods in Tanzania. Lewiston, NY: Edwin Mellen Press.

Population Reference Bureau (1991) 1991 World Population Data Sheet. Washington, DC: Population Reference Bureau.

Reddy MA, ed. (1994) Statistical Abstract of the World. Detroit: Gale Research.

Schearer SB (1981) The value of focus group research for social action programs. *Studies in Family Planning* 12:407–408.

Schoenmaeckers R, Shah IH, Lesthaeghe R, Tambashe O (1981) "The Child Spacing Tradition and the Postpartum Taboo in Tropical Africa: Anthropological Evidence." In: Child Spacing in Tropical Africa. Traditions and Change. HJ Page, R Lesthaeghe, eds. London: Academic Press, pp. 25–71.

Singh K, Ratnam SS (1990) "Family Planning: Clinical Aspects." In: Health Care of Women and Children in Developing Countries. HM Wallace, K Giri, eds. Oakland, Calif: Third Party Publishing Co., pp. 204–218.

Sombo N, Kouassi L, Koffi AK, Schoemaker J, Barrère M, Barrère B, Poukouta P (1995) Enquête Démographique et de Santé, Côte d'Ivoire 1994. Calverton, Md: Institut National de la Statistique et Macro International.

Stycos JM (1981) A critique of focus group and survey research: the machismo case. *Studies in Family Planning* 12:450–456.

Tafforeau J, Timyan J (1987) Analyse. Enquête quantitative. Bouaflé (Unpublished report).

Timyan J (June 1987) Report: Focus Group Discussions. Community Primary Health Care Project, Bouaflé, Côte d'Ivoire. New York: Columbia University, Center for Population and Family Health.

USAID (1990) Proposal for integrating MCH/FP activities into the CCCD Project in Côte d'Ivoire. Abidjan, Côte d'Ivoire/Washington, DC: US Agency for International Development, October.

USAID (1991) Project identification document (PID) for the family planning and health project in Côte d'Ivoire. Abidjan, Côte d'Ivoire/Washington, DC: US Agency for International Development, April.

US State Department Bureau of Public Affairs (1990) Background Notes. Côte d'Ivoire. Department of State Publication 8119. Background Notes Series. Washington, DC: US Government Printing Office.

Van Willigen J, Dewalt BR (1985) Training Manual in Policy Ethnography. Washington, DC: American Anthropological Association.

Wilson RP (1991) Technical Report. Policy Ethnography for Family Planning, Côte d'Ivoire, 1991. Atlanta: Centers for Disease Control and Prevention, International Health Program Office.

WHO (1991) Maternal Mortality. A Global Factbook. Geneva: World Health Organization.

World Bank (1987) Financing Health Care Services in Developing Countries. Washington, DC: World Bank.

13

Integrating Mental Health Care and Traditional Healing in Puerto Rico: Lessons from an Early Experiment

JOAN D. KOSS-CHIOINO

In response to resolutions passed in 1977 by the Thirtieth World Health Assembly and by the WHO meeting on "Promotion and Development of Traditional Medicine" (WHO, 1978), the journal *Social Science and Medicine* explored the "Utilization of Indigenous Healers in Health Delivery Systems" (Maclean and Bannerman, 1982). This issue recognized that "traditional medicine is still an established and lively manifestation of culture" (Maclean and Bannerman, 1982:1815). Neumann and Lauro (1982) detailed the positive aspects of linking Western biomedicine and traditional ethnomedicines as better access to high-quality care; more appropriate referral for severe or special cases; opportunities for traditional healers to increase their skills; relief of high demand on biomedical health care services; and low-cost expansion of public health care.

More than 10 years later there has been little progress toward the goal of integrating traditional ethnomedicines with biomedical health care in the public health domain (Chi, 1994). Since the Aro project in Nigeria (Ademuwagun et al., 1979; Lambo, 1978) there have been only a few reported programs intended to link ethnomedical health care with biomedical mental health care (or prevention) at the community level (Bergman, 1973; Bibeau, 1985; Chi, 1994; Ruiz and Langrod, 1976). There is, however, a growing anthropological and psychiatric literature that addresses the importance of integrating traditional or folk treatment into mental health care delivery (e.g., Gaines, 1992; Hughes, 1996; Kiev, 1972).

Healing practices not included within Western biomedicine, categorized as both traditional and alternative (i.e., newly emergent), have been studied for at least three decades (see, for example, Ademuwagun et al., 1979; Kleinman, 1980; Lebra, 1982; Nichter, 1992; Snow, 1993). Complex relationships, including informal patient referrals between traditional medicine and biomedicine, have been documented in a number of societies, particularly in Latin America and sub-Saharan Africa (Ballay, 1986; Ezeji and Sarvela, 1992; Finkler, 1985; Harwood, 1977; Koss-Chioino, 1992, 1995; Oyebola et al., 1981). However, relatively few studies describe and/or evaluate programs focused on linking or integrating traditional (or alternative) medicine with public health institutions.

Most programs that focus on traditional healers have been either informal and unsystematic or short-lived experiments with inconclusive outcomes (e.g., Bergman, 1973; Ruiz and Langrod, 1976). Many have simply not been well documented and, unfortunately, there has been little exploration of the reasons for negative outcomes or lack of continuity of programs.

To examine the context of the success or failure of such programs critically, this chapter begins by describing the sociopolitical, religious, and medical contexts of the planning and organization of an experimental project in Puerto Rico carried out some 20 years ago (1976–1979).[1] The Therapist-Spiritist Training Project was officially focused on mental health care in the community as part of the community mental health initiative. Although there have been some lasting effects, the project did not become formally institutionalized within the public health system when its three-year tenure ended, a common fate for projects that seek to introduce systemic changes. A description of the methods used in developing the project, including methods of evaluation, follows. The ways in which the project was organized, its successes and failures relative to formal and informal aspects of organization and process, are discussed next. To understand the lack of continuity when the experiment ended, we then consider details of how the project worked for individual participants and describe aspects of its conceptualization, organization, and eventful course. Intended and unintended outcomes are described next, and some of the complexities of this particular model for bridging traditional and contemporary biomedical healing systems are assessed. A final section summarizes salient issues and prospects associated with the formal integration of ethnomedical healing systems and public health and mental health care, as reflected both in the literature and the Puerto Rican experience.

Background: The Social, Political, and Religious Context of Traditional Healing and Mental Health Care in Puerto Rico

Puerto Rico's political and economic status has been tied to the United States since the Treaty of Paris in 1898, a result of the Spanish-American War. Approximately 3.75 million people inhabit the island and migrate at will to the

United States, mainly to densely populated cities in the Northeast, often returning as fortunes allow. Despite this continuous contact, identity remains specifically Puerto Rican, persisting even in third- and fourth-generation "NeoRicans" born on the mainland (Rodriguez Cortes, 1990).

From its founding as a Spanish colony to its present status as a "free associated state" under benevolent US domination, Puerto Rico has always been a place between, more of a crossroads and a way station than a place focused on itself. Puerto Ricans are caught in the cross-streams of two cultures, Euroamerican and Latin American, subject to extensive cultural change yet maintaining a distinct core of cultural traditions. They are also heirs to two very different worldviews, which might be labeled "scientific" and "spiritual."

One example of this seeming contradiction is the widespread religious-healing cult of "Spiritism" (*Espiritismo*). Its ritual is centered on "working" with spirits in hundreds of small, household-based *centros* (and a few larger temples), presided over mostly by female mediums who hold two or more weekly sessions with an audience of 25 to 100 persons. The mediums, sitting around a table, become possessed by spirits and experience visions in order to heal (*sanar*) the supplicants, who bring a variety of health and social problems (Garrison, 1977a, 1977b; Harwood, 1977; Koss, 1975, 1977; Rogler and Hollingshead, 1961). Variations on this form of religious healing (found in parallel forms in all of Latin America and much of the Mediterranean) have developed extensively over the past 30 years, incorporating features of the Afro-Cuban cult of *Santería* on both the island and the continent.

Although historical evidence indicates that Spiritism has been in Puerto Rico since at least 1873, its practice has continually met varying degrees of opposition from both the Catholic Church and the biomedical establishment since its introduction (Koss, 1976). In the mid-1970s most Spiritist centers followed the teachings of the books of Allan Kardec, the pen name of a French scholar, Hippolyte Denizarth Leon Rivail (1803–1869). Spiritism, considered by its French intellectual advocates as the exploration of a newly discovered realm of beings, was introduced into Puerto Rico as the new "psychological" science by elites who studied in France and Spain. It almost immediately met opposition by the medical boards established by Spain in its colonies. In the latter part of the nineteenth century, however, important government officials were known to be believers (Koss, 1976). With medical acculturation due to the presence of, and subsidies from, the United States, and ongoing modernization of public institutions patterned after those in North America, Spiritism gradually went underground yet maintained a large base of adherents among the poor as well as the elite (still including, it is rumored, government officials).

At the same time, the community mental health movement grew in popularity in the United States, destined like many other public health programs to be adopted—with sponsorship from the United States Public Health Service—in Puerto Rico.[2] Before the 1960s, in most states, as well as in Puerto Rico, public mental health meant either long-term residential treatment in a state mental hospital or inpatient care and outpatient emergency clinics in acute care hospital settings. However, ideas about the causes of mental illness had expanded by the 1960s to include interpersonal relations, family influences, emotional traumas, and other psychosocial phenomena. New psychotropic medications were so promising that persons with severe mental illness were expected to have long periods of remission from dysfunctional states. Community-based institutions, such as day hospitals, halfway houses, and 24-hour emergency services, were needed to permit the mentally ill to leave hospitals and live in the community.

These concerns and newer ideas about mental illness as directly related to behavioral and social factors opened the way for social scientists to take part in the community mental health movement, since they were knowledgeable about social relations in communities. This period was also a time for the maturation of ideas about US ethnic minority group needs and rights, following upon epidemiological studies which concluded that immigrants were at greater risk for mental illness than the resident population. In the early 1970s, newly instituted approaches to mental health led to the National Institute of Mental Health (NIMH) funding projects which explored the characteristics and use of traditional healing practices in ethnic minority communities.

In Puerto Rico 11 community mental health centers were established during the 1960s and 1970s. Community assessments in preparation for their establishment frequently noted that Spiritist centers were a widespread healing resource. Aspects of the relationship between Spiritism and persons with severe psychiatric illness had been described by Rogler and Hollingshead (1961, 1965), who viewed Spiritism as an important source of support for the mentally ill and their families, as well as a means to explain etiology and the course of the illness within an indigenous frame of reference. During the ensuing period I carried out studies of psychosocial aspects of Spiritism in Philadelphia, Pennsylvania (Koss, 1965, 1975, 1977), as did Garrison (1977a, 1977b) and Harwood (1977) in New York City. Following almost six years of research into Spiritism in Puerto Rico and a consultancy with the mental health division of the Puerto Rican Department of Health, I was informed of interest within the Division of Manpower, Research and Training of the National Institute of Mental Health in a project that would formally link traditional healing in the community with the Department of Health's Division of Mental Health.

Method and Design of the Project

Understanding Two Systems of Mental Health Care

From 1968 to the conceptualization of the project in 1974, I carried out a series of ethnographic studies of Spiritist practices, practitioners, and clients in large urban *centros* in four different sectors of the San Juan metropolitan area. Two of the Spiritist centers were attended mostly by middle-class persons, the others by lower-income persons. After collecting data through unstructured interviews and hundreds of hours of observations in the metropolitan area, I sampled centers in small Puerto Rican towns and rural barrios recommended by Spiritist adherents, friends, or colleagues. The studies provided information on the range and variation in Spiritist practices across the island of Puerto Rico.

One of the larger temples in San Juan offered weekly training classes in mediumship, and, at the urging of the president of the temple, both my research assistant and I enrolled to gain better understanding of Spiritist practice and belief. Our training experiences underscored the great differences in the experience of treating emotionally distressed or disordered persons with a biomedical tool kit of knowledge and medications, compared to the intimacy, in Spiritism, of sympathetically experiencing a client's distress within one's own body and then allowing spirits to take possession of it to diagnose and heal (Koss-Chioino, 1992, 1995, 1996.)

Several conclusions from earlier studies became important in planning the Therapist-Spiritist project. For example, it was clear that all of the small centers and the larger temples were autonomous, almost entirely dependent on a single individual, the leader or president. This person was usually the organizer of the *centro*. Sessions were held in his or her home, in special rooms built or set aside for this purpose. Moreover, the small *centros* often did not endure over long periods but were subject to divisiveness, then abandoned when serious conflict arose between a medium and the president, if the latter's hegemony and spiritual faculties were questioned (Koss, 1977). The implication of this hierarchical arrangement for the planned linkage project was that we knew in advance that *centro* leaders had to be recruited individually. Subsequently, an introduction to their mediums might be forthcoming, and they too might be recruited.

I also learned that at least three-fourths of the mediums were women, many of whom were also *centro* presidents. However, a number of men were also *centro* presidents. When married couples, siblings, or other relatives worked together, the man was almost always the leader, even if the woman was the most prestigious, active medium. An understanding of gender, age, and occupation among Spiritist practitioners was important to project planning in order to recruit participants in each of the project communities. Moreover, the survey of Spiritist centers on the island provided information about which communities had Spiritist practitioners (especially presidents) willing to participate in a program to formally link them with mental health care professionals and public health institutions. They became a "community advisory group" and some were seminar lecturers in years two and three.

During the first studies I was well aware that Spiritist practices intended relief of distress in both supplicants and mediums (who are always former supplicants), but I had not yet fully appreciated Spiritism as an ethnomedical system. This appreciation came as a result of two events. First, I led a group of students in a study of the community adjacent to a mental health center in a small town. We asked about physical and emotional distress, and help seeking, using a semistructured interview and the Cornell Medical Index (Brodman et al., 1956; Koss, 1975). We found that the women who were interviewed, who were the only persons available during the daytime, reported a very large number of symptoms (relative to standards set for the Cornell Medical Index). In reporting where they sought help for emotional distress it became clear that Spiritist mediums, priests, and older women relatives were more often consulted than the mental health personnel available to the community. We also concluded that particular symptoms were associated with particular sources of help, and that help-seeking paths were influenced by prior successes or failures in finding relief. The linkage project was later able to describe systematically the types of complaints that were brought to the mental health system in contrast to those brought to Spiritists, and how both could be utilized in a complementary way in treating an episode of distress (Koss-Chioino, 1992, 1995).

The second event occurred in conjunction with my work as a consultant with the Health Department. In discussing patients with the therapists, ambivalences expressed by the mental health professionals alerted me to the many contradictions between biomedical mental health care delivery and spirit healing. Differences in practice between the two systems indicated two very different sets of world- and self-views, which mental health professionals from families involved in Spiritism found irreconcilable when dealing with patients from the same background. This commonly led to discomfort and denial on the part of the mental health professionals, but also motivated them to understand enough about Spiritism to compare the systems, each on its own merit.

In turn, the Spiritists uniformly voiced their desire to understand biomedical approaches to mental illness (particularly neurophysiology and psychotropic medications), in part potentially to adopt some techniques (in their usual eclectic style), but also to acquire knowledge of when and how to refer clients whom the spirits could not help. These two positions (therapists' and Spiritists') were keys to designing the content of the seminars and led to the perspective we eventually advocated, that each of the healing systems was unique, yet partial parallels could be bases for valid comparisons. To reinforce the dual-perspective approach, case review conferences were also designed to compare "matched cases" treated in each system (which proved more difficult).

Designing an Integrated System

As originally conceived, the Therapist-Spiritist Training Project had three general goals:

1. To establish a forum for the meaningful exchange of information between Spiritist mediums and mental health professionals (physicians, psychologists, nurses, social workers, and mental health technicians; primary care physicians in training were later added).
2. To offer a training curriculum to transfer knowledge and skills across the two healing systems.
3. To develop new psychotherapeutic approaches from a synthesis of the most relevant and effective healing techniques in both systems.

The training program had specific objectives: to (1) augment the therapeutic skills of practitioners from both systems; (2) augment knowledge of the psychological basis of behavioral disorders for both groups; (3) develop referral networks between the two systems; (4) provide practitioners with a guided training experience that would increase clinical effectiveness; (5) provide trainees with information about community health resources and the lifestyles and patterns of interpersonal relationships among patients and clients; (6) promote mutual understanding and cooperation between therapists and Spiritists; and (7) encourage use of community mental health services by the Spiritists, and outreach activities on the part of therapists.

It was decided to run the program in three different communities, one community each year over a three-year period, to explore possible differences in community response and issues of replication.

Our experience with the two healing systems that we planned to link in a systematic way showed us that careful consideration had to be given to the construction of a framework for the project. The NIMH division that was interested in funding it focused on manpower and training; therefore, the project was officially classified as a "training project." This focus was adopted because it seemed most likely to work, given a number of conditions and constraints. First, there was the problem of acceptance of the Spiritists as colleagues by the mental health professionals, given considerable distance in social status between them. Second, Spiritists often harbored deep feelings of distress resulting from the denigration they knew existed and sometimes experienced, both as individuals and as a group. There was also some anxiety regarding possible legal consequences of their healing practices, even though there was no evidence of anyone being prosecuted, at least during the preceding 10 years. A third condition was the very different ways in which "training" routinely took place in the two systems: in biomedicine most training is formal and legally regulated, whereas Spiritist training is accomplished through mentoring and apprenticeship and is regulated by custom. It is influenced by ideas and concepts of individual practitioners. This rather important difference needed to be considered and overcome as a "constraint."

Framing the program as "continuing medical education" (CME) for the mental health professionals and as training in mental health diagnosis, etiology, and treatment for the Spiritists seemed to have good potential for bridging these differences. The CME approach was possible because of the sponsorship and interests of the Health Department and was also a way for that institution to justify the project by "educating" traditional healers about mental health and encouraging screening and referrals of their clients to mental health services. This suited the Spiritists, since they believe that lifelong learning (about the spirit world and its role in the lives of incarnate persons) is not only essential but also built into the healer persona. At the least, a "training" label and framework for the project included a format for the exchange of ideas based on the very different paradigms about illness and healing; at best it legitimized the inclusion of traditional healers in public mental health programs as "community resources" who play a potentially important role in community health.

This framework affected a number of decisions of immediate relevance, such as where to hold the meetings. The original plan was for groups of Spiritists and mental health professionals to meet twice per week, once at a designated health department facility and once at the *centro* of a Spiritist participant. Meetings in health department facilities were held at the same location for one year, then moved to another town. Meetings in *centros* rotated each week among different volunteered *centros*, because each of the Spiritists traditionally worked independently. In fact, a certain degree of competition and suspicion among Spiritists made cooperation difficult. We felt we had to recognize their rather fierce independence at the same time that the project advocated cooperation among them, as well as with the mental health professionals, in the goal of mutual education.

The plan of meeting weekly in the Spiritist centers had to be abandoned, in part because of scheduling and notification difficulties, but also because the first group of therapist participants found that the plan did not accord with the idea that they were participating in continuing medical education. The groups did meet a few times a year at Spiritist centers in order to attend a healing session. Although the hoped-for leveling in social status between the health professionals and Spiritists was not achieved through a balancing of meeting locales, locating the seminars in a public mental health facility made the project appear more legitimate to those who denigrated the Spiritists.

Recruitment of participants had to follow different guidelines for each system. In each of the three communities, prior ethnographic fieldwork provided the knowledge of how to assess Spiritist "popularity" in terms of the continuity of a *centro* over time and an expected number of regular attendees. Spiritists who had practiced five or more years and were well known in the community were invited to participate. In the recruitment of mental health participants, prior knowledge of the community mental health centers guided the selection of communities and institutions; criteria included receptivity to Spiritist practices on the part of persons in leadership roles in medical settings and a promise of cooperation on the part of the medical director of the institution. Dossiers of information (i.e., personality inventories, sociodemographic data, Profile of Mood States) and life histories were collected prior to attendance at the seminars for each person who agreed to be a "participant."

Evaluation

The project proposal outlined three evaluative measures, and others were added as the project progressed.

1. Attempts to gauge changes in the attitudes of participants regarding belief and understandings about mental illness were made with two questionnaires, one based on Spiritism and the other on psychotherapy and psychopathology, which included yes–no statements about values, ethics and cosmologies, and illness etiologies.
2. Detailed questionnaires were completed about the expected results and outcomes of treatment for 100 new patients, one from each participant (Koss, 1987).
3. To assess changes in management and treatment, histories of new patients with similar types of emotional distress—typical of the caseload of each participant—were recorded in detail during the baseline and follow-up periods of each project year.

Sessions with targeted community mental health center (CMHC) patients were videotaped; we taped entire sessions for the Spiritists because they most often treated clients in a group.

The project seminars were evaluated in two ways. First, an 11-item questionnaire was designed to measure satisfaction with the lectures and lecturers, including the type and quality of knowledge gained. Second, informal evaluation discussions accompanied by socializing were held at the completion of each half of the seminar programs each year.

In addition, yearly evaluations were made by three consultants from the United States and two from Puerto Rico (one anthropologist, four physicians), as well as the directors and some unit heads of the CMHCs and hospitals where we held programs.

The project proposal did not specify measurement of change in treatment outcomes from the beginning to the end of the study; as a training project it focused on changes that occurred among Spiritist and therapist participants and their readiness to share knowledge and link the healing systems. (Given the current body of information on treatment research, I would design the project rather differently today and examine outcomes of treatment in addition to outcomes of training.)

Initial Responses and Planned Organization

An unexpected incident shaped the project's organization and reception: I sought sponsorship first from the Department of Sociology and Anthropology at the University of Puerto Rico (where I was on the faculty), but the proposal was summarily rejected on the rationale that the study of Spiritism as a community mental health resource was not a proper social science topic because it dealt with "superstition." In great frustration I appealed to the subsecretary for mental health, who had requested my earlier consultation on the community mental health centers. A psychiatrist himself, he recalled that his wife's uncle, in emotional distress on his return from Vietnam, had been cured by a Spiritist medium after several psychiatrists had failed. He agreed to sponsor the project, which ultimately led to its approved training status.

Balance between therapists and Spiritists was integral to the structure of the seminar programs; the first session each week was equally divided between mental health professional and Spiritist lecturers. Specific topics were scheduled in advance and dual perspectives on each topic were discussed. Although the Spiritists were accustomed to volunteering their time and expertise because they considered healing an avocation, they were paid to lecture at the same rate as the health professionals.

Topics included concepts of "health and illness" and approaches to community care; human development and illness; diagnostic techniques; therapeutic techniques; psychopharmacology compared with herbal medicine; referral systems (including the Spiritists' informal referrals to physicians); organic brain syndromes and Spiritist concepts regarding somatic illness etiologies (the role of the central nervous system, trance, and possession); and "psychosomatic" illness, including Spiritist ideas of illness causation.

The second weekly session consisted of patient reviews, one from each group, with specific patients arranged in advance matched by type of distress and/or age and gender. In the beginning the Spiritists organized their presentations as they saw fit without the restrictions of a standard format. After several months of presentations some Spiritists began to adopt and modify the format used by the therapists. Discussions about the paired patients permitted comparison of treatments for similar problems across the two very different systems.

A desire to minimize status distinction between Spiritists and health professionals led to a decision to label all participants as "healers." Participants were informed of the anthropological approach to "ethnomedicine," in which healing systems in any setting, biomedicine as well as Spiritism, could be compared. (Films about traditional healing in other societies were shown during the seminars.) At first the health professionals were not happy being labeled "healers," but they became more accepting as the seminar year progressed. As mentioned earlier, many had prior experience with Spiritist healers and a few had come from homes where Spiritism was practiced. Their responses to these earlier experiences were quite mixed, their ambivalence fairly intense. During the first year of the program two mental health technicians spoke out about their unease: in one case a young mental health technician, raised by a mother who practiced Spiritism, confessed that she often worked "spiritually" with her patients but had never mentioned the fact to her supervisors (one of whom was present). Another young therapist talked at length of how his mother and her sisters had a Spiritist center in their home into which he had been drawn when younger. With subsequent training in counseling psychology, however, he felt both embarrassed and conflicted about his relationship with his mother and with Spiritism. At the end of the project year he reported that much of his sense of conflict had been relieved, and this had led to a reconciliation of differences with his mother.

Community Responses and Internal Processes

Overall, the proposed plan worked well over three years in three communities. Numbers of therapists, Spiritists, and visitors attending the seminars almost doubled each year. (During the rather difficult first year, between 11 and 40 persons participated over 29 sessions; the numbers grew to between 22 and 67 in the final year.) The program captured professional attention to the extent that we subsequently carried out three similar versions of about four months' duration for physician trainees at the request of the health department.

The basic pedagogical approach to engaging healers (of both types) appeared to be successful in leveling status differences, not only between Spiritists and mental health professionals but also among mental health professionals of differing statuses. This was assessed by observations of the pattern of participants' relationships during the seminars (i.e., reports on who exchanged ideas most frequently or supported other participants' notions, who became friends and spoke of seeing the other participant outside of the seminar). However, it was not a smooth road; there were a few difficult problems stemming from reactions outside the project, as well as conflicts that arose among participants.

Community Reactions

Shortly after the public announcement of the project by the health department (but prior to the project's initiation) a popular daily paper in San Juan ran an article entitled "Escuela de Curanderos en Salud" ("School for Folk Healers in the Health Department"). It featured a cartoon in which an African-looking medicine man is showing a chicken's claw and a small glass of a (supposed) herbal infusion to a medical doctor as a prescription for a rather brutish-looking (mental) patient. The burlesque tone of the article indicated a lack of belief that the health department would sponsor a project involving traditional healers. The health department did not seem to feel terribly threatened by what they labeled an "erroneous form" of description of their intent. In addition, several letters supportive of the project were addressed to the subsecretary for mental health by prominent Spiritists, who sent copies of articles from Spiritist newspapers and newsletters about "psychic therapy" as analogous to spirit healing, thus explaining the relationship of spirit healing to mental health treatment. After the project had run for four months, an article in a prestigious newspaper, *El Mundo*, gave an evenhanded account. In subsequent years (1977–1979), two-page spreads about Spiritism in other newspapers described the project in a favorable light.

The Catholic Church responded to the program only in its third year. Church resistance to the program was based on reports from the priest at the public hospital at which the seminars were held. He had been at that hospital only a few years but had previously undertaken to study Spiritism. He asked to sit in on our seminars. His studies of Spiritism were reported in the periodical *El Visitante de Puerto Rico* on May 21, 1978. In answer to a question about the church's attitude toward Spiritism, he wrote: "The church totally rejects Spiritism, because it develops hate, distrust, suspicion, lack of responsibility, contact with the devil and fear of God" (Guevera, 1978:8). Unknown to the project's director and participants at the time, during his observation of the integrated seminars, the priest was in a state of high agitation. When he could sit no more he endeavored to have the project director and me excommunicated through a local campaign. His campaign began with a series of extremely damning articles in the local Catholic press. In response, a small number of health professionals stopped attending the seminars.

Spiritism was originally conceived by Allan Kardec in opposition to established religion and its role in appointing priests who intercede for the laity. Our response was to seek out the priest's Superior, who, it turned out, had been trained in psychology. Discussions with him focused on research and on training in social science and psychology as the goals of the seminars. Shortly afterwards the Superior managed to pacify our opponent and we encountered little further resistance in the few months left to the project.

In the period following our confrontation with the antagonistic priest, several other priests and nuns, as well as a few local politicians, attended the seminars.

Reactions among Project Participants

The first and most serious conflict among participants occurred barely three months into the program. Attendance dropped off dramatically and we discovered several undercurrents of gossip. The conflict largely affected the Spiritists but was spearheaded by a therapist, the director of the CMHC where we were based. He had aligned himself with one of his therapists who was also a believer in Spiritism and a member of a sect within the Spiritist movement (followers of an Argentine, Joaquin Trincado). These therapists claimed that the practices of the other Spiritists were merely superstitions; they looked for ways to discredit the Spiritist mediums by calling them "witches." At the same time a rumor was circulating that the project was an attempt by the government to register all Spiritists for commitment to the insane asylum; this rumor caused all of the mediums from one center to withdraw from the project. The hostility of the director of the CMHC toward the less-educated members of other Spiritist sects seemed to validate this rumor. Moreover, many of the therapists who had families involved with Spiritist practices feared that their credibility as mental health professionals might be damaged by identification with healers who were not involved with "scientific" Spiritism (a term coined by the director of the CMHC), a missionary sect whose adherents promote the idea that they practice "rational" Spiritism, possess the "truth," differentiate themselves from those who use ritual paraphernalia such as candles and images of saints and spirits and seek an ecstatic state of possession while in trance.

To resolve the conflict I managed to get the two therapists immediately below the director in the administrative hierarchy—the director of the Outpatient Unit and the director of the Child Unit—to counter his opinions in the seminars and support those Spiritists whom the director and his therapist friend had deprecated. The Outpatient Unit director had an intellectual interest in the psychological aspects of Spiritism (he became director of the Therapist-Spiritist Project after that first year); the Child Unit director wanted to understand more about Spiritism because of her husband's involvement. The CMHC director desisted from further interference because he needed the goodwill of his two unit directors, realized that the project was important to the subsecretary, and had been warned to improve his job performance. Following three weeks of intense and conflict-ridden discussions, threats to leave the project, and many absences, attendance returned to what it had been before the conflict escalated. (We encountered a similar problem in the second year but with much less friction.)

The question then arose, however, of whether a Spiritist center, which it was rumored we intended to establish, would be located in the CMHC or in the regional hospital next door. We assured the group that establishing a Spiritist center was not a goal of the project, and most of the original participants settled into the seminars for the remainder of the year.

The conference room at this mental health center was adjacent to the locked ward, which had a large window. Patients would gesture at the window when anyone passed. Given Spiritist belief in bad spirits as the cause of "craziness," the mediums were distressed by the "bad vibrations" they encountered each time they attended a conference and felt this influenced the seminar proceedings and led to some of their distress. This distress was diminished by a Spiritist lecturer's presentation on how to practice Spiritism in a hospital. She described such practices as very different from those that take place at one's *centro*. She suggested that hospital practice required more "control" (appeals to protector spirits) in the absence of the "table" and water container (i.e., spirit fluids) common to Spiritist practice.

A crisis occurred in year two of the project. A mental health technician participating in the project, who had experience with Spiritism through her schizophrenic mother, made a suicidal gesture. She was rescued by a boyfriend, who took her to a health center in a town they were visiting. The attending physician had been at the seminars and agreed with her plea that she be referred not to mental health services but instead to a well-known Spiritist who also participated in the project. She told the physician that she was afraid she would lose her job if treated in a mental health setting. He felt that she might get better care (i.e., protection against another attempt) from the Spiritists since he was dissatisfied about the attention given another patient at the CMHC emergency service. When the crisis had passed, the mental health technician called a meeting of her colleagues and supervisor at the home of the Spiritists who had cared for her and whose sessions she was still attending. Under the thin disguise of an anonymous recording as a "training" vehicle, she told the story of her psychological crisis. Since the Spiritists had diagnosed her as "obsessed" (i.e., taken over by a spirit), she could claim lack of awareness of her actions and thus lack of responsibility; therefore, she did not expect negative sanctions. Her plan worked. It illuminated the dilemma faced by mental health professionals who feel they cannot seek help from their colleagues for emotional crises. This incident had the beneficial effect of suggesting the feasibility of formalizing referrals between mental health professionals and Spiritists.

Outcomes

To compare changes in diagnosis and treatment over the course of the project, written records and/or videotaped sessions of client/patient cases were collected from each core participant before and after their nine months in the project. We were able to chart differences in diagnostic procedures resulting from the project; for example, when Spiritists utilized the new etiology of "psychic cause" and referred a patient to the CMHC, or when a therapist explored a patient's belief in Spiritism and suggested a conference with the Spiritist whose center the patient was attending.

Systematic comparisons between therapist and Spiritist cases were attempted as follows. Presenting complaints of the aggregated (990) cases of women were compared across the healing systems (Koss-Chioino, 1992). The comparison yielded interesting findings. (1) In this opportunistic, clinical sample, over 47% of the Spiritist cases could not be assigned a psychiatric diagnostic label. The cases were comprised of three main physical complaints—headaches, leg aches, and fatigue—and one psychosocial complaint—family problems. It seems that the healers were as frequently seen for general sociosomatic malaise as for emotional disorders. (2) No Spiritist cases could be classified as a "schizophrenic disorder," largely because the Spiritist interpretation of causality did not include "hallucinations or delusions" as diagnostic signs of emotional distress or disorder. Instead, Spiritists consider "visions" to be "normal" experiences of spirits. These findings illustrate the difficulties involved in carrying out comparisons over two very different medical systems.

In participants' written evaluations of the seminars, overall trends showed high satisfaction (percentages of positive answers on questionnaires never were lower than 53% and averaged 82% across three years). Positive answers were somewhat higher for Spiritists than therapists. Appreciation for the case review sessions was expressed by both groups. At the oral evaluation sessions, when dropouts were invited and questioned, we learned why approximately half of the therapists and one-fourth of the Spiritists who had originally committed to participate had dropped out. Most said (out of politeness?) that the time required (evenings or Saturdays) proved difficult for family or educational reasons. But one-third of the dropout therapists reported that the Spiritist lectures and case discussions were too repetitive and boring. Some Spiritists with little formal education reported that the therapist lectures were hard to understand due to unfamiliar terms describing health and mental health topics. Bridging differences in education and interest made program planning quite difficult. However, a fair number of participants from both groups, including a few physicians, became attached to the project and traveled considerable distances to attend seminars in years two and three. In retrospect, the most effective bridge was informal socializing and the opportunity for personal contact in which friendships were formed between healers from both groups.

The project was judged workable and successful by both the visiting and Puerto Rican consultants (as well as by members of the health department). Success was facilitated by the open-ended approach we used (i.e., lecture topics were suggested by the participants each year, and the timing of the programs and special events was decided by the participants). Project planning was based on an attitude that events that emerged each year would lead to shaping and arranging subsequent programs. The outside consultants remarked on the number of visitors from local communities. The consultants' reports were generally positive about meeting our goals, and took note of good attendance and the atmosphere of the seminars in which interchange was most often lively. Their later reports focused on how the project might be institutionalized. Toward this end the principal investigator and the project's director gave talks in almost every medical training setting in Puerto Rico, sometimes accompanied by Spiritist lecturers.

During year one, four therapists and eight project staff persons, particularly one therapist participant who became a lecturer as well as one of our most active supporters, consulted four of the Spiritists about patients. In years two and three, referrals to the mental health professionals by Spiritist participants, and by mental health professionals to Spiritists, for themselves or family members, were reported (we knew about four therapists and six doctors, with four Spiritists seeing physicians in the mental health system for their own problems). The Spiritists said that they referred their patients to the CMHC for "psychic or mental causes" (instead of "material" or "spiritual" causes) once they understood more about mental illness. We tracked 10 cases of cross-referrals of patients, and 10 additional referrals were reported by therapists and Spiritists.

A report on these informally initiated referrals, developed from descriptions by the participants and from cases directly observed by the project director or me, resulted in creation of a unit to refer patients or clients in both directions. It was organized at year two's CMHC site during year three. The initial success of this unit was due to the positive interest of the director of the CMHC (who was a psychologist) and the participation of the Outpatient Clinic director and several of her staff. At least nine healers became involved and about 26 patients received dual treatment, responding to the consensus of a governing committee made up of therapists and Spiritists (Koss, 1980). Outcomes of treatment for the referral patients were assessed by how quickly they returned to their pre-episode level of functioning so that they would not have to receive temporary hospitalization in some cases or long-term residential care in others. All but two of the patients were sent home. We could only follow three patients for approximately 18 months and they were not hospitalized again during that period.

Because one of the main reasons for referral to the unit was discomfort on the part of the therapists over sending patients into long-term residential care, the Department of Health promised to create staff positions for the unit so that it would be permanently supported. Although the medical director of the region initially appointed a psychologist to be in charge of the referral unit, and it continued for a year beyond the life of the project, the position was not funded again when the subdivision heads of the Department of Health were replaced following the change in majority political party that came with the gubernatorial election that year. For at least five years after the project ended, however, we received reports of referrals from Spiritists to mental health professionals and from mental health professionals to Spiritists.

Some Lessons Learned and Some Limitations

Relatively few systematic programs aim to link or integrate traditional healers into biomedical clinical care (see Good et al., 1985). A number of reports describe how traditional healers have been invited into mental health or primary care clinics to work with patients in a special project. A few well-organized programs had significant problems, such as cooptation of the healers or lack of support from the biomedical institution (e.g., Good and Good, 1981; Ruiz and Langrod, 1976). In my experience on the faculty of a department of psychiatry that espoused the need to consider the cultural backgrounds of its patients, even sporadic opportunities to involve traditional healers directly in biomedical health care were difficult to carry through. In the United States in general, direct involvement of nonbiomedical practitioners in clinical care may even be looked upon as potentially unethical. It may be possible when the patient or family requests it, but this takes full support and often a special intervention on the part of attending physicians.

There are exceptions to the prevailing attitude, however, as reported for some Indian Health Service hospitals, where there are special rooms arranged as traditional dwellings for healing ceremonies—largely on the Navaho reservation (Goldstein, 1986). The most inclusive programs for integrating traditional healers into clinical contexts (including their concepts and techniques) have occurred in China, Taiwan, and more recently Thailand (Bibeau, 1985; Chi, 1994; Jilek, 1993; Jingfeng, 1988; Koss-Chioino et al., in preparation; Rosenthal, 1981). The Chinese model for integration insists on full cooperation between Western medical doctors and practitioners of traditional Chinese medicine, but this has not been implemented to reflect total integration, a combination of parts into a whole (Bibeau, 1985; Rosenthal, 1981).

In reviewing the model for linkage and possible integration that was developed in the Puerto Rican study, the following approaches appeared successful:

1. The rule of flexibility that permitted the project director and me to respond to the views and suggestions of the participants, leading to ongoing changes and additions to the plan.
2. The scheduled opportunity to exchange views informally and form friendships through socializing, overcoming several social barriers.
3. The opportunity for discussion in an environment as free of judgment as possible, in which ideological differences could be transcended.
4. The opportunity, especially for the therapists, to admit the validity of Spiritist beliefs and practices considered suspect by many health professionals and labeled "craziness," superstition, or black magic.
5. The pedagogical framework which provided a structure (and idiom) for the leveling of status differences, which in turn facilitated (and was crucial to) the exchange of ideas.

On the other hand, certain failures must be acknowledged in the interest of revising the model. The project was never fully integrated into the health department and was not sustained. The referral unit, a potential opportunity for continuity, was closed. Both the lack of continuity of the project and the demise of the referral unit after two years were related to the politics of health in Puerto Rico, in which the heads of government departments, including health, always change when political leadership changes. (In addition, I left Puerto Rico to work elsewhere, as did the project's director.)

Further, the last of our three main goals was not met: the synthesis of treatments and/or diagnostic techniques from both healing systems into new psychotherapeutic approaches was never formalized or tested. This was partly because the Spiritist healers did not enter into intense exchanges of ideas and techniques with the therapists. Whether or not their reaction reflected the difficulties of decreasing the not inconsiderable ideological distance between them, it seemed that the Spiritists continued to feel subordinate to the therapists. They appeared reluctant to openly share their most closely held ideas and techniques— perhaps in fear of cooptation. Suspicion about the effect of giving up secrets (a deeply rooted aspect of Spiritism) is an inheritance from their earlier persecution and a response to ongoing discrimination (Koss, 1977).

There is little doubt that, following the project, there was a newer consciousness and open public acceptance of Spiritism as a healing system—which persisted over many years. This was evidenced by newspaper and magazine articles that mentioned the project as well as by numerous invitations by universities, physicians, and therapists to lecture. That this was only due to the project is doubtful. The idea of possible integration seems to have lasted longer in the Spiritist community, as suggested by discussions in its journals. At present it appears that Spiritism is not nearly as widely practiced as it was 15 to 20 years ago. A number of the larger centers no longer exist. Many persons have turned to the newly emergent healing alternatives in which a number of the former participants in the Therapist-Spiritist Training Project play active roles. Yet small Spiritist *centros* persist despite the fact that many of the older Spiritists have died. Healing with spirits, in whatever form, will probably last forever. Can it or should it be integrated into public mental health services as a viable healing alternative? Further research and experimentation are needed to answer this question.

Notes

1. The Therapist-Spiritist Training Project in Puerto Rico was funded by the National Institute of Mental Health (MH 14310–03; MH 15210) and sponsored by the Department of Health of Puerto Rico, to whom I am still grateful. Dr. Hector Rivera Lopez, Ms. Fredeswinda Román, Mr. Edgardo Rivera Saez, and numerous mental health professionals (especially, Drs. José Gomez, Juan Moran, and Michael A. Woodbury) and Spiritist healers (especially, Don Jorgé Quevedo, Doña Guané Clara de Millan, and Doña

Dominga Vasquez, among many others) were wonderfully wise and giving colleagues during the project's tenure. They deserve my deepest appreciation but are in no way responsible for my interpretation of the project's development and career.

2. In 1963 the US Community Mental Health Act was passed by Congress, motivated by the idea that all persons were entitled to optimal mental health treatment services in their local communities. The federal government defined the essential tasks of a community mental health center and how states (and Puerto Rico) could ensure comprehensive service delivery. The act mandated a research and development unit charged with assessing community needs and planning and carrying out preventive measures.

References

Ademuwagun VA, Ayoade JA, Harrison I, Warren DM, eds. (1979) African Therapeutic Systems. Waltham, Mass: Crossroads Press.

Ballay YB (1986) Doctors and healers in Africa: the example of southeast Nigeria. *Impact of Science on Society* 36:287–295.

Bergman RL (1973) A school for Medicine Men. *American Journal of Psychiatry* 130:663–666.

Bibeau G (1985) From China to Africa: the same impossible synthesis between traditional and western medicines. *Social Science and Medicine* 21:937–943.

Brodman K, Erdman AJ, Wolf HG (1956) Cornell Medical Index Health Questionnaire Manual. New York: Cornell University Medical College.

Chi C (1994) Integrating traditional medicine into modern health care systems: examining the role of Chinese medicine in Taiwan. *Social Science and Medicine* 39:307–321.

Ezeji PN, Sarvela PD (1992) Health-care behavior of the Ibo tribe of Nigeria. *Health Values* 16:31–35.

Finkler K (1985) Spiritualist Healers in Mexico. New York: Bergin and Garvey.

Gaines AD, ed. (1992) Ethnopsychiatry. The Cultural Construction of Professional and Folk Psychiatries. Albany, NY: SUNY Press.

Garrison V (1977a) Doctor, espiritista or psychiatrist? Health-seeking behavior in a Puerto Rican neighborhood of New York City. *Medical Anthropology* 1:64–185.

Garrison V (1977b) "The Puerto Rican Syndrome." In: Espiritismo in Case Studies of Spirit Possession. V Crapanzano, V Garrison, eds. New York: John Wiley & Sons, pp. 383–449.

Goldstein MJ (1986) Expressed emotion to relatives, maintenance drug treatment, and relapse in schizophrenia and mania. *Psychopharmacology Bulletin* 22:621–627.

Good BJ, Good MD (1981) "The Meaning of Symptoms: A Cultural Hermeneutic Model for Clinical Practice." In: The Relevance of Social Science for Medicine. L Eisenberg, A Kleinman, eds. Dordrecht: Reidel, pp. 165–197.

Good BJ, Herrera H, Delvecchio-Good MJ, Cooper J (1985) "Reflexivity, Countertransference, and Clinical Ethnography: A Case from a Psychiatric Cultural Consultation Clinic." In: Physicians of Western Medicine. Anthropological Approaches to Theory and Practice. RA Hahn, AD Gaines, eds. Dordrecht: Reidel, pp. 193–221.

Guevera VR (1978) Iglesia y Espiritismo. *El Visitante de Puerto Rico*, May 21, pp. 8–9.

Harwood A (1977) Rx. Spiritist as Needed. New York: Wiley.

Hughes CC (1996) "Ethnopsychiatry." In: Medical Anthropology: Contemporary Theory and Method, rev. ed. CF Sargent, TM Johnson, eds. Westport, Ct: Praeger, pp. 131–150.

Jilek WG (1993) Traditional healing against alcoholism and drug dependence. *Curare* 17:145–160.

Jingfeng C (1988) Integration of traditional Chinese medicine with western medicine: right or wrong? *Social Science and Medicine* 27:521–529.

Kiev A (1972) Transcultural Psychiatry. New York: Free Press.

Kleinman A (1980) Patients and Healers in the Context of Culture. Berkeley: University of California Press.

Koss JD (1965) Puerto Ricans in Philadelphia: Migration and Accommodation. PhD dissertation. Philadelphia: Department of Anthropology, University of Pennsylvania. Ann Arbor, Mich: University Microfilms.

Koss JD (1975) Therapeutic aspects of Puerto Rican cult practices. *Psychiatry* 38:160–170.

Koss JD (1976) Religion and science divinely related: a case history of spiritism in Puerto Rico. *Caribbean Studies* 16:22–43.

Koss JD (1977) Social process, healing and self-defeat among Puerto Rican spiritists. *American Ethnologist* 4:453–469.

Koss JD (1980) The Therapist-Spiritist Training Project in Puerto Rico: an experiment to relate the traditional healing system to the public health system. *Social Science and Medicine* 14:373–410.

Koss JD (1987) Expectations and outcomes for patients given mental health care or spiritist healing in Puerto Rico. *American Journal of Psychiatry* 144:56–61.

Koss-Chioino JD (1992) Women as Healers, Women as Patients. Mental Health Care and Traditional Healing in Puerto Rico. Boulder, Colo: Westview Press.

Koss-Chioino JD (1995) "Traditional and Folk Approaches among Ethnic Minorities." In: Psychological Interventions and Cultural Diversity. JF Aponte, RY Rivers, J Wohl, eds. Boston: Allyn and Bacon, pp. 145–163.

Koss-Chioino JD (1996) "The experience of spirits: ritual healing as transactions of emotion (Puerto Rico)." In: Yearbook of Cross-Cultural Medicine and Psychotherapy, vol. 1993. W Andritzky, ed. Berlin: Verlag für Wissenschaft und Bildung, pp. 251–271.

Koss-Chioino JD, Pornsiripongse S, Subcharoen P (in preparation) Ethnomedicine and public health in Thailand: Traditional healing, integration and co-optation.

Lambo TA (1978) Psychotherapy in Africa. *Human Nature* 1:38–40.

Lebra TS (1982) "Self-Reconstruction in Japanese Religious Psychotherapy." In: Cultural Conceptions of Mental Health and Therapy. A Marsella, G White, eds. Dordrecht: Reidel, pp. 269–284.

Maclean U, Bannerman RH (1982) Introduction: utilization of indigenous healers in health delivery systems. *Social Science and Medicine* (special issue) 16:1815–1816.

Neumann AK, Lauro P (1982) Ethnomedicine and biomedicine linking. *Social Science and Medicine* 16:1817–1824.

Nichter M (1992) Anthropological Approaches to the Study of Ethnomedicine. Philadelphia: Gordon and Breach.

Oyebola DDO, Bannerman RH, Bibeau G (1981) Professional associations, ethics and discipline among Yoruba traditional healers of Nigeria. *Social Science and Medicine* 15B:87–92.

Rodriguez Cortes C (1990) Social practices of ethnic identity: a Puerto Rican psychocultural event. *Journal of Behavioral Sciences* 12:380–396.

Rogler LH, Hollingshead AB (1961) The Puerto Rican spiritualist as psychiatrist. *American Journal of Sociology* 67:17–21.

Rogler LH, Hollingshead AB (1965) Trapped. Families and Schizophrenia. New York: John Wiley & Sons.

Rosenthal MM (1981) Political process and the integration of traditional and western medicine in the People's Republic of China. *Social Science and Medicine* 15A:599–613.

Ruiz P, Langrod J (1976) Psychiatry and folk healing: a dichotomy? *American Journal of Psychiatry* 133:95–97.

Snow L (1993) Walkin' over Medicine. Boulder, Colo: Westview Press.

WHO (1978) The Promotion and Development of Traditional Medicine. WHO Technical Report Series 622. Geneva: World Health Organization.

14

Project Community Diagnosis: Participatory Research as a First Step toward Community Involvement in Primary Health Care

MARK NICHTER

> Although many national and international agencies claim to be committed to a
> participatory approach to helping the rural poor, little is known about how to trans-
> late ambitious plans into effective action. The record of earlier community devel-
> opment and cooperative efforts is largely a history of failures, resulting more often
> in strengthening the position of traditional elites than in integrating poorer ele-
> ments into the national development process. Current calls for involvement of the
> rural poor in the development process often seem little more than wishful think-
> ing, inadequately informed by past experience as to the investments in institutional
> innovation required to give reality to an important idea. (Korten, 1979:1)

In the 1970s–1980s, the themes of community participation and bottom-up planning became fashionable in international health and development circles.[1] High-
ranking health officials in developing countries were exposed to the rhetoric of
health democratization and encouraged to develop primary health care programs
having a participatory component. These programs typically incorporated provisions for community health workers (CHWs) and community health committees (CHCs). The planners of such programs made assumptions about what
constitutes a "community" as well as the extent to which, in the name of health,
democratic ideals could be fostered within social structures based on norms and
values that are not democratic.[2] More specifically, assumptions were made about
how CHWs should be selected, trained, and supported; how CHCs should be

organized and for what social unit(s); and the manner by which a "community's felt needs" could be identified. Rarely examined (Mackay, 1981) was the issue of whether the rural poor wanted CHWs or CHCs at all, or whether they viewed them as poor substitutes for trained government primary health center field staff.

In South Asia, government-sponsored CHW programs were often introduced in haste following political fanfare. By and large, they were poorly monitored and failed to mobilize participation of impoverished sectors of the society, the very populations for whom they were intended. The failure of these programs in India was documented within a few years of implementation and was linked to political factors (Sussman, 1980; Walt, 1988).

In this chapter, I describe the Community Diagnosis (CD) project, a formative research project initiated in Karnataka State, South India, in 1979–1980 to examine what the poor felt their health priorities were and to document their response to a CHW scheme about to be implemented in this region. Five aims of formative research are to: (1) inform those developing interventions about what local populations are doing, thinking, and saying about focal issues, behaviors, and the like; (2) identify and critically assess intervention possibilities; (3) investigate motivations and opportunities for change as well as resource- and non–resource-related constraints; (4) provide information about how best to implement an intervention (who, when, where, how); and (5) monitor community response to interventions over time, enabling midcourse correction.

The CD project was designed as an exploration in how participatory research could be used as a first step in fostering the poor's involvement in formative research toward the end of improving primary health care. The general aims of the project were to: (1) document local health concerns, self-treatment practices, and patterns of seeking health care; (2) provide baseline data on how the poor viewed government health services; (3) gather data on their impressions of the impending CHW program and how it should be implemented; and (4) create listening posts in two districts of Karnataka State capable of monitoring community response to the CHW program. While the first three goals of the project were realized, the fourth was not, due to lack of funding and a change in political leadership in Karnataka State in 1980–1981.

It is beyond the scope of this chapter to discuss the dynamics of project implementation in great detail (Nichter, 1980a; Nichter and Nichter, 1980). Following a brief discussion of participatory research and the Community Diagnosis project, I will use two examples from the project to show how participatory research can be conducted and prove useful in primary health care program planning, implementation, and monitoring. The first example illustrates how participatory methodologies were used to elicit data on local health concerns and perceptions of "folk epidemiology" in Karnataka. The second example describes how the Community Diagnosis project was able to elicit community members' ideas about the CHW and CHC schemes and how they should be implemented.

The Community Health Worker Scheme: A Brief History

Although the need for involving the community in health care delivery had been discussed in India since the 1950s, it was not until the mid-1970s that community participation became a program goal. In 1975, the Srinvastasa Committee called for the creation of a community health worker (CHW) program. At this time, Kerala State was being heralded as an international success story for lowering infant mortality rates to a level comparable to Western countries. This success was attributed to the political will of a literate public which was proactive in monitoring health center activities (Chopra, 1982; Franke and Chasin, 1992; Nag, 1988, 1989; Panikar, 1979; Ratcliffe, 1978).[3] Some health planners suggested that community participation could be mobilized elsewhere by community health workers.

According to national CHW guidelines, one CHW was to be chosen by each village having a population of 1,000 or more. This CHW would then be trained at a local primary health center for three months. After training, the CHW was to receive a medical kit and backup support from primary health center workers. The CHW would be given a token monthly government honorarium for two to three hours of community health service a day, during which time he or she was to attend to simple medical problems, mobilize community involvement in health programs, and assist in health education.

An underlying rationale for creating a health functionary outside the formal health infrastructure was to bridge the communication gap between the community and the primary health center. The CHW was expected to know the "felt needs" of the community and facilitate appropriate services and organization. As envisioned, the CHW was to be responsible to the community.

The CHW plan was initiated in India in late 1977 in all but four states (Karnataka dissented for political reasons), and by 1978 it had been implemented in 28 districts around the country. One of the major problems in implementing the CHW program was that it was largely administered through the primary health center. The primary health center controlled CHW resources (honoraria and medical supplies) and technical knowledge. In many areas the primary health center medical officer was responsible for the selection of CHWs. According to several reports, CHWs were viewed by primary health center staff as their aides and subordinates, mobilized to reduce their workload and help them perform their duties. Maru (1980:1) studied the opinions of primary health center (PHC) staff toward formal control of CHWs. He notes:

The expressed desire for control was inversely related to the level of bureaucracy. The desire for formal control was the strongest among the lowest level field workers who interact with the CHWs on a regular basis. It decreased as we moved up to the district and state levels. Our study of PHC–CHW interface revealed that a large majority of PHC staff favored PHC controls over both the selection and the day to day activities of CHWs.

According to Maru, many PHC field staff believed that "control of CHWs is a must because people are dishonest; there is no love without fear, without our supervision they will not comply with our demands as many of them are leader-type" (Maru, 1980:2). These views illustrate the tendency of the health care bureaucracy to resist innovations which undermine preexisting power structures. Instead of being encouraged to develop culturally sensitive health education messages responsive to local resources and health practices, CHWs were given a diluted form of standard paramedical instruction (Srivastva, 1978). The CHW program in the mid-1970s did little more than create another cadre of paraprofessional health workers responsible to the health center, not the community.

By 1979 it was clear that formative research was needed to operationalize the CHW program and identify locally appropriate selection criteria and processes. K.G. Rao of the National Institute of Health and Family Welfare has addressed the vital need for such research:

> There is a need for continuous research to evolve suitable criteria for selecting community health workers, insuring optimal community involvement in the selection process. Probably, changes in selection procedure need to be worked out for each state in India based on the local situation. . . . The idea of village level (health) committees has been suggested. But there is no research to provide guidelines on such aspects as the composition of such committees, inclusion of politician leaders/community workers, etc. The formulation and substance of useful, lively, dynamic health committees . . . need to be evolved through research. (Rao, 1979:1)

Could the CHW scheme be more effectively implemented to fulfill envisioned program goals? This was a core research question raised in 1979 as the state of Karnataka considered adopting its own version of the CHW scheme.

Social Science and Participatory Research

> A major weakness of our planning has been the neglect of microanalysis at the grassroots level. Insufficient and inaccurate data are largely due to the inadequacy of painstaking field research. Lack of detailed analysis of the social and economic microcosm continues to plague the planning process. This has resulted in broad aggregates and generalizations, blurring the human factor, and mystifying the effect of our plans on the poor. (Chorpande, cited in Srinivas, 1979:11)

In 1980, India had a population of more than 600 million people, 80% of whom lived in rural areas, in approximately 560,000 villages. These villages comprised 390 bureaucratic districts having a population of over 1 million to 1.5 million each. Sixteen national languages and countless dialects coexist as well as multiple caste and tribal subcultures. Given the vast social and cultural diversity, the question arises: Who can carry out the type of region-specific research needed by development planners?

Within India there are relatively few social scientists whose research and training are health-oriented and who are committed to the arduous life of rural development work. For those who choose such a vocation, there are few opportunities for sustained research which offer any measure of job security or advancement. Although it is true that development agencies have increasingly required social science research as a part of program development, project managers commonly use social scientists "for confirmation, to gild the lily" after a project has already been designed (Cochrane, 1979). In other cases, social science research is contracted out to organizations (e.g., social marketing firms) which have no sustained interest in a particular problem, project, or population.

A decade before the proliferation of nongovernmental organizations (NGOs) fostered by funding for AIDS research, Srinivas criticized data produced by development entrepreneurs[4] deriving profit from conferences on poverty and the increasing number of "social surveys" required by international development agencies:

> Low qualifications, poor involvement with the community, harsh working conditions, and lack of sympathy with the aims of the surveys they conduct, often characterize field investigators. The results are commonly of dubious value. (Srinivas, 1979:11)

In the health and development field, there has been an overreliance on survey methodologies by planners who blindly believe that larger samples net greater truth. The dubious value of surveys—designed in the capital instead of developed in the field following careful ethnographic research—has been aptly demonstrated by researchers such as Campbell et al. (1979). These seasoned ethnographers and a team of experienced Nepalese assistants readministered a battery of survey questionnaires used by development agencies in rural Nepal. Their study revealed that the data collected during the original surveys had yielded a distorted impression of villagers' behavior and knowledge. Distortion resulted far less from sampling than from nonsampling errors: errors in the linguistic and conceptual intelligibility of survey questions, problems with interview questions involving culturally sensitive topics, informants' fears of repercussions for responding negatively to questions posed by outsiders, the dynamics of image management, and so on. As one reviewer of the study poignantly noted:

Because of the inappropriateness of the surveys for collecting data and because of the culturally inappropriate ways those surveys are designed, people are deprived of meaningful participation (in development) at even this minimal level. (Blustain, 1982:20)

On the basis of this study, Campbell and colleagues argued for the use of in-depth participant observation as a means of developing culturally sensitive survey instruments, identifying when surveys are and are not appropriate means of collecting data, and evaluating the trustworthiness of data collected.

Similar arguments have been made more recently by those advocating rapid assessment procedure (RAP) studies of health problems, which employ in combination a wide range of field methods as a substitute for (or a step preceding) large-scale knowledge, attitude, and practice (KAP) surveys (e.g., Bentley et al., 1988; Manderson and Aaby, 1992a, 1992b; Scrimshaw and Gleason, 1992; Scrimshaw and Hurtado, 1987). However, while the quality of baseline data generated by RAPs is significantly better than that produced by KAPs, local participation in RAP research remains limited, with neither procedure fostering a process of local problem solving. Participatory research creates an environment in which new knowledge is not just learned but thought about and incorporated in a problem-solving process which entails the generation and consideration of several possible courses of action (Cornwall and Jewkes, 1995).

What is required for community participation in health planning and implementation is for the local beneficiaries of programs to participate in the collection and analysis of information enabling the generation and assessment of possible interventions. A weighing of opportunity costs and relative benefits associated with each option, as proponents of participatory research have argued, requires not just better extractive data collection, but a process of learning which facilitates critical examination (deKoning, 1996; Fernandes and Tandon, 1981; Hall, 1981, 1982; Perez, 1997; Tandon, 1981). Participatory research (1) fosters an alliance between professional researchers and lay representatives affording the latter the opportunity to contribute to the process and direction of enquiry; (2) challenges assumptions made by planners and decision makers providing a check to the incompleteness and time-bound nature of expert knowledge and placing the opinions of stakeholders center stage; and (3) enables dialogue by translating popular knowledge into a form that planners and decision makers understand as well as translating expert knowledge into a form the lay population can understand.

Project Community Diagnosis and Research Setting

At the time the CD project was being conceptualized, international support was being marshaled for health paraprofessionals in developing countries. As a medi-

cal anthropologist working in the field of international health, I argued that social science paraprofessionals also were needed to engage their communities in
problem solving through participatory research. What needed to be explored
was (1) how CD teams could be organized and social science paraprofessionals
trained to collect data and foster such a community problem-solving process and
(2) what ongoing support for CD teams would be needed from social science
professionals to make CD teams sustainable.

In 1979, I was able to obtain funds from the Indo-US Subcommission on
Education and Culture to initiate an exploratory community diagnosis of health
based on the principle of participatory research. The project took place in two
rural districts of Karnataka State. The health status of the population of Karnataka
State was reported to be midway between that of Uttar Pradesh (the state with
India's highest infant mortality) and Kerala (the state with India's lowest infant
mortality). Two field sites within Karnataka (North and South Kanara, located
approximately 300 kilometers apart) were chosen because of contrasting patterns of residence, social organization, and kinship, as well as overall health status. The field site in South Kanara District was characterized by dispersed mixed-
caste settlements, some of which are matrilineal, others patrilineal. In 1978, the
Bangalore-based Population Institute ranked South Kanara "healthiest" out of
the state's 19 districts. By contrast, the field site in North Kanara District was
characterized by centralized villages, composed of single caste, largely patrilineal
hamlets; North Kanara was ranked eleventh in health status among the state's
districts.

The health care arenas of both districts are pluralistic and composed of a variety of practitioners (Nichter and Nichter, 1996). Both regions have a number
of different types of traditional practitioners including folk healers, practitioners
of ayurvedic humoral medicine, exorcists and spirit mediums, and astrologers.
Government primary health centers staffed by practitioners trained in allopathic
medicine are situated to serve populations of approximately 100,000. Private
practitioners of allopathic medicine are located in nearly every town having a
population greater than 10,000, with the number of doctors in South Kanara far
exceeding North Kanara.

Poor to lower-middle-class rural households were targeted for CD project
activities. Most participants were small landholding agriculturists who also engaged in daily wage labor, fishing, or some small-scale industry such as the hand
rolling of *bidi* cigarettes. Sample selection for in-depth interviews and follow-
up surveys was based on the distinct characteristics of each region. In South
Kanara, 82 very poor households from 8 villages were selected to participate in
the CD project by a cluster sampling procedure sensitive to caste divisions and
proximity to a crossroads town. In North Kanara, 200 households from 14 villages were selected by a cluster sampling procedure with the size of caste samples
weighted to accord with the local demographic pattern. Each CD household

participated in several rounds of research activities. CD project research activities took place over a five-month period in each district. The purposes of these activities were:

1. To organize local teams of community diagnosis investigators composed of young male and female residents of the communities in which research was to be carried out. They would seek the opinions of a group of older, more experienced community advisers in matters of health and development activities.
2. To explore the extent to which these lay investigators could be taught basic anthropological skills (e.g., participant observation, structured observations, interviewing, group discussion) through training exercises and active modeling by experienced social science instructors.
3. To conduct a diagnosis of community health care priorities, patterns of health care utilization and expenditure, and health-related issues identified by both health care providers (public health officials, etc.) and the local population.
4. To document community response to government health personnel, services, and a newly proposed community health worker scheme.
5. To identify innovative approaches to health education which would be sensitive to lay health concerns and cultural communication styles.

Methods training was a major aim of the project. CD investigators were taught to (1) use a mix of ethnographic methods to enhance the validity (Maxwell, 1992) and trustworthiness (Lincoln and Guba, 1985) of qualitative data collection, and (2) use data collection as a first step in raising community consciousness about health problems. Research was carried out as an iterative process, each step building on previous research findings, fostering critical review. In-depth interviews were carried out with villagers over several months. As rapport and trust developed, several key informants assumed the role of community advisers and were asked to play a more proactive part in project discussions. Focus groups enabled CD researchers to engage informants selected according to common characteristics (age, gender, caste, etc.) in a communication environment designed to foster interaction and encourage a consideration of differences of opinion. Focus group participants were presented common scenarios and health care–seeking dilemmas to elicit and assess differences in response related to group characteristics. Scenarios were developed from local illness stories and personal narratives. Focus groups were also used to pretest survey questions and other research methods.

The collection of qualitative data through participant observation and the aforementioned research methods preceded the development and pretesting of several surveys used in the project. Ethnographic data were collected to document the range of local experiences, ideas, and practices, while complementary survey instruments were developed to measure consensus. Caste and village meetings were held both to discuss project findings and to consider the strengths and weaknesses of alternative ways of solving problems, such as the selection of a community health committee and community health worker.

Use of Participatory Research to Elicit Local Health Concerns

Methods

It was reasoned that, to establish rapport and gain community cooperation, the CD team would have to focus on a series of health problems deemed locally important and to provide a concrete example to community members of how they might benefit from participating in the research project. Project staff called public attention to the recently publicized, but little understood, CHW plan the Karnataka State government was about to implement. The CD team presented its mission to the community as collecting data on existing health problems and people's opinions about the CD plan as well as how it might best be implemented in their setting. Data collection on common health problems and patterns of health care utilization preceded data collection on the activities of government health outreach workers and the CHW plan. Data on health problems were justified to the community as useful for health planners when making decisions about resource allocation and health staff/CHW training. Community diagnosis research was responsive to the data needs of public health officials, but research agendas were not imposed on the CD team. Research activities responded to local interests and practices.

To elicit perceptions of common health problems, a "free listing" exercise was initiated, followed by a methodology adapted from rapid rural appraisal studies in agriculture (see Chambers, 1992; McCracken, 1989). Informants were asked first to list separately common illnesses experienced by children and adults and then to indicate which were the most troublesome, expensive to treat, and serious. Using grains of rice to trace out a crude histogram, informants were then asked to compare local illnesses four or five at a time in terms of relative severity and commonality (by age, season, etc.). Each illness was designated by a symbol (a physical object or an image). These histograms were then used as a visual prop for discussion with other members of an assembled group (separate groups of men, women, elders, etc.). Each group member was asked to modify the order indicated by the preceding member in terms of his or her own experience. The exercise proved useful in gaining a rough approximation of the range of perceptions of illness prevalence and severity and the degree of consensus. However, as some community members pointed out, these exercises provided only generalities; some illnesses rated as less severe than others could become very serious for a particular person and prove fatal if not attended to properly.

CD members were encouraged to explore (1) perceived associations between types of illnesses and factors rendering individuals and groups vulnerable, (2) factors thought to cause particular illnesses, and (3) practices thought to prevent illness and the relative utility of such practices. Attention was paid to the details of "folk epidemiology"—causal relations derived by community members from a combination of empirical observations and analogical reasoning. These data were collected to better understand popular health practices and the concerns and concepts which guided them.

In several instances, it was found beneficial to sequence research topics in a manner that made sense to the local population and to place on hold topics health officials wanted researched. For example, early in the CD project, a regional health official expressed interest in obtaining information on the age at which breastfed infants were introduced to various types of solid foods. Wanting to gain his support, I agreed to develop a survey on this issue. Community members responded poorly to the survey. Two community advisers suggested that the CD team first focus on diet in relation to children's illnesses. Emphasis was shifted to children's illnesses associated with dietary behavior. Following questions about diet and illness, respondents were more willing to engage in conversation about routine dietary practices including breastfeeding and the relationship between these practices and health status.

Findings

In South Kanara, the following illnesses were identified by these methods as particularly troublesome and dangerous for children: fevers (especially fevers with chills which resulted in febrile fits); diarrhea (especially diarrhea with vomiting and blood in stools); respiratory complaints (especially noisy, labored breathing associated with both acute lower respiratory infections and asthma); and skin diseases (especially those which were recurrent, resulted in swelling, and were thought controllable only by injections). Among adults, illnesses identified as dangerous were fevers with chills, respiratory complaints (including TB and asthma), and gynecological complaints associated with weakness (see Bang and Bang, 1994). Preferred treatments for these complaints varied by illness and included ayurvedic as well as allopathic medicine.[5] Considerable concern was also expressed about folk dietetics—foods deemed appropriate and inappropriate to eat when ill, vulnerable, or convalescing.

During observations of practitioners in both field sites, it was observed that a common question asked of both ayurvedic and biomedical practitioners was: What foods are appropriate to consume during different types of illness *and* with different types of medication? Recognizing that diet during illness was a common health concern and that malnutrition among children following illness was an important public health problem, the CD team took up this topic as a focus of inquiry.

An observation which emerged during research on folk dietetics was that opinions about food were framed not only in relation to specific illnesses (e.g., states of poor digestion, etc.), but also in terms of an individual's constitution (*prakṛti*) and the lifestyle and dietary habits of particular castes. These observations were used to further explain the purpose of CD research. A question asked by nearly all persons interviewed was: "Why do you ask me questions about diet and health— I know little. Why don't you ask your questions to 'so and so' esteemed people in the area?" The following explanation was offered in return:

> Do all people have the same constitution, habits, the same diet or tastes, the same ability to digest different types of food, the same needs? Knowing the experience of a rich man, does that help us understand the experiences of the poor? When purchasing a cock, does one consult a Brahmin [a local proverb]?

Examples of five folk epidemiological associations identified during CD research illustrate the logic behind popular health concerns.

1. Children have more problems with worms than adults; children eat more sweet things, which produce more phlegm, which produces an environment conducive to the proliferation of worms. Once children are able to consume bitter and pungent foods, worms are more easily controlled.
2. Children have more diarrhea at the time of teething; their humors are unbalanced at this time of sudden bodily change.
3. Wounds become infected because of impurities in the blood; more attention is thus paid to purifying the blood and eating foods which are not toxic or aggravating for the blood, than to keeping a wound externally clean.
4. If a mother increases her consumption of food during the latter months of pregnancy, this may impair the baby's health; it will leave less space for the baby to grow since the fetus shares the same bodily space as food.
5. Those who roll *bidi* cigarettes (a cottage industry in South Kanara) are more likely to become afflicted with TB; just as smoking leads to lung problems, inhaling tobacco dust as an occupational hazard leads to lung problems.

Participatory Research as the Basis for Designing Appropriate CHW and CHC Programs

Methods

Key informant interviews and focus groups were conducted to gather local opinion about various aspects of implementing the CHW plan. Four rounds of surveys were conducted to generate quantitative data on a subset of questions entailing choices among options identified during qualitative research. It was critical to conduct this component of the CD project following qualitative research on popular health culture. Questions related to the CHW scheme were asked only after data were collected on health concerns and existing patterns of health care utilization, power relations among community factions were explored, and rapport was established with members of each faction. Had a survey of community opinion about the CHW program been conducted before or without building such rapport, it is doubtful that community members would have been so forthcoming or frank with their opinions.

Although news of the new CHW scheme had sporadically appeared in regional newspapers, few people in North and South Kanara had heard of it prior to the CD project. When the CHW role was described to villagers, some asked whether this was an alternative to increased primary health center field staff involvement in the region. One of the first CD surveys polled community preferences for CHWs. Individuals were asked who should be selected for this position and how. A second survey assessed conditions requiring treatment, priorities, and desired treatment methods. A third survey explored how CHWs should be selected. A fourth survey looked at ways of improving access to common medicines.

Findings: Responses to the CHW scheme

First Survey: Preferred Characteristics of CHWs. Respondents were asked, "Would you prefer more government health workers to visit your village or local people trained to treat minor ailments and give advice about health, diet, and how to prevent illness?" The idea of a CHW was popular among the rural poor in both districts (see Table 14.1 for survey response data). When asked about the preferred sex of a CHW, South Kanarese respondents preferred females, but many preferred males or had no preference. The greater preference for females in South Kanara may be associated with the matrilineal kinship system prevalent in this region. Matrilineality accords South Kanaran women greater freedom and status than women in North Kanara, which is patrilineal. Support for female CHWs also came from the Muslim community, which viewed CHWs primarily as health providers for women and children, and the Christian community, famous on the Malabar Coast for producing nurses. In North Kanara, a strong preference was voiced for male CHWs. A sense of impropriety was associated with women traveling between caste hamlets. Furthermore, several high school–educated, unemployed young males were found in the community. It was strongly felt that they should be given "service work." As one informant noted:

> There are educated youth from the households of the poor here. The government encouraged their families to educate these youth, and now they have no

Table 14.1 Selected Responses from First Survey: Preferences in Choice of CHWs

QUESTION	OPTIONS	SOUTH KANARA (N = 82), %	NORTH KANARA (N = 200), %
Staffing: Would you prefer more government health workers to visit your village, or local people trained to treat minor ailments and give advice about health, diet, and how to prevent illness?	More government workers	29	2
	Local people trained as CHWs	71	98
Characteristics: If only one CHW could be trained in your place (*uru*), should this be a male or a female?	Prefer male	28	76
	Prefer female	42	24
	Either	30	NA
Age	25–35	NA	85
	20–30	66	NA
Education	Must be literate	97	90

work which dignifies their new educational status. If others are to follow them, they should be given this new work. Let others see they are recognized as youth leaders, our future.

In North Kanara, 85% of informants considered 25–35 years an appropriate age range for a CHW; in South Kanara, two-thirds of the total sample identified 20–30 years as an appropriate age range. The preferred age range of 20–35 corresponds with a growing trend in rural South India of the young taking up positions of leadership in local government.

In North Kanara, 90% of informants stated that a CHW should be at least literate, while 43% thought a high school education was desirable. In South Kanara, 97% of informants deemed literacy mandatory, with 64% stating that a high school education or above was desirable for male CHWs (87% of interior village informants). For women CHWs, however, 45% of the total sample (63% of interior village and 32% of town informants) deemed literacy sufficient. Thus literacy was perceived to be a basic requirement for a CHW, but higher education was considered to be a more important criterion for male than female CHWs.

Second Survey: Desired Focus and Specialization of CHWs. While some scholars (e.g., Banerji, 1985) have noted that child survival programs may allocate medical resources to groups the community does not feel warrant special attention, to the neglect of others, Community Diagnosis research found strong support for giving special attention to child survival programs (Table 14.2). Over two-thirds of community members polled in both districts supported child health as a CHW's primary responsibility. Special services for the elderly were also recognized as a growing health service need, albeit better served by primary health center workers and doctors (allopathic and ayurvedic) than CHWs.

Respondents were also asked, "Of the different types of health care available (allopathy, ayurveda, homeopathy, herbal medicine) which type(s) of therapy should a CHW be trained to use?" Most people interviewed thought that CHWs should be trained in the use of a mix of practices, based on perceived efficacy and cost.

Informants were asked to list those health problems and illness states for which a CHW should learn to use herbal medicines. In both districts, children's illnesses associated with malnutrition, skin rashes, and pregnancy/postpartum problems were mentioned by at least 50% of respondents. In the case of skin diseases, many people expressed the opinion that curing these ailments required allopathic and herbal medicine in combination. Allopathic medicine dried infected wet sores and wounds and reduced swelling; herbal medicine cleaned the blood.

Notably, in North Kanara, 40% of those persons identified as making a good CHW were already administering some form of traditional medicine or came from a family renowned for medical knowledge. In South Kanara, 34% of males identified as good CHW candidates and 50% of female candidates came from families renowned for knowledge of herbal medicines.

Table 14.2 Selected Responses from Second Survey: Preferred Types of Programs and Treatment Methods

QUESTION	OPTIONS	SOUTH KANARA (N = 82), %	NORTH KANARA (N = 200), %
Is the primary responsibility of a CHW child health?	Agree	>67	>67
What type of therapy should CHWs be trained to use?	Allopathy only (biomedicine)	5	20
	Homeopathy/ ayurveda/local herbal medicine only	16	1
	All of the above	79	79

Third Survey: Selection of a CHW. A third round of surveys inquired about how a CHW should be selected. Intra- as well as interregional differences of opinion emerged (Table 14.3). For example, a significant number of informants (37%) from roadside villages in South Kanara favored CHWs being selected by primary health care doctors, but few informants from interior villages concurred. Differences in opinion were tied to (*1*) varying perceptions of the commitment of local government bodies (*panchayat*) and primary health center staff, and (2) regional styles of decision making associated with differences in social structure. In North Kanara, few people supported CHW selection by health center doctors. A common concern voiced by informants was that ad hoc open meetings to identify CHW candidates might foster factional politics. An idea suggested during focus groups in both districts was having a smaller health committee identify appropriate candidates.

Table 14.3 Selected Responses from Third Survey: Selection of a CHW and Membership of CHC

QUESTION	OPTIONS	SOUTH KANARA (N = 82), %	NORTH KANARA (N = 200), %
How should a CHW be selected?	Appointed by *panchayat*	27	9
	Selected by PHC doctor, from community suggestions	20	2
	Selected at open village meetings	2	5
	Selected by CHC	42	84
Who should be responsible for organizing a CHC?	Each village or large hamlet	43	92
	Each *panchayat*	55	8
How should members in the CHC be chosen?	Appointed by *panchayat*	20	14
	Selected at open meetings	46	76
	Selected by meetings of caste representatives	34	10
Should there be an economic "ceiling," so that all members of a CHC earn less than that amount?	Yes	96	92

The third survey asked how a Community Health Committee (CHC) might be organized and who its members should be. In rural South Kanara, where households are scattered, the *panchayat* was deemed a credible body for selecting an appropriate mix of community members to serve on a health committee. In North Kanara, single-caste hamlets are common and a tradition of caste meetings exists. A preference for health committees organized by hamlet was really a preference for caste committees. Members of the same caste living in nearby hamlets expressed interest in forming a caste health committee based on social ties and not geographic proximity per se. Of those North Kanarese informants who opted for hamlet/village health committees, half favored this type of committee organization.

Preferred membership selection procedures also differed by region in accord with local social organization. In North Kanara, a vote for open hamlet meetings was actually a vote for intracaste selection by dominant castes. In South Kanara, a region undergoing land reform in the mid-1970s, the poor hesitated to articulate their needs in an open meeting for fear of intercaste politics.

Inclusion and Exclusion Criteria. During focus groups preceding the third round of surveys, opinions were voiced that upper-class villagers would make little use of CHWs but might try to dominate health committees. Community advisers suggested that committee membership be limited by a household economic ceiling (Rs.6,000–7,000 per year; US$1,000). When polled, 96% of South Kanarese and 92% of North Kanarese rural poor informants supported such an economic ceiling as a criterion for committee membership. Another issue was whether or not government development workers, medical practitioners, and the wealthy should be invited to be members of CHCs. In North Kanara no government servant, local practitioner (traditional or allopathic), schoolteacher, large landowner, or merchant was supported for honorary committee membership by more than 20% of the sample. In South Kanara, medical practitioners received slightly greater support for membership (35%). In both North and South Kanara, government development workers in the fields of health, nutrition, and agriculture were deemed important committee resources, but few people wanted them to be standing members of the CHC. Notably in North Kanara, 55% of households expressed opposition to including local schoolmasters on the health committee, as they were considered representatives of the rich. Such an opinion was expressed by few people in South Kanara.

Overall, the rural poor saw a successful health committee as one that was not dominated by government development workers, health practitioners, the wealthy, or formal community leaders. There were, however, regional variations in opinions about committee membership. For example, in South Kanara, *panchayat* members were supported as committee members by 45% of households polled, while in North Kanara they were supported by only 16%. Planners often assume that local government servants should mobilize community action. This may not always be the case. For example, health planners have commonly discussed the role of schoolteachers in mobilizing community involvement in health. In South Kanara, this appeared to be appropriate. One-third of the sample supported the idea that the schoolmaster be a CHC member and 92% said that he or she should be an adviser. By comparison, in North Kanara only 5% wanted the schoolmaster to be a committee member and 40% an adviser.

What should the role of a Community Health Committee be beyond choosing a CHW? Other possible functions of a CHC emerged during community meetings when household health expenditure data were presented. This sparked dialogue about the need for a more immediate supply of basic medicines. At one memorable meeting in South Kanara, lively discussion emerged from a consideration of the following CD data (Nichter, 1980b):

1. Approximately 20% of an interior villager's total health expenditure is for transportation to a practitioner or source of medication.
2. More than 25% of patients frequenting a nearby village primary health center are sent to a town an hour away by bus to fill a medical prescription. Patients receiving medication at the primary health center are given only a two-day supply of medication at a time. This makes frequent, time-consuming trips back to the health center necessary.
3. Primary health center field staff are trained in the use of a number of basic medicines, but they do not have ready access to any of these medicines. One-half to two-thirds of patients seen at primary health centers could be cared for at home by health center field staff or CHWs if they had access to appropriate medical supplies.
4. Medicines purchased in small quantities by patients were over 25% more expensive than medications purchased in bulk.

Impressed by such data and visual demonstrations of cost differences in purchasing large and small quantities of common medicines, community members engaged in a discussion of alternative means for improving access to common medicines. Two suggestions emerged from such group discussions relating to community financing. A fourth survey was conducted to poll the popularity of each of these ideas and the role of CHCs in ensuring that even the poorest could have access to basic medicines.

Fourth Survey: Access to Basic Medicines. The first question involved having the primary health center stock commonly needed medicines for sale, with bulk rate prices posted. Free medicines would be reserved for the "poorest of the poor," a status determined by CHCs based on agreed upon criteria. This concept was supported by 90% of South Kanarese and 84% of North Kanarese informants (see Table 14.4). When asked about the creation of local medical cooperatives that would stock basic nonperishable medicines (for use by CHWs and health center field workers, and to be sold at bulk rate prices), 100% of South Kanarese and 98% of North Kanarese informants stated that they would be willing to pay a small household levy each year (during harvest season) to be members of such cooperatives. Moreover, 90% of South Kanarese and 92% of North Kanarese informants thought medicine should be sold at a small (5%) profit beyond the bulk rate cost to subsidize free medicines given to the poor. The posting of a medicine price list was supported as a means of increasing consumer knowledge. There were mixed feelings about whether levies on medicines should supplement honoraria given to CHWs. Some community members noted that this might be an incentive for CHWs to prescribe. Others questioned what type of medicine would be stocked. Some expressed a lack of faith in the efficacy of government-purchased generic medicine. Most people polled felt that overseeing provision of basic medicines would strengthen the role and increase the status of the CHC.

These data suggest that the concept of community financing for health was supported by the poor in the form of cooperative purchase of medicines. This was more popular than general "user fees" being levied for services provided. Also supported was turning over to CHCs the decision of who receives free care.

Table 14.4 Selected Responses from Fourth Survey: Improving Access to Common Medicines

QUESTION	OPTIONS	SOUTH KANARA (N = 82), %	NORTH KANARA (N = 200), %
Should the primary health center stock and sell commonly needed medicines, posting the bulk prices publicly?	Yes	90	84
Should local medical cooperatives be established, which would stock basic nonperishable medicines to be sold at bulk prices? And would you be willing to pay a small levy each year to be a member of such a cooperative?	Yes	100	98
Should the medical cooperatives mark up the price of medicines about 5%, to finance free medicine for the "poorest of the poor"?	Yes	90	92

It has been argued that community involvement in health financing enhances people's sense of belonging and commitment to community services.[6] CD data suggest that community members are interested in deciding who pays what for health care and how funds collected are to be used. Proactive community financing programs may be contrasted with passive schemes where levies are imposed from above to support health services and where CHCs have little control over how the funds are spent.

Discussion

> We have to step out of our professional egocentrism and establish a partnership between the health system and the community. No group of professionals should take over the people's right of decision because this creates dependency rather than self reliance. The health system's major responsibility should be to increase the capacity of the community and of individuals to solve their own health problems. The best of intentions lead only to frustration unless practical programs result. (Taylor, 1968:161)

Reliable, up-to-date information on popular health cultures, the availability, distribution, and maximization of health care resources (both public and private), and knowledge of the microeconomics of health care seeking are essential to the planning, implementation, and evaluation of primary health care programs as envisioned at Alma-Ata (Berman, in press; WHO, 1978).

The importance of such data has been widely acknowledged in the international health literature, yet relatively few primary health care programs have made provisions for formative research which remains in touch with the pulse of the community. Such research needs to be ongoing, enabling midcourse corrections as programs are tailored to changing local realities. In this chapter, the possibility of developing regional paraprofessional community diagnosis teams supervised by a network of professional social scientists has been discussed. Such teams could provide ongoing community feedback about health and development programs at various stages of planning and implementation.

Project Community Diagnosis was a fledgling attempt to explore the feasibility of mobilizing such participatory research teams in rural areas of India. The project ran into its fair share of difficulties—problems in selecting appropriate team members, establishing an identity, and sustaining community interest in participatory research. More critical, the Karnataka State government changed political leadership just as the project was finishing; the new government introduced the CHW program in Karnataka in great haste, and CD project staff had little contact with newly appointed officials. Thus Project Community Diagnosis had no effect on the implementation of Karnataka State's CHW program. The CHW program was short-lived and largely unsuccessful due to poor administration, inappropriate candidate selection, and training not responsive to local health culture. A valuable organizational lesson was learned during the project: in order to be effective, CD teams needed to communicate regularly with a liaison person within the health infrastructure having access to sympathetic health officials at all levels.[7]

Despite these difficulties, the project experience was promising enough to suggest further exploration of the regional participatory research team concept as a contribution to community-based public health efforts. What remains to be tested is whether such teams, once organized and trained, can function independently with a limited amount of support and supervision from professional social scientists (and health educators, etc.). Indigenous social scientists will further need to consider the ethical and political difficulties involved in developing such teams in concert with or opposition to state agenda (Madan, 1982; Paul and Demarest, 1984; Uberoi, 1968).

Research data generated by the CD project illustrate the kind of information regional participatory research teams might collect. The data indicate how regional differences in settlement patterns, kinship systems, social structure, health culture, and past experience with primary health center staff influence the response of the rural poor to health programs designed to involve them. The reasoning of villagers and planners is often quite different. For example, the emphasis of health planners on female CHWs, logical in terms of a CHW's scope of activities, may not be deemed appropriate locally. What needs to be considered are the social and economic ramifications of participation in different settings (UN, 1977). Training illiterate CHWs may make sense in one area but not in another, where high school or college graduates work as daily wage laborers and the community has begun to question the value of higher education. Schemes to involve schoolteachers in mobilizing community involvement in health may be appropriate in some areas but not in other areas, where teachers are the relatives of favored caste leaders and are viewed as paid government employees, not community servants. The same is true with respect to administering health programs through local government. In some areas of India, local government bodies are viewed by the poor as responsive political institutions committed to rural development; in other areas they represent vested interests of the rich to the detriment of the poor. Such issues need to be considered before plans are made to involve the community; otherwise what is planned to assist the rural poor may turn out to be assistance for the elite in the name of the poor (Ferguson, 1990; Morgan, 1993).

There are two other reasons why it would be advantageous to develop a network of participatory research teams as part of the primary health care process. The first involves bridging the gap between a comprehensive (community-oriented) primary health care model and a selective disease–oriented primary health care model (Mull, 1990). A community diagnosis approach to primary health care could (1) identify problems in need of outreach services involving both technical resources and social support (e.g., the monitoring of chronic illness and care of the elderly), and (2) remind those in public health about how populations respond to symptoms common to several diseases requiring the coordination of vertical health programs. A better understanding of community response to fevers, illnesses of the lungs, reproductive health, and so on, might lead those in public health to consider productive areas where programs might work cooperatively—such as acute respiratory infection (ARI), dengue, and malaria; ARI and TB; or reproductive tract infections, sexually transmitted disease, HIV, and family planning.

A second reason for supporting a participatory research agenda involves improving health and medical education. Lack of understanding of popular health behavior impedes health education. The creation of culturally appropriate approaches to health education and behavior change constitutes an area where CD teams could make a significant contribution. Up-to-date information on popular health culture(s) and changing patterns of lifestyle (e.g., consumption patterns), self-treatment, and so on, could facilitate more targeted approaches to health communication which focus on existing behavior patterns and recognize diversity in practice among heterogeneous populations. Banoo Coyagi, director of one of the more successful primary health care pilot projects in India, has spoken to this point:

> The rural audiences are not an amorphous whole but several diverse groups of people with different values and aspirations. The message—be it health, family planning or anything—must be designed differently to reach these different groups. This requires an empathetic approach with the combined insight of social and behavioral scientists, media specialists, extension workers, community health workers, and a most important source of inspiration, the people themselves. (Coyagi, 1980:8)

A Swahili proverb states that when one is walking it is difficult to see the soles of one's feet. While involved with the routine struggles of day-to-day life, it is difficult to step back and reflect. This is one reason why eliciting community needs has been so difficult. Participatory research fosters a process of discovery and critical thinking, enabling community members at once to recognize and think beyond their individual needs and positions. For "experts" such as myself, such research reminds us to reexamine our own assumptions while enabling us to be privy to local ways of solving problems.

Notes

1. Ideological reasons behind the promotion of community participation are discussed by Ugalde (1985) and Morgan (1990). Community participation has recently regained popularity in regions of India such as Kerala where the decentralization of

health planning is currently underway. Under the newly envisioned *Panchayat Raj* system, "communities" draw up proposals and submit them to the state ministry of health for funding. Missing from the system is local level research enabling community members to critically assess their needs. Facilitators of participatory research are clearly needed.

2. See Woelk (1992), Cornwall and Jewkes (1995), and Jewkes and Murcott (1996) for critical reviews of conceptual and practical difficulties related to the definition of community and the interpretation of community participation. Communities have been defined as: (1) people living in one location and sharing values, culture, and problems; (2) people sharing common interests at one point in time; (3) those sharing health risks within and beyond spatial boundaries; and (4) a set of power relations within which people are grouped. See Southall (1970) and Schwartz (1981) for a critical assessment of the way the concepts of tribe and community have been used and misused by social scientists and those in the development community. See Morgan (1993) for a critical discussion of the primary health care movement and the political ideology of participation.

3. It is popular to cite Kerala as a "good health at low cost" success story and make it seem that political will and primary health services are largely responsible for lower mortality rates and better overall health. While state health facilities are largely responsible for immunization and family planning success, this explanation may be overly simplistic given that a large majority of "community" members seek most of their health care from private practitioners.

4. I am not suggesting that all NGOs in India tailor their activities to match funding opportunities. For a recent review of some of India's best NGO activity in public health see Pachauri (1994).

5. Banerji (1981) has questioned the popularity of indigenous medicine, i.e., ayurveda, in India, suggesting that what people want is more effective health services. While I would agree with him in part, data such as these suggest that, despite the rising popularity of allopathic medicine, indigenous medicine is still valued. This is true not only among the poor, but also among the middle and upper classes, for a variety of reasons (Nichter and Nichter, 1996).

6. Several NGO-sponsored projects in India have demonstrated that communities are willing and able to contribute financially toward health care costs. The Ford Foundation (1990) has recently published four relevant case studies. See also Berman (1991).

7. Regional health educators (assigned to groups of villages and primary health centers) seemed to be the most appropriate people to work as liaisons between community diagnosis teams and the health ministry. This assessment contributed to the development of South Asia's first field-based master's degree (M.A.) curriculum in health education developed in Sri Lanka in 1983–1985 with WHO sponsorship.

Acknowledgment

An earlier version of this chapter was published in *Social Science and Medicine* (1984) 19:237–252.

References

Banerji D (1981) The place of indigenous and western systems of medicine in the health services of India. *Social Science and Medicine* 15A:109–114.

Banerji D (1985) Health and Family Planning Service in India. An Epidemiological, Socio-Cultural and Political Analysis and a Perspective. New Delhi: Lak Paksh.

Bang R, Bang A (1994) "Women's Perceptions of White Vaginal Discharge: Ethnographic Data from Rural Maharashtra." In: Listening to Women Talk about Their Health. Issues and Evidence from India. J Gittelsohn et al., eds. New Delhi: Har-anand Publishers, pp. 79–94.

Bentley ME, Pelto GH, Strauss WL, Schumann DA, Adegbola C, de la Peña E, Oni GA, Brown KH, Huffman SL (1988) Rapid ethnographic assessment: applications in a diarrhoea management program. Social Science and Medicine 27:107–116.

Berman P (1991) Health Economics, Health Financing and the Health Needs of Poor Women and Children in India. New Delhi: Ford Foundation.

Berman P (In press) Rethinking health care systems: private health care provision in India. World Development.

Blustain H (1982) Review of: The Use and Misuse of Social Science Research in Nepal. Rural Development Participation Review 3(2):20.

Campbell JG, Shrestha R, Stone L (1979) The Use and Misuse of Social Science Research in Nepal. Kathmandu: Center for Nepal and Asian Studies.

Chambers R (1992) Rural Appraisal: Rapid, Relaxed and Participatory. Brighton: Institute for Development Studies Discussion Paper No. 311.

Chopra P (1982) The paradox of Kerala. World Health Forum 3:74–77.

Cochrane G (1979) The Cultural Appraisal of Development Projects. New York: Praeger.

Cornwall A, Jewkes R (1995) What is participatory research? Social Science and Medicine 41:1667–1676.

Coyagi B (1980) Health communication with rural audiences. Communicator 15(1):1–8.

de Koning K, Martin M (1996) "Participatory Research in Health: Setting the Context." In: Participatory Research in Health: Issues and Experiences. K de Koning, M Martin, eds. New Delhi, India: Vistaar Publishing House.

Ferguson J (1990) The Anti-Politics Machine. Cambridge: Cambridge University Press.

Fernandes W, Tandon R (1981) Participatory Research and Evolution. Experiments in Research as a Process of Liberation. New Delhi: Indian Social Institute.

Ford Foundation (1990) The Costs and Financing of Health Care. Experiences in the Voluntary Sector in Four Regions of India. New Delhi: Ford Foundation.

Franke R, Chasin B (1992) Kerala State, India: radical reform as development. International Journal of Health Services 22:139–156.

Hall BL (1981) Participatory research, popular knowledge and power: a personal reflection. Convergence 14:6–17.

Hall B (1982) "Breaking the Monopoly of Knowledge: Research Methods, Participation and Development." In: Creating Knowledge: A Monopoly? B Hall, A Gillette, R Tandon, eds. Toronto: International Council for Adult Education, pp. 1–13.

Jewkes R, Murcott A (1996) Meanings of community. Social Science and Medicine 43:555–563.

Korten DC (1979) Community Social Organization in Rural Development. Resource paper for the Ford Foundation, Yogyakarta, Indonesia, October.

Lincoln Y, Guba E (1985) Naturalistic Inquiry. Beverly Hills, Calif: Sage Publications.

Mackay DM (1981) Editorial. Journal of Tropical Medicine and Hygiene 84:93–94.

Madan TN (1982) "Anthropology as the Mutual Interpretation of Cultures: Indian Perspectives." In: Indigenous Anthropology in Non-Western Contexts. H Fahim, ed. Durham, NC: Carolina Academic Press, pp. 4–18.

Manderson L, Aaby P (1992a) An epidemic in the field? Rapid assessment procedures and health research. Social Science and Medicine 35(7):839–850.

Manderson L, Aaby P (1992b) Can rapid anthropological procedures be applied to tropical diseases? *Health Policy and Planning* 7:46–55.

Maru R (1980) Community health worker: some aspects of the experience at the national level. *Medical Friends Circle Bulletin* 51, March:1–5.

Maxwell J (1992) Understanding and validity in qualitative research. *Harvard Educational Review* 62:279–300.

McCracken J, Pretty J, Conaway G (1989) An Introduction to Rapid Rural Appraisal for
Agricultural Development. London: International Institute for Environment and
Development.

Morgan L (1990) International politics and primary health care in Costa Rica. *Social
Science and Medicine* 50:211–219.

Morgan L (1993) Community Participation in Health. Cambridge: Cambridge University Press.

Mull D (1990) "The Primary Health Care Dialectic: History, Rhetoric and Reality."
In: Anthropology and Primary Health Care. J Coreil, D Mull, eds. Boulder, Colo:
Westview Press, pp. 28–47.

Nag M (1988) The Kerala formula. *World Health Forum* 9:258–262.

Nag M (1989) Political Awareness as a Factor in Accessibility of Health Services. A Case
Study of Rural Kerala and West Bengal. New York: Population Council, Population
Centered Working Papers, No. 3.

Nichter M (1980a) Community Health Worker scheme: A plan for democratization.
Economic and Political Weekly 15:37–43.

Nichter M (1980b) Health Expenditure Data for North and South Kanara Districts,
Karnataka. Project Community Diagnosis Data Report, Section 2. New Delhi:
USAID, pp. 1–62.

Nichter M, Nichter M (1980) Project Community Diagnosis Baseline Data Reports and
Methodological Guide to the Organization and Training of Community Diagnosis
Health Teams. New Delhi: USAID Office of Health, Nutrition and Population.

Nichter M, Nichter M (1996) Anthropology and International Health. Asian Case Studies. Amsterdam: Gordon and Breach.

Pachauri S, ed. (1994) Reaching India's Poor. New Delhi: Sage Publications.

Panikar P (1979) Resource not the constraint on health improvement: a case study of
Kerala. *Economic and Political Weekly* 14:1803–1809.

Paul BD, Demarest WJ (1984) Citizen participation overplanned: the case of a health
project in the Guatemalan community of San Pedro la Laguna. *Social Science and
Medicine* 19:185–192.

Perez C (1997) The colors of participation. *Practicing Anthropology* (special edited
edition) 19 (Summer).

Rao KG (1979) Innovative research for primary health care. Paper presented at the 18th
Annual Conference of the Indian Association for the Advancement of Medical Education. New Delhi: February.

Ratcliffe J (1978) Social justice and the demographic transition: lessons from India's
Kerala State. *International Journal of Health Services* 8:123–144.

Schwartz NB (1981) Anthropological views of community and community development.
Human Organization 40:313–322.

Scrimshaw NS, Gleason GR, eds. (1992) RAP. Rapid Assessment Procedures. Qualitative Methodologies for Planning and Evaluation of Health Related Programmes. Boston: International Nutrition Foundation for Developing Countries.

Scrimshaw SCM, Hurtado E (1987) Rapid Assessment Procedures for Nutrition and
Primary Health Care. Anthropological Approaches to Improving Programme

Effectiveness. Los Angeles: University of California, Latin American Center Publications.

Southall AW (1970) The illusion of tribe. *Journal of Asian and African Studies* 5:28–50.

Srinivas MN (1979) Reflections on rural development. *Mainstream* 11, May 12:11.

Srivastva RN (1978) Evaluating Communicability and Comprehensibility of the Manual for CHWs, vols. 1 and 2. New Delhi: UNICEF.

Sussman GE (1980) "The Pilot Project and the Choice of an Implementing Strategy: Community Development in India." In: Politics and Policy Implementation in the Third World. MS Grindle, ed. Princeton, NJ: Princeton University Press, pp. 103–122.

Tandon R (1981) Participatory research in the empowerment of people. *Convergence* 14:20–29.

Taylor C (1968) "The Health Sciences and Indian Village Culture." In: Science and the Human Condition in India and Pakistan. W Morehouse, ed. New York: Rockefeller University Press, pp. 153–161.

Uberoi JPS (1968) Science and swaraj. *Contributions in Indian Sociology* 2:119–127.

Ugalde A (1985) Ideological dimensions of community participation in Latin American health programs. *Social Science and Medicine* 21:41–53.

United Nations Protein Food Advisory Group (1977) Report on Women in Food Production, Food Handling and Nutrition. New York: UNICEF.

Walt G (1988) CHWs: are national programmes in crisis? *Health Policy and Planning* 3:1–21.

Woelk G (1992) Cultural and structural influences in the creation of and participation in community health programmes. *Social Science and Medicine* 35:419–424.

WHO (1978) Primary Health Care. Report of International Conference on Primary Health Care, Alma-Ata, USSR, September 6–12. Geneva: World Health Organization.

VI

HEALTH INSTITUTIONS

15

Neglect of Cultural Knowledge in Health Planning: Nepal's Assistant Nurse-Midwife Program

JUDITH JUSTICE

Assistant nurse-midwives, women trained in maternal and child health care, are considered core paramedicals in community-based primary health care programs in many countries. The primary health care approach, a high priority in international health policy since the late 1970s, is based on the premise, among others, that health services are most effective when tailored to fit specific needs and the socioeconomic environment of particular populations. Developing countries receive extensive assistance for community-based primary health care from international donor agencies whose policy statements and reports repeatedly emphasize the need for local input in health planning, including information about local customs and beliefs.

Since the 1960s, United Nations agencies, especially the World Health Organization (WHO), the United Nations Children's Fund (UNICEF), United Nations Fund for Population Activities (UNFPA), and bilateral aid agencies, including the United States Agency for International Development (USAID), have developed and funded training programs for assistant nurse-midwives (ANMs) as part of national maternal and child health programs. This has been justified on the grounds that in many countries, Nepal among them, women could be more effective than men in providing maternal and child health care and assistance in family planning. Increasing education and employment opportunities through the ANM program were also viewed as ways of enhancing women's social status. Initially designed as part of the basic health services approach to providing care in clinics, the ANMs' role was later redefined by international donor agencies and many national governments to include promotive and preventive services, a change meant to ensure community-based primary health care.

To stimulate the development of ANM programs and nursing in general at the country level, WHO has sponsored intercountry workshops, provided long- and short-term consultants on nursing to national governments, and provided international fellowships to strengthen national nursing administrative and educational capacity. WHO and UNICEF also have donated supplies and equipment for the support of nursing education and services, and bilateral aid has been used for fellowships, curriculum development, and construction of training campuses.

Yet in Nepal, as in many other parts of the world, the ANM program has not worked as international agencies and governments expected. Often the assistant nurse-midwife has not been able to work effectively because traditional expectations about women conflict with her health role as designed by health planners. This chapter examines the problems faced by the ANM program in Nepal, at both the local and planning levels, and suggests how it might be made more effective.

Research Methods

To examine the planning and implementation of community-based primary health care in Nepal, beginning in the late 1970s, I started at the international level and progressed through the national and district levels to the delivery of services at the local level, the rural Nepali village. By using traditional anthropological methods—in-depth, open-ended interviewing and participant observation—I studied the activities of international planners involved with Nepal, the formulation of government priorities and programs in Kathmandu (Nepal's capital), and the delivery of health services in outlying districts and villages. Interviews were both formal and informal, using structured and unstructured formats with a guideline of topics. Interview and observation notes were written up daily. Key issues were identified and used as a guide for sorting and analyzing the descriptive, qualitative data.

The first research challenge was to gain access to the international and national health bureaucracies involved with Nepal's community health program to understand how planners work and how their perceptions and social interactions influence the decisions they make. My previous experience working in international agencies (one year with the United Nations in New York and two years with UNICEF in India) had provided me with some understanding of the internal structure of international aid agencies and their interaction with national governments.

To find out who the planners were and how they worked, I made contact with the major international agencies supporting rural health programs in Nepal in the late 1970s, including WHO in Geneva and New Delhi, UNICEF and the United Nations Development Program (UNDP) in New York, USAID and the World Bank in Washington, the Canadian International Development Agency (CIDA) and the International Research Development Centre (IRDC) in Ottawa, nongovernmental organizations such as the Britain Nepal Medical Trust (BNMT), and consulting groups contracted for the Community Health Program under USAID. I visited the headquarters and regional offices of these agencies to review documentation and interview staff members who formulated agency health policy or were associated with work in Nepal. I also interviewed staff social scientists. I wanted to find out from them what their roles had been in planning the donor agency's assistance to Nepal's health program, what kinds of social and cultural data had been available, and how they were used.

In Nepal, I interviewed Nepali officials in the Ministry of Finance, the Planning Commission, and the Ministry and Department of Health in Kathmandu, including personnel in the assistant nurse-midwife and other health programs. I met with people who had worked on Nepal's long-term health plans as well as those implementing community health services. I also interviewed staff members and consultants with the various international agencies and reviewed available documents.

To understand the actual workings of the community health program and the role of the ANM, I interviewed government officials, administrative health officers, health service practitioners, ANMs, and patients, and I observed activities at the district and health post levels over a period of 12 months. For this last step, I visited 10 districts that had different geographic characteristics and represented different phases of the community health program. During these visits I familiarized myself with government activities at the district level, the role of the local and district *panchayats* (government councils), health post committees, health facilities, and the local operation of the community health program.

In addition to interviewing health officers and administrative officials in the district centers, I visited 24 health posts to meet ANMs, other health workers, and those using the services. It took several days of walking to reach many of these locations. I spent a number of days at each post, accompanied ANMs and other health workers on their home visits, and made follow-up visits to the homes of patients who came to the post. I also visited several small community health projects sponsored on a pilot basis by religious missions such as the United Mission to Nepal and nongovernmental organizations such as Save the Children UK, which provided support for ANM programs. On some of these field visits I was alone or with my Nepali research assistant, a young Thakali man from the western hills. On others I was accompanied by ANMs and other local health workers, by officials from the central or district level, or by foreign health advisers. The latter visits enabled me to understand what information health officials sought and how they obtained it. By moving back and forth from the local to the national level, I was able to observe how information was transmitted in both directions and what factors facilitated or constrained the flow. Although I tried to understand the functioning of the health programs I observed, I was not in a position to evaluate their medical effectiveness, and this was not my intention. My aim was to see how appropriate the ANM and other health programs were to the local culture.

By visiting rural health posts and accompanying ANMs and other health workers on their daily rounds, I acquired some understanding of local conditions and the problems faced by health workers, usually of urban origin, in an isolated rural environment. The difficulties of travel and communication made me more sensitive to the obstacles encountered by Nepali and foreign planners based in Kathmandu in obtaining information at the local level.

During this research, my original question—What kinds of information do health planners need, and when do they need it?—evolved into a new question: What contribution can an anthropologist make to health planning? The answer must come from an understanding of the planning process—the complex cultural settings in which policies and plans filter down through stages of implementation to interact with cultures at the local level. Using the traditional anthropological approach of studying a culture through the perceptions of participants, I hoped to enhance our understanding of this process and thus to find more effective ways of assisting planners in their difficult undertaking of designing programs, such as the Assistant Nurse-Midwife Program, that may eventually provide services to all.

The Nepalese Situation

Nepal is a Hindu kingdom, governed as a partyless monarchy until 1990 when it became a constitutional monarchy. It is located in the Himalayas, north of India and south of China and Tibet; it is about 500 miles long and 100 miles wide. In 1982, some 96% of its ethnically diverse population of approximately 14 million lived in rural areas and practiced subsistence agriculture under extremely difficult conditions. The high mountainous terrain, divided by three river systems, isolates the rural population from the central government in the Kathmandu Valley and has hindered the development of transportation, communication, and other infrastructure, including health facilities. Many rural areas can be reached only by walking hilly trails for hours or days.

Since the 1950s, when few modern health facilities existed, Nepal has expanded its health services. By the early 1980s, the health system included nearly 70 hospitals ranging from 15 to 300 beds; approximately 450 medical doctors, of whom only 25% were located in rural areas; 350 nurses, with 14% in rural areas; and 550 health posts staffed by paramedical workers, located throughout Nepal's 75 districts. The health posts, which are the heart of Nepal's rural health program, were theoretically to have a health assistant, one or two auxiliary health workers, one or two ANMs, two to six village health workers, and a peon, whose official job would be to do custodial work and run errands. But many health posts had only a health assistant, village health workers, and a peon. Each post served between 10,000 and 30,000 people, depending on geographic location and population density (WHO, 1978).

While much had been accomplished in Nepal in combating some health problems, such as the eradication of smallpox and control of malaria, morbidity and mortality rates were still very high, especially for infants and children. Childhood diseases ranked as the country's major health problem. Although the accuracy of available statistics was questionable, it was estimated in 1980 that 54% of all deaths were among children under 5 and that between 134 and 260 infants per 1,000 live births died in their first year, one of the highest infant mortality rates in Asia. Because of the high infant mortality, life expectancy at birth was low: 46 years for males and 43 years for females (WHO, 1979).

The main causes of infant and child death were diarrhea from impure water and foodborne diseases, nutritional deficiencies, pneumonia, other communicable diseases, and injuries. Many of these conditions are curable, if not preventable, as are the major causes of maternal morbidity and mortality: poor nutrition, frequent pregnancies, lack of proper prenatal care, complications of pregnancy and delivery, and medically unsupervised abortions (Ministry of Health, 1979b). On the basis of the 1976 National Fertility Survey, the crude birth rate per 1,000 population in Nepal was estimated at 43.6—again one of the highest in Asia. Nepal's population growth rate in 1976 and in 1992 was over 2.5% per year because women marry early and continue having children throughout the fertile years. Because sons were strongly preferred, couples had many children (6.8 per married woman; United Nations Children's Fund, 1978), in the hope that at least one or two sons would survive to adulthood. Few couples knew about or had access to modern means of contraception, despite government attempts to promote family planning. Conditions in Nepal indicated a compelling need for maternal and child health services.

The assistant nurse-midwife program in Nepal offered two years of training for females who were at least 16 years old and had at least an eighth-grade education. Its stated purpose was primarily to deliver maternal and child health (MCH) services to the rural population. Based in health posts, the ANMs were responsible for prenatal care, birth assistance, postnatal care, family planning, and limited infant and child care. They were expected to conduct MCH clinics, including vaccinations and health education sessions, and to make home visits to pregnant women, families with young children, and couples eligible for family planning services.

Although as early as 1965 there were 16 ANMs working in hospitals (United Nations Children's Fund, 1982), it was not until 1973 as part of the pilot project for Integrated Community Health Care, later redefined as community-based primary health care, that they were first assigned to rural health posts and outreach clinics and expected to make home visits on a regular basis. The number of ANMs increased rapidly during the 1970s. By 1977, it had grown to 404 (Ministry of Health, 1980). By 1980, the five ANM training campuses, located in Tansen, Kathmandu, and three Terai cities near the border with India, had trained 1,049 females (WHO, 1978). By then the ANM was considered a core worker in Nepal's rural health program, and approximately 60% were assigned to rural health posts (Ministry of Health, 1980).

Although ANMs were supposed to be trained to work in health posts as outreach workers for MCH, rather than to serve as staff nurses, by the 1970s the curriculum was primarily in curative medicine. This was more appropriate to clinical settings than to community responsibilities, which were primarily preventive and promotive health. Many ANMs, although technically assigned to health posts and paid as if working there, actually worked in hospitals. That they preferred this assignment was understandable, as that is where 90% of their training took place. Here, they filled a gap because there was no government funding for the services they provided in hospitals. Although the 1980 Health Manpower Survey indicated how many ANMs had been trained and assigned to hospitals, health centers, and health posts, it did not show how many were actually on duty. According to government reports, all ANM positions in health posts were filled; however, official estimates were that only 30% of the ANM health post positions actually had ANMs working in them at any one time (Ministry of Health, 1980).

Difficulties at the Local Level

Most ANMs never reached the remote areas to which they were assigned, and those who did rarely remained long. Why? The answer is clear: it is socially unacceptable in Nepal for girls and women to travel and live alone, as ANMs were expected to do. Although there are differing social practices, economic opportunities, and degrees of freedom among the various ethnic and religious groups in Nepal, conservative Hindu values dominate the Nepalese view of women: their roles are limited primarily to those of wife and mother. Traditionally, women do not work outside the family but contribute labor to the household and to domestic and agricultural production. Since a woman's status is determined by her marriage, and virtually all women marry, parents are concerned with protecting the reputations of their daughters until they can make good matches for them.

ANMs typically came from urban areas, since girls in rural areas, with limited educational opportunities, seldom met the minimum requirement of an eighth-grade education. In Nepal in the early 1980s, the literacy rate for females aged 10 years and above was 3.7%, in contrast to 24.7% for males. For females in rural areas, the rate was 2.7%, compared with 26.4% for those in urban centers (Acharya, 1979). Although rural educational facilities were increasing, village parents were less willing than urban parents to send girls to school, and rural girls who did go were sent for a shorter time. In addition, some urban families had a more liberal attitude than rural families toward the employment of women outside the home. Although ANM training was viewed as an avenue to salaried work, and perhaps to a better marriage, the parents were often unaware of the working situation for which the girls were being prepared.

Many of the rural health posts to which ANMs were assigned were located in isolated villages, several days' walk from the nearest district center or a road adequate for use by motorized vehicles. Far from home and family, ANMs had to live on their own. If accommodation was available at the health post, it usually was occupied by the health assistant, so ANMs had to find housing in the community. In addition, they were usually the only women working at the post; the other staff workers were almost always men. Therefore, as the only women, the ANMs were especially vulnerable to local criticism and abuse. It was against all sociocultural values for a young, unmarried woman to live on her own in a village or with male staff in a health post. Male workers in rural health posts were also discontented because of the working conditions, especially their isolation from urban areas, but they were not vulnerable in the same sense as women, and their reputations were not at stake.

The social difficulties the ANMs faced were easy to understand in the 24 health posts in 10 districts which I visited. For example, when I arrived at a post in the Terai, in a culturally conservative district of strong Muslim influence, bordering on India, I found two ANMs, 17 and 18 years old, standing together at some distance from the male health workers. They gave the impression of being unsure of their role and afraid. Both were from Kathmandu. They were very unhappy at the post and described their situation as difficult. Initially they had no place to live and were not accepted by the villagers. They described ways in which the male health workers and villagers had tried to take advantage of them. For example, the senior health assistant expected the ANMs to serve as his assistants in the health post and as personal maids. The young women were also fearful of sexual advances. Although they felt fortunate in having each other for support and now shared a rented room in a nearby house, it was difficult for them to adjust to living without piped water, electricity, and other amenities available in urban areas.

In Nepal's hierarchical society, the urban ANMs were regarded by rural residents as alien and socially superior. Villagers described their white-and-blue nursing uniforms as "fancy saris" and made remarks about their city shoes, thus accentuating the social distance and communication problems experienced by the ANMs. Acceptability in the community was influenced not only by urban–rural differences, but by regional differences and attitudes, language barriers, and ethnic and caste distinctions. All outsiders were viewed as strangers, especially members of a different caste and ethnic background. Reluctant to call on strangers for help, the villagers continued to rely on family members for pregnancy care, resorting to the health post only when serious problems occurred. But even local women who were only 16 years old would be inappropriate as ANMs, because unmarried women without children were viewed as too young and inexperienced to inspire confidence as midwives.

A district doctor who was sensitive to the problems ANMs were having said that those in his district were from urban areas and had great difficulty in adjusting to rural life. He recognized their vulnerability and the obstacles they faced in living and working alone. Those who stayed for a year usually adjusted, he observed, but the only ones who stayed that long were those who needed to work and could not afford to go home. He cited the lack of training in rural settings as another cause of the ANMs' problems.

A nursing consultant also observed that ANMs lacked training in rural areas. At the ANM campuses, she said, they were treated as though they were in an isolated religious convent, which fitted with Nepali expectations. They then were sent out to work, completely on their own, in total contrast to those expectations. Furthermore, the consultant stated, ANMs were not trained to work independently or to organize and manage their own work, though their job description clearly required these skills.

In the 1979 Mid-Term Review of Nepal's health services, health post records indicated few prenatal or postnatal clinic activities, family planning services, or home visits (Ministry of Health, 1979a). Although primary health care programs stressed the ANMs' role in the community, there was little incentive for ANMs to leave the safer environment of the health post to visit villages. ANMs rarely had access to transportation, even when it was available to others at the post, since they were at the bottom of the health staff hierarchy.

ANMs were supposed to be supervised by the District Public Health Nurse (PHN), but in 1979 only eight of Nepal's 75 districts had PHNs. One PHN told me that she had visited each of the 11 health posts in her district only once during her two-year assignment. In another district, where many health posts were accessible by road, the PHN said she was unable to visit the ANMs because she had no means of transportation and was afraid of being robbed. This PHN was very unhappy in her job. She hoped to be transferred to the capital, where she could arrange for further training abroad, which would qualify her for an administrative position in the central Ministry of Health. It was not possible, she said, to lobby for training or promotion from the district. The district doctor, her supervisor, confirmed that she spent most of her time sitting in the district health office complaining and arranging for a transfer back to Kathmandu, and that she was rarely involved in MCH services, even in the district clinics.

Like the ANMs, most PHNs had difficulty adjusting to rural conditions, even in district centers, where adequate accommodations were provided in district hospitals. Even though PHNs usually were older than ANMs and married and therefore had a higher status and greater social acceptance, it was extremely difficult for them to travel on foot or by road to health posts without suitable transport, porter services, and protection. The result was that ANMs received little support or supervision. Those ANMs who did go to rural areas had no choice but to rely on their own limited resources or to give up their jobs and return home.

In addition to the social problems faced by the ANMs, their job description often contradicted local customs in relation to pregnancy and child care. For example, as part of WHO's program to upgrade the skills of traditional birth attendants (TBAs), ANMs were instructed to teach pre- and postnatal care and safe methods of delivery to local birth attendants. But in many regions of Nepal, there were no *sudenis* or *dhais* (TBAs). Only 10% of women received any kind of formal health care during pregnancy (American Public Health Association, 1980; Ministry of Health, 1979b). Except in the case of complicated deliveries, for which ANMs received no training, neither ANMs nor TBAs were typically called upon by village women, who relied on themselves and family members for routine delivery and postnatal care (Parker et al., 1979). In the few areas where there were TBAs, they were mostly older women. It was unlikely they would welcome suggestions from young, unmarried ANMs. Consequently, assigning ANMs to teach TBAs had limited relevance in most of Nepal.

Difficulties at the Planning Level

In 1978, a task force was appointed by Nepal's Institute of Medicine to review the ANM program. Although the task force did not tackle the underlying problem—that, because of social and cultural conditions, the program was inappropriate—some of the practical problems were listed in the report: (1) women of urban origins were unwilling to go to rural areas; (2) ANMs received no supervision; and (3) women and children were not being served in rural areas. The report suggested a solution: existing ANMs should be offered upgraded training to enable them to work in hospitals, while the present rural program should be replaced by a new health auxiliary program which would recruit women from the same areas in which they would ultimately work. The curriculum should be redesigned and a pilot training program carried out. However, at the time of this study, these sensible recommendations had not been implemented.

Even though in 1979 the Ministry of Health knew that the ANM program was not working as planned, it permitted the Institute of Medicine to proceed with plans to expand the program and open new ANM training campuses. Discussion of expanding the ANM's role in primary health care continued in Kathmandu, just as though the ANMs were functioning satisfactorily.

It is not only planners in Nepal who push ahead despite known obstacles. When I visited WHO headquarters in Geneva in June 1979, physicians and planners asked how primary health care was working in Nepal. I discussed the problems of the ANM program with them. Most indicated that they knew of similar problems from personal experience in South Asia and in their own countries. Even in countries with a traditional birth attendant program, ANMs as young unmarried women usually found it difficult to gain respect for themselves and their services. One planner was revising policy guidelines for ANM training. I felt that our discussion was unlikely to influence those guidelines significantly, because the unwelcome evidence, if fully considered, would threaten the very existence of the program.

If the ANM program was in many ways ineffective and culturally antithetical, why was it organized and subsequently continued? Health officials in Kathmandu, including Nepalis from urban areas, were all well aware that it was socially unacceptable for women to travel and live alone; there were also the general difficulties of working in remote areas. Nevertheless, this program was part of the WHO-UNICEF support package in response to the government's request for assistance. Accepting it provided a variety of benefits for the government. Especially since 1975, International Women's Year, international, national, and private forces had exerted pressure for greater employment of women in Nepal. Except for nurses and some women doctors, most positions in the Nepali health service were filled by men. In the rural health program, men were hired to be family planning motivators, village health workers, and health assistants. The ANM program offered the government an opportunity to show that it was also developing careers for women. Moreover, the foreign assistance funds provided for establishing ANM training schools were difficult to refuse.

To these reasons must be added others that reflect aspects of the international and national bureaucratic cultures. One aspect is the momentum of international health policy, which inundates local realities as it sweeps downward from policy-making circles to planners in Kathmandu. In a sense, the prevailing health policy—in this case, the promotion of ANMs in community-based health care—is part of the bureaucratic culture of the international donor agencies. Another aspect is the insulation of policymakers from the outcomes of their programs. Since neither Nepali nor foreign planners are involved in implementation of the ANM program, they are shielded from daily reminders of local realities. Still another aspect is the value system of the Western health bureaucracies, which filters out "soft" (i.e., subjective and nonquantitative) social and cultural information from the planning and evaluation process.

A final aspect is the reward system within health bureaucracies. Although Nepali civil servants at the Central Secretariat level are aware that many of the plans promoted by the donor agencies, like the ANM program, are unworkable, they can expect no rewards from either the government or the agencies for voicing their reservations. If they at least appear to cooperate, they can expect rewards in the form of job security and travel to international conferences. At the same time, they may find ways to obstruct programs they do not believe in or ways to redefine them to fit personal or bureaucratic priorities. Foreign planners and consultants, for their part, see themselves as being responsible to offices in Geneva and Washington. Although they may be aware that programs need to be changed, they do not want to make mistakes or take actions that might jeopardize their positions in Nepal or their prospects for advancement. Often they are specialists who are assigned certain tasks over a relatively short term. Their reward lies in successful completion of these tasks, not in criticizing entire programs.

Suggestions for Changing the ANM's Role

If the ANM program has not proven effective in providing maternal and child health services in rural areas, it has nevertheless made a variety of positive contributions, both manifest and latent, to hospital care; the development of nursing cadres; the expansion of training institutions; female employment and government manpower lists; individual social status; increasing purchasing power; and to international agencies, including the provision of jobs for international advisers. Considering the benefits it brought to the individual, society, government, and international agencies, a complete dismantling of the ANM program was unlikely. An alternative was to change the program, so that it would be more appropriate to local conditions and needs. By 1979, some steps had already been taken in this direction. Nepali health officials had dealt informally with the ANMs' problems by permitting many ANMs to work in hospitals, even though their names remained on the rosters of the health posts where they were officially assigned and paid. While this solution made use of the skills ANMs had acquired, it unfortunately bypassed the larger problem of meeting the critical need for maternal and child health services in rural Nepal.

The recruitment of older married women from the areas where they would be posted certainly would be a culturally appropriate alternative to the practice of hiring young unmarried urban women. ANMs could then live at home and be available at local health posts and to the nearby community, even though it would still be difficult to travel to more distant areas alone. Arranging for two or more women to be posted together, even when they live with families, would provide additional support. Furthermore, communities would feel responsible for their own women and would help ensure their protection.

Unfortunately, employing older rural women would require lowering the educational requirements for ANM candidates—a change that health officials would be unlikely to make, given the trend to upgrade and professionalize all health workers. Therefore, I believed that adjusting the existing ANM program to improve its cultural appropriateness gradually was a more realistic strategy. A first step would be to include in the training program an extensive field placement in a rural area for ANM training of both faculty and students, allowing them to become familiar with local conditions and customs. At one ANM training campus I visited, each student group had a four-week field placement in a village. A foreign nurse who worked with the government as an ANM tutor lived with the students in the village, where they met with local leaders, talked with women about local practices for delivery, learned about birth and infancy taboos and rituals, and provided supervised maternal and child health services at the local health post and in mobile clinics in surrounding villages. This was the only such program I observed, but it appeared to be an excellent example of how field experience could be incorporated into the training program. It also illustrated the importance of experience in rural areas for health educators and trainers themselves. Unfortunately, long-term village residence is in some ways easier for a single foreign woman to undertake than it is for her Nepali counterpart. Most female Nepali doctors, nurses, and educators are married women whose husbands work in urban centers; when they go to rural areas, they encounter the same cultural expectations and conflicts as do the ANMs.

Another strategy would be to study traditional birth practices, which vary among ethnic groups and regions, and the role of local women who are called on to assist in delivery, including older family members and traditional birth attendants. ANMs could incorporate information learned from these women into their own work with patients.

The few ANMs who have been able to work effectively in rural health posts should be studied to learn what factors contributed to their success. This information would be useful in determining recruitment criteria as well as for revising training programs. Finally, simplifying the ANMs' job description to limit their responsibilities to those tasks that are most essential and can be competently done with the available resources would increase their confidence and self-esteem.

Sociocultural Information and the Health Planning Process: The Anthropologist's Role in Planning

My goal in undertaking this research was to find better ways for health planners and social scientists to work together. In the course of my work I found that preconceived impressions often intensified misunderstandings. For example, it is commonly thought that anthropologists are interested in studying only traditional medical practices and practitioners. But many anthropologists share with planners an interest in providing effective health care within a given cultural milieu and in solving the problems faced by rural health workers. Planners frequently interpret anthropological reports as providing a negative perspective on local conditions. From the anthropologist's point of view, such information, even if its implications might seem negative, is directed toward the constructive result of understanding a situation from the perspectives of all participants.

The planners and administrators I interviewed in Nepal and in the headquarters of donor agencies often described social and cultural information as "soft" data, saying that it was too descriptive, too wordy and confusing, and too difficult to evaluate. They considered anthropologists' reports to be full of jargon, unwieldy, and unusable; anthropological studies were described as being "written for the university" and too narrow in scope. Many planners stated that, when designing a new program, they could not be concerned with the detailed information on which they feel anthropologists focus. Since meeting deadlines is very important in the donor agencies, planners tend to see the gathering of anthropological data as too time-consuming, and there is resistance to reports that are longer than a few pages. Some agency administrators said that length was not the issue, however, because they simply did not have time to read *any* background information. Foreigners did not claim to be familiar with anthropological information about Nepal. Some Nepali planners and administrators said that they were knowledgeable about rural Nepal's culture, but they agreed with advisers that such information is often irrelevant to health planning at the central level. Faced with the task of formulating a plan for all of rural Nepal, planners do not focus on the complexities of information specific to each local area and group. To take this detailed information into account would make their task much more complicated, and thus they tend to disregard such potentially confusing information.

National and international economic and political considerations are just as important in shaping health policy and the plans for specific programs as are the health goals themselves. The kinds of information that planners perceive as useful are determined in part by the structure and procedures of the government and international bureaucracies. Since meeting deadlines is critical to fulfilling agency demands, planners feel that they cannot wait for new studies to appear or spend time reading lengthy reports and books. Though organization policy often requires reports by anthropologists and other social scientists, planners and administrators feel that they need quantitative "hard" data, primarily statistical facts, to justify expenditures. To them cultural data are impressionistic, not quantifiable, and hence largely useless.

The planner's point of view has considerable validity. Many social science topics are inconsequential to the needs of bureaucrats, social science research does take time, and often relevant information may be buried in scholarly reports. In an earlier paper on the peon's role in the health service (Justice, 1983),

I explored the barriers to obtaining and incorporating socially relevant information into the planning process for Nepal's community health volunteer program. But the example of the assistant nurse-midwife demonstrates that the problem is not confined to the difficulty of obtaining cultural information. In this case, the information is available, but it is not being used.

The low-level peon, "the invisible worker," is the most accessible worker in Nepal's rural health service, despite the fact that his contribution is overlooked by national and international planners. Ironically, the ANM, whose role is designed and emphasized by national and international planners, is ineffective, since the social and cultural barriers to her success have also been overlooked. As discussed, everyone knows that young unmarried women cannot live and travel alone in remote villages in Nepal. Several international and government reports recognize that the ANM program does not produce useful health workers for the rural areas.[1] Yet these observations and recommendations are not reflected in plans and proposals. Thus it is not the availability or unavailability of information that determines whether it will be used.

Conclusion

The case of the ANM program in Nepal offers a key lesson for social scientists and health planners: the availability of relevant information in itself is not sufficient to ensure culturally appropriate health programs. The relevant cultural information is available—in fact, is common knowledge—yet it still does not influence health planning. Therefore, the question is how anthropologists and planners can work together more fruitfully to gather pertinent sociocultural information and incorporate it into planning and programs. If anthropologists tend to write for themselves and their fellow academics, it can also be said that planners tend to plan for themselves and their fellow planners. Each group needs to understand the other's point of view. Anthropologists need to understand the conditions under which planning is done and the limited alternatives available to planners trying to adapt policies and programs to local conditions. They need to present their information in a form that planners can use. For their part, planners need to understand that sociocultural information is vital and worth the time and money invested in examining it. Such collaboration could contribute to making the roles of the assistant nurse-midwives and other health workers more appropriate to the social and cultural setting.

Postscript

Many changes have taken place in Nepal since this study was originally written in 1982, including the dramatic but relatively peaceful transition from a partyless monarchy to a constitutional monarchy with a multiparty elected parliament. The population has grown from 14 million to 21 million. The health sector has seen the expansion of health facilities and the establishment of the Institute of Medicine for in-country training of medical and nursing professionals, along with the expansion of training for paramedicals. Health status has improved slightly, as reflected by increased life expectancy at birth, to 55 years for males and 52 years for females. By the 1990s, health facilities had expanded to 131 hospitals, 97 health centers, 755 health posts, and 3,300 sub–health posts (Dixit and Maskay, 1995). Medical doctors in government service included 334 in urban areas and 583 in rural areas.

Nevertheless, little has changed with respect to the assistant nurse-midwives, who remain central to the successful delivery of health services at the health center, health post, and community level. Although some of the changes recommended in 1982 have been incorporated into health planning in Nepal, traditional attitudes and practices relating to the status of women continue to influence what ANMs and other categories of female health workers can do. For example, local women were recruited to work as community-based health volunteers, but this program also encountered many problems related to the status and expectations of women. This situation is not unique to Nepal. ANMs are the backbone of community health programs in many countries, including neighboring India, where their services are also limited by unrealistic plans and by local cultural factors which lead to a misfit between international and local expectations. Thus the lessons learned from an examination of Nepal's Assistant Nurse-Midwife program continue to be relevant today.

Although the number of ANMs increased from 1,049 in 1980 to 1,751 in 1995, the need for maternal and child health services has not decreased as childhood diseases remain Nepal's major health problem and infant mortality rates are still among the highest in Asia (infant mortality rate of 79 per 1,000; under-5 mortality rate of 118 per 1,000). Maternal mortality rates are also among the highest in Asia (Thapa, 1996). Reports indicate that problems continue in the delivery of rural and community health services, including the functioning of the ANM (Aiken, 1994; Gautam and Shrestha, 1994; Liverpool Associates in Tropical Health, 1995; Ministry of Health, 1995–1996, 1997; Purdey et al., 1994). As predicted, the ANM program has become more professional with the entry criteria raised from completing eighth grade to completing tenth grade. Training of ANMs was transferred in 1994 from the Institute of Medicine to the Council for Technical Education and Vocational Training and affiliated private schools. This shift has resulted in poorly monitored education programs and inadequately trained ANMs.

A career ladder has also been created for ANMs, who now have supervisory responsibilities for the new categories of community health workers, including maternal and child health workers and female community health volunteers. Both of these positions were created in an attempt to address some of the problems identified by my study and in other reports, primarily that women health workers would be more effective if they were from the local area and worked near their family homes. These new health workers, however, have not functioned as well as expected, in part for the same reasons identified when studying the ANMs in the late 1970s. In addition to their low status as women, which places them at the bottom of the health system hierarchy, the chain of supervision from the top down remains extremely weak. Although there are more trained nurses in Nepal, still only a few districts have public health nurses to provide supervision for ANMs. Without supervision from above, ANMs are poorly equipped to provide guidance and support for the female health workers under them. Many rural health facilities are still without ANMs, as ANMs prefer to work in hospitals and urban centers. Although Nepal still receives large amounts of external assistance for health (including assistance for the ANM program) from a range of international health organizations, most donors have not addressed the problems related to establishing an effective system of supervision for ANMs, as this does not fit with their bureaucratic structures and procedures.

Certainly the need to improve the status of women has received attention, particularly after the 1994 International Conference on Population and Development and the 1995 Conference on Women in Beijing. The growth in rhetoric about women, however, has not always resulted in increased financial assistance, especially at the local level and for strengthening ongoing paramedical health programs designed to provide essential services to mothers and children. Often support is channeled to new activities which are more attractive and better fit the current international priorities, without first solving the problems identified in earlier programs, such as the role of ANMs.

What do the ongoing problems of the ANM indicate about the contribution of anthropology to health planning? In the case of the ANM program, the availability of information failed to prevent a culturally inappropriate design from being implemented, revised, and maintained for many years; nevertheless, such information may still contribute to making the program more effective. Although sociocultural information cannot ensure culturally appropriate programs, it remains an essential ingredient. Anthropologists make a direct contribution to health planning by sharing their approach, which is to study a situation from the perspective of the participants. This provides a missing link between planning and implementation. At the same time, we need to work harder to collaborate more effectively with health planners who hope to improve the planning process and existing programs, and thus better meet the needs of local communities.

Note

1. Problems in Nepal's assistant nurse-midwife program are noted in the following reports: Mid-Term Review (Ministry of Health, Nepal, 1979a); Planning for Health

Manpower (Ministry of Health, Nepal, 1980); Assistant Nurse-Midwife Task Force Report (1978); An Evaluation of AID-Financed Health and Family Planning Projects in Nepal (American Public Health Association, 1980).

Acknowledgments

I would like to thank Elizabeth Colson, Ruth Dixon, George Foster, Ellen Hershey, and Betty Webster for their constructive comments on earlier drafts of this chapter. Tony Bondurant and Ivan Somlai provided valuable information and assistance with revisions for the chapter in 1997. I am indebted to colleagues in Nepal and Geneva who helped with the research and the paper.

Earlier versions of this chapter were published in Social Science and Medicine (1984) 19, no. 3:193–198, and in Policies, Plans and People: Culture and Health Development in Nepal (Berkeley: University of California Press, 1986).

References

Acharya M (1979) Statistical Profile of Nepalese Women: A Critical Review. The Status of Women in Nepal, vol. 1, pt. 1. Kathmandu: Centre for Economic Development and Administration, Tribhuvan University.

Aiken J-M (1994) Voices from the inside: managing District Health Services in Nepal. International Journal of Health Planning and Management 9:309–340.

American Public Health Association (1980) An Evaluation of AID-Financed Health and Family Planning Projects in Nepal. Washington, DC: American Public Health Association.

Assistant Nurse-Midwife Task Force Report (1978). Unpublished mimeographed report. Kathmandu.

Dixit H, Maskay BD, eds. (1995) Medical Education in Nepal. Kathmandu: Nepal Medical Council and Nepal Medical Association.

Gautam M, Shrestha B (1994) Health Sector Review—Nepal. Kathmandu: For His Majesty's Government/Ministry of Health (HMG/MOH).

Justice J (1983) The invisible worker: the role of the peon in Nepal's Health Service. Social Science and Medicine 17:967–970.

Liverpool Associates in Tropical Health, UK and HURDEC (1995) ANM Study. Liverpool: Liverpool Associates in Tropical Health.

Ministry of Health, Nepal (1979a) Mid-Term Review 2035: Research and Evaluation of Health and Health Services Mid Fifth Plan Period (2013–2036). Kathmandu: Ministry of Health.

Ministry of Health, Nepal (1979b) Nepal Country Health Programming Exercise for the Preparation of the 6th Plan Programme Proposal for Health Ministry (1980–1985), vol. II. Kathmandu: Planning Unit, Ministry of Health, His Majesty's Government.

Ministry of Health, Nepal (1980) Planning for Health Manpower. Kathmandu: Institute of Medicine and Ministry of Health.

Ministry of Health, Nepal (1995–1996) Annual Report 2052–2053. Kathmandu: Department of Health Services.

Ministry of Health, Nepal (1997) Second Long Term Health Plan 1997–2017. Kathmandu: Ministry of Health.

Parker RL, Shah SM, Alexander CA, Neumann AK (1979) Self-care in rural areas of India and Nepal. *Culture, Medicine and Psychiatry* 3:3–28.

Purdey AF, Adhikari GB, Robinson SA, Cox PW (1994) Participatory health development in rural Nepal: clarifying the process of community empowerment. *Health Education Quarterly* 21:329–343.

Thapa S (1996) Challenges to improving maternal health in rural Nepal. *Lancet* 347:1244–1246.

United Nations Children's Fund (1978) Annual Report on Nepal. Kathmandu: UNICEF.

United Nations Children's Fund (1982) Children of Nepal: A Situational Analysis. Kathmandu: UNICEF.

WHO (1978) A Decade of Health Development in South-East Asia 1968–1977. New Delhi: Regional Office for South-East Asia, World Health Organization.

WHO (1979) Country Health Profile. Kathmandu: World Health Organization.

16

Bureaucratic Aspects of International Health Programs

GEORGE M. FOSTER

Since the end of World War II, great strides have been made in meeting health needs, particularly in Third World countries, which historically have lagged behind industrialized regions. Death rates have fallen significantly, longevity has markedly increased, environmental sanitation has improved, maternal and child health facilities have multiplied, immunization programs increasingly protect children against common childhood diseases, and the incidence of many other diseases, such as malaria, has been notably lowered.

At the same time, enormous health problems still confront most of the world, and it is highly unlikely that "Health for All by the Year 2000" will be achieved (WHO, 1979). Why should this be? In public health we have long since acquired the skills needed to provide pure water and environmental sanitation, to immunize against the common childhood diseases, to design nutritionally balanced diets, and to teach personal hygiene and food safety. These skills, as Ramalingaswami notes, "were largely responsible for the great transformation in health that took place in the industrialized world at the time of the First Industrial Revolution" (Ramalingaswami, 1986:1097). They are also the skills that can effect a comparable revolution in Third World health conditions. But we are failing fully to utilize these skills, according to Ramalingaswami, because of political, cultural, ethical, and bureaucratic factors.

These factors are marked by a common characteristic: they are all sociocultural. Not one is primarily medical. In other words, medical knowledge and medical research alone cannot bring health for all. Our problems lie in the fields of politics and commitment, of planning for health needs, and of administration of programs and projects.

This is not the first time in history that administrative and planning talents have been called on to help meet perceived health needs. Perhaps the earliest "international" health agencies were the Public Health Boards established by north Italian city-states to meet the threat of the Black Death (1347–1351). Not only did the boards monitor the incidence and progress of illness within their boundaries; they also exchanged information with their counterparts in other cities with a view to establishing quarantine measures. Considering the low level of medical knowledge at that time, it is perhaps not surprising that "the rise and development of the Health Boards and of related health legislation were not so much the brainchild of the medical profession as they were the products of the administrative talents of Italian Renaissance society. . . . From their beginnings the Boards were in the hands not of the medical men but of administrators who, of course, made use of the knowledge and skills of physicians and surgeons whenever the situation demanded" (Cipolla, 1976:20–21).

History repeats itself today, for knowledge and skills beyond those of medicine alone are needed to make progress in meeting health needs. Specifically, administrative, political, economic, sociocultural, and ethical factors must be taken into account in the planning and conduct of health programs. Within the field of international health this fact is appreciated in varying degrees. Thus it is generally agreed that knowledge of the sociocultural characteristics of recipient groups is essential to the best planning and execution of health programs. Less widely accepted is the fact that the structural and dynamic characteristics of health agencies profoundly influence the planning and mode of operations of international health programs. Health bureaucracies are therefore just as logical objects of scientific investigation as traditional communities.

To study bureaucracies, of course, is hardly a novel idea. Since the time of the German sociologist Max Weber (1864–1920), social scientists have studied administrative organizations to understand how their structure and dynamics influence the societies of which they are a part. Empirical research has confirmed the obvious: informal relations and unofficial practices are widespread in all bureaucracies, and are essential to their activities. Far from detracting from the efficiency of the organization (as Weber's model postulated), these relationships and practices often contribute to more efficient operations (e.g., see discussion of Simmons, below).

Although the health field has provided the arena for a number of studies of bureaucracies and the health professions within national boundaries, relatively little research on health agencies—in contrast to the communities they serve—has been carried out in the international setting. Among exceptions is Simmons's early analysis of the clinical team in a Chilean health center, which revealed the highly useful but unofficial function health center nurses performed in mediating between doctors and patients (Simmons, 1955). When in a routine administrative shift of duties the nurses were assigned full-time to home visiting, communication between doctors and patients virtually broke down. Equally revealing is Philips's review of the Rockefeller Foundation's hookworm campaign in Ceylon from 1916 to 1922 (Philips, 1955). The study is important because it demonstrates how the physicians' misconceptions about appropriate innovative roles and their lack of knowledge of what their activities meant to the tea coolies were responsible for the failure of the program. Practically all of the problems in planning and operating international health programs encountered 50 years later in the post–World War II period emerged during those six years.

Methodology

This study is based on information acquired through participant observation. In common anthropological usage, the term implies that researchers speak the language of and participate as fully as possible in the life of the members of a group— a peasant community, urban ghetto residents, staff of a hospital, or a government agency—with specific goals in mind, such as writing a scientific monograph, a popular book, or a committee report. Information gathered in this fashion tends to be "interpreted" rather than "analyzed." Anthropologists ask of their data, "What does this all add up to? What do the data tell us about human behavior, about social organization and culture?" Competing interpretations are the rule; there are no ways to repeat a study under controlled conditions duplicating the first anthropologist's work, no simple way to prove or disprove a hypothesis. The interpretation that seems most plausible to most anthropologists is generally accepted until and unless a more plausible hypothesis appears.

Reflection upon 40 years of personal observations and experiences in the field of technical aid, especially international health programs, augmented by examination of the published record and discussions with colleagues in many fields, has led to the conclusions in this study. During my professional life I have observed and participated in the development of a number of international multi- and bilateral technical aid programs, beginning in 1943 when, as a "social science analyst," I joined the US Institute of Inter-American Affairs (IIAA), which had been established a year earlier to help Latin American countries develop their agricultural, health, and educational systems. The IIAA was the forerunner and prototype of today's United States Agency for International Development (USAID). In 1946, after two years as a Smithsonian Institution (SI) visiting professor in Mexico City, I returned to Washington. There, in 1951, my contact with the IIAA was renewed when SI colleagues in several Latin American countries and I carried out an initial study of aspects of the institute's work in public health. Our report (Foster, 1951), which stressed the cultural and social "barriers" that inhibited acceptance of much of the American program, was enthusiastically received by IIAA health personnel. It appeared to answer many questions that had puzzled them, especially why new public health centers failed to attract the clients for whom they were designed. As a result, the SI anthropologists were invited to join an IIAA evaluation team formed to appraise the results of the first 10 years of its health programs (Foster, 1953, 1982a).

In 1953 I accepted a professorship in the Department of Anthropology at the University of California, Berkeley, where, during the following 30 years, I served as consultant in a number of overseas technical aid projects and programs: for USAID in community development and health education in India, Pakistan, the Philippines, Indonesia, Afghanistan, Nepal, and Northern Rhodesia (today Zambia), for periods of several weeks to six months; for UNICEF and, especially, WHO, for periods of two weeks to three months in Geneva, Indonesia, India, Sri Lanka, Malaysia, Thailand, and the Philippines, with shorter stays in Nepal, Nigeria, Cameroon, and Kenya.

A considerable number of stateside and international workshops, committee memberships, and meetings also gave me opportunity to interact with international health specialists, and to observe them in action. All these experiences added to my understanding of the bureaucratic aspects of international health agencies and programs.

Types of International Health Agencies

Organizations working in the international field may be classified as follows:

1. Multilateral organizations, exemplified by the specialized United Nations agencies such as the World Health Organization (WHO) and the United Nations Children's Fund (UNICEF). The critical characteristic of these agencies is that membership is open to all countries, whose representatives collectively set policy.
2. Bilateral governmental agencies such as the US Agency for International Development (USAID), based on working agreements between the donor organization and the ministries of health of recipient countries. Although improved health is also the goal of such agencies, basic policy is set largely by the donor organization, and its activities constitute an arm of the foreign policy of the supporting government.
3. Private secular organizations such as the Rockefeller, Ford, and other large, multipurpose foundations, and myriad smaller and more specialized groups that depend on charitable contributions for support. Historically, these

organizations have stressed preventive medicine and public health measures rather than clinical activities.

4. Private religious organizations such as the medical missions that have been
supported by Western European and North American Christian denomi-
nations for a century and a half. Historically, medical missions have been
more concerned with curative activities than with preventive measures.
They differ from the other organizations in that meeting health needs
often is not a primary aim in itself, but rather a strategy to help achieve
the ultimate goal of making converts. Medical missions and private secular organizations are usually grouped under the rubric private voluntary
organizations (PVOs) or nongovernmental organizations (NGOs).

This chapter focuses on the multi- and bilateral organizations. Although distinctive in important ways, as huge bureaucracies conforming essentially to the
procedures of governments, they are sufficiently similar to one another to permit joint analysis and comparison. Almost without exception they conform to a
"donor–recipient" pattern in which specialists from technologically advanced
countries work with "counterparts" in less developed countries in improving
health services in the latter regions. This pattern is largely a product of the past
50 years.

By the end of World War II it was clear that war-ravaged Europe required
major financial help to rebuild. This came largely in the form of Marshall Plan
aid from the United States. It was also clear that during the war the rest of the
world had changed significantly, and that even greater changes were an immediate prospect. European colonies were soon to become independent. They, and
other countries little if at all industrialized, would need major financial and technological help in their developmental efforts, essential to achieve higher standards of living and, it was hoped, political stability. Thus was born the concept of
huge technical aid programs in such fields as health, agriculture, and education,
as a major arm of foreign policy of the industrialized countries, and as a field of
cooperation within the United Nations and its specialized agencies (Basch, 1978).

Evolving Models of Technical Aid

From their beginning, technical assistance programs have been based on underlying assumptions judged to be self-evident by the program personnel. Tendler
states the basic assumption: "Development assistance was established on the
premise that the developed world possessed both the talent and the capital for
helping backward countries to develop. Development know-how was spoken
about as if it were like capital—a stock of goods capable of being transferred
from its owners to the less privileged" (Tendler, 1975:10).

From this it logically follows that if some people have "know-how" and others do not, those with the know-how are the proper ones to plan and execute the transfer. Technical aid and developmental planning in general are, as Korten and Alfonso point out, "based on an organizational model which assumes that the major planning decisions will be made centrally based on economic analyses prepared by highly trained technicians. . . . The decisions are made by experts far removed from the people and their needs, and implemented through structures intended to be more responsive to central direction than local reality" (Korten and Alfonso, 1981:2).

Premises change over time. This is as true of premises underlying international health organizations as of other large bureaucracies. Over the past 50 years three sequential models of the perception of problems encountered in delivering technical aid can be identified: the "silver platter" model, the sociocultural model, and the bureaucratic model.

The Silver Platter Model

In the early years of technical aid, planners and technical specialists—health personnel included—felt that their task was to attack problems with the techniques and institutional forms that worked well in industrialized countries. Although speaking only of higher education in (then) British Africa, Ashby aptly described the picture for all technical aid:

> Underlying British enterprise in providing higher education for her people overseas was one massive assumption: that the pattern of university appropriate for Manchester, Exeter and Hull was ipso facto appropriate for Ibadan, Kampala, and Singapore. . . . As with cars, so with universities: we willingly made minor modifications to suit the climate, but we proposed no radical change in design, and we did not regard it as our business to enquire whether French or American models might be more suitable. (Ashby, 1966:244)

The result was universities often poorly suited to the needs of developing countries.

In the history of international health programs, the same underlying assumption repeats itself continually: the health strategies that have served the West are universals, equally suited to Boston or Bombay. Health programs have been seen as exercises in the transfer of techniques, in the implantation of educational, preventive, and curative services based on the biomedical model, in which the major challenge is to persuade people to abandon their traditional beliefs and practices in favor of the new. As with British higher education, this assumption often has produced inappropriate and ineffective health services in Third World countries.

It was further assumed that people in less developed countries, the recipients of help, would immediately appreciate the advantages of the new ways, once exposed to them, and that given the opportunity they would quickly adopt them. The errors underlying this "transfer of techniques" approach are beautifully illustrated by the early health program of the US Institute of Inter-American Affairs, established in 1942. The centerpiece of the program was American-type public health centers, emphasizing preventive activities in such fields as maternal and child health care and environmental sanitation. Initially these centers failed to attract anticipated patronage. Behavioral research revealed that in countries where people have limited access to modern health care, they are uninterested in prevention until their first priority (treatment of illness) has been satisfied. Only after curative services—initially lacking—were added did health centers begin to play an important health role (Foster, 1952).

The Sociocultural Model

By the mid-1950s this early ethnocentric view of technical aid began to give way to a new approach which postulated that the major problems in the transfer of advanced technologies, including those of the health sciences, are rooted in the society and culture of the recipient peoples, and that programs and projects aimed at redressing poverty, poor health, inefficient agriculture, and illiteracy must be designed to fit the needs and expectations of these people. The populations toward whom these programs are pointed, it is argued, want to raise their standards of living and are willing to modify their behavior when they perceive advantage in the new ways. But psychological, social, and cultural "barriers" inhibit these changes. Consequently, if these barriers can be identified through sociocultural research, and if the motivations to change can be identified, then developmental assistance can be presented in such a way that client peoples will eagerly accept it. This model represents an enormous advance over the silver platter model. As far as it goes, it is correct. Without an understanding of the local community, its worldview, and its comprehension of the innovative alternatives presented to it, planners and technical specialists are working blindly.

The Bureaucratic Model

Even the most sophisticated applications of the sociocultural model, however, often failed to produce the desired results. Little by little we have come to realize that not only is it important to understand the recipient's culture, but it is equally important to understand the sociocultural forms of innovating organizations. Just as barriers to change are found in peasant communities, so are they found in the structure, values, and operating procedures of development bureaucracies, and in the individual personal qualities of planners and change agents. In other words, the bureaucratic model says that to develop the most effective aid programs it is essential to understand the culture of the agency developing and guiding a program, as well as the national and international assumptions (both conscious and unconscious) that shape bureaucratic cultures.

For many reasons, the bureaucratic model has been less completely accepted than the sociocultural model; many health personnel still reject it, insisting that the community, and the community alone, is the problem. It is easy to see why the sociocultural model has been so readily accepted: it is nonthreatening to agency personnel, for the problem is defined as "out there," away from the centers of policy, planning, and program operations. No one in the innovating organization need feel responsible, or on the spot, in accepting this model.

Even for those who realize the validity of the bureaucratic model, it is often psychologically difficult to admit that "we are a part of the problem." Not all reluctance to attempt the innovative action that the bureaucratic model calls for, of course, is psychological. Staff members of bureaucracies fully understand the limits of their organizations, of their inherent rigidity, and of the many constraints they place on reflective thinking and action. Since efforts to bring about major organizational changes so often seem futile, staff members find it easier to accept organizational norms as a given, and to place their hopes on changes in community forms that will make clients more receptive to their programs. Perhaps they are realistic in taking this position. Certainly the changes in traditional communities since the end of World War II suggest that they can indeed change more rapidly than entrenched bureaucracies.

Bureaucracies as Sociocultural Systems

In their structural and dynamic aspects, bureaucracies are much like communities. Normally they are composed of people of both sexes and different ages, organized in a hierarchy of authority, responsibility, obligations, and functional tasks. They also have social structures that define the relationships, roles, and statuses of their members. Through formal and informal educational methods, new members of bureaucratic societies learn appropriate role behavior and the values, routines, and premises that guide the organization.

Bureaucracies further resemble communities in that they are integrated, functional units in which the parts fit closely together; consequently, no change occurs in isolation, without rearrangement in the role relationships of the members, without increasing the responsibilities and authority of some and diminishing those of others. Like community members, the personnel of large organizations jealously guard their traditional perquisites and privileges; they do not easily surrender their vested interests, except in exchange for something as good or better. They rationalize their positions by assuring themselves that what is good for them is best for the organization.

Bureaucracies also resemble communities in that, within norms of behavior and values, individual members exhibit great variation in ability, character, personality, views, and judgment. The personnel of bureaucracies are not simply carriers of their organizational cultures; they are also psychological beings needing ego gratification and satisfaction from their performances. They are characterized by emotional securities and insecurities, likes and dislikes, hopes and doubts. Sometimes they feel successful in their accomplishments, and at other times they feel threatened or rejected. To understand the working of bureaucracies, it is essential to pay attention to the ever-present psychological dimension of personnel.

Evaluating International Health Agencies

The identification and evaluation of the strengths and weaknesses of international health organizations is a highly subjective exercise. A pessimist will look at the world's unmet health needs and conclude that, a half century after their founding, these agencies fall far short of what was expected of them. An optimist, comparing contemporary world health levels with those prevailing at the end of World War II, can only conclude that the agencies have accomplished much more than might have been anticipated. For the fact is, as pointed out earlier, enormous strides have been made in meeting the world's health needs, particularly in developing countries. That much remains to be done is more an indication of the magnitude of the task than of the shortcomings of health organizations.

International health agencies have helped significantly in raising world health levels by a variety of means: they have attracted able and dedicated administrators and technical specialists and they have drawn on the latest biomedical knowledge of the world's medical research institutions. By means of travel grants, traineeships, and fellowships for Third World health personnel, they have helped strengthen indigenous ministries of health and health care facilities in the countries concerned.

It is widely assumed that multilateral agencies have major advantages over bilateral ones. In the case of WHO, for example, all member nations can feel that this is *our* organization, no longer dominated (as in the early years) by the West. In the WHO annual General Assembly there is opportunity for broader input and discussion of a wider variety of concerns and ideas than in any bilateral program. Moreover, the continuing interaction of personnel from many countries in the same office permits dialogue on a wide spectrum of ideas that cannot be achieved in an organization largely representing a single cultural tradition.

Worldwide campaigns such as smallpox eradication, immunization against childhood illnesses, and oral rehydration therapy to treat infant diarrheal diseases can be pursued with a vigor and degree of support impossible for any bilateral agency. And, with respect to educational and legal efforts to persuade mothers to nurse rather than bottle-feed their infants, the multilateral organizations do not suffer the political constraints imposed on some of the bilateral agencies. There are problems, of course, as when member nations insist that specific diseases are not found within their borders. For example, when the first cases of AIDS were recognized in 1983, many African governments refused to acknowledge cases within their borders. Yet it has proven easier for WHO to persuade these countries that they must be involved in AIDS control than it would have been for any bilateral agency.

For reasons like these, increased channeling of health aid through multilateral institutions has emerged as an attractive solution to many of the problems encountered in bilateral programs. Yet the evidence is not all one-sided. Basch states the problem: "This step, it is asserted, would reduce many of the tensions and obligations implicit in bilateral arrangements, distribute aid on the basis of need rather than political loyalty, and make assistance contingent on policy reforms backed by world opinion." Yet, he continues, "while this may be so, multilateralization introduces into the ODA [official development assistance] picture at least a third bureaucracy with its inherent red-tapism, delay, and administrative expense, and it blurs the special relationships and specific mutual interests of the parties concerned" (Basch, 1978:339). Moreover, at times, bilateral organizations can innovate in ways that the multinational organizations, for all their strengths, cannot attempt for policy reasons.

Problems Encountered in International Health Agencies

In considering the problems encountered in international health agencies, and in looking for ways in which their effectiveness may be increased, we are dealing with "the art of the possible" (Ramalingaswami, 1986:1097). Some of the factors that prevent health agencies from realizing their full potential are inherent in all bureaucracies and little can be done about them. Other problems, however, seem self-imposed; with innovative action from within the organization they can be significantly reduced, to the benefit of the agency and its clients. Examples of both follow.

Rationalizing Budgets

Agencies never have all the financial resources they believe they can spend profitably. Hence officials of all bureaucracies do the natural thing: in requesting funds for future activities they cast their past achievements in the best possible light and describe future plans in the most glowing terms. International health agencies are not immune to this exercise. To justify their budget requests they need quick results, especially results that can be counted: numbers of latrines installed, children vaccinated, and family planning methods demonstrated. Long-range strategies that take time to produce results suffer in comparison to programs such as these. Again, the need to show that the organization is forward-looking creates pressure to generate new projects simply for their own sake, often without adequate research and evaluation of all of the implications of the proposal. Moreover, the launching of new projects may necessitate the dropping of promising ongoing projects before they have had time fully to demonstrate their potential.

Limited Corporate Memories

Health agencies, like other corporate groups, often seem marked by what can be called a "limited corporate memory"; only with difficulty do they learn from their own past, and they fail to draw on the relevant prior experience of others. For example, by the end of World War II the history of medical missions, and data from the early Rockefeller international health programs and other cross-cultural health activities, contained invaluable information about strategies most likely to produce results in designing and carrying out health projects in developing countries. Yet when the major multilateral and bilateral agencies began their work 50 years ago, they paid little attention to this wealth of experience. Consequently, they repeated mistakes made many times in the past, mistakes which might have been avoided.

More recently, the concept of primary health care (PHC) offers a similar picture: the reinvention of the community development (CD) wheel of 20 years earlier. In this process international health agencies have made many of the same mistakes and suffered the same disappointments as the earlier enthusiastic CD advocates (Foster, 1982b; Muhondwa, 1986). As Bichmann writes,

> There are surprising analogies between the PHC and the CD approach . . . but in the documents promoting the PHC-strategy, no clear reference to this fact is given. . . . As PHC with its comprehensive approach encompasses sector-external health-related subjects like agricultural development, road infrastructure, education, etc. so did the CD programmes of the fifties and sixties aim at integrated rural development including health-related activities. . . . Generally speaking, CD did not yield the expected results on a nation-wide scale. . . . Why then should PHC produce a better outcome than CD? (Bichmann, 1983:7)

It is difficult to tell whether failure to consider prior relevant experience is inherent in bureaucratic structures, or whether it reflects a reluctance of personnel to diminish the appearance of their creativity by giving credit to others. Whatever the explanation, in contrast to budgeting problems, which appear insoluble, appropriate research resources *can* improve the corporate memory problem. After all, learning from experience is commonplace.

Constraints Imposed by Agency Doctrines

Bureaucracies usually must develop policy in the absence of much of the information that ideally should be available. The dangers inherent in this situation can be guarded against partially by periodic reviews of progress and by keeping policy as flexible as possible so that course corrections can be made as needed. Policies, like engineering designs, should not be frozen until all the problems have been solved. In international health agencies, however, it sometimes looks as if ideologically attractive but untested policies are raised to the level of doctrine more because of the enthusiasms and special professional interests of those in a position to make such decisions than because of objective consideration of what is known. And, once policy becomes doctrine, it is the rare staff member who can afford to question it. The life expectancy of whistle-blowers in bureaucracies is not long.

The concept of community participation (CP) as a major component in primary health care strategies illustrates this point. First broached as a promising PHC approach in 1975 in WHO's widely quoted *Health by the People* (Newell, 1975) and in the study *Alternative Approaches to Meeting Basic Health Needs in Developing Countries* (Djukanovic and Mach, 1975), CP was elevated to the level of doctrine on the basis of the 1977 UNICEF–WHO Joint Committee on Health Policy report, "Community Involvement in Primary Health Care. A Study of the Process of Community Motivation and Continued Participation" (WHO, 1977).

This study illustrates a common bureaucratic practice: the use of "research" to legitimize previously decided-upon policies rather than to provide data for judging the desirability of the policies. There are good things about the study. It analyzes, and draws conclusions from, case studies of projects in each of nine countries in which it can be argued that the community had indeed been "involved." However, a tenth case study was excluded from the final draft because its findings were contrary to the desired conclusions. In fact, in no sense was the sample random, and no serious effort was made to consider negative evidence. The study disingenuously notes that "time did not permit an exhaustive study," and the methodological weaknesses of the report are made clear. In spite of these obvious limitations, the report was accepted as the solid evidence on which the role of CP was spelled out in the 1978 Alma-Ata Conference on Primary Health Care (WHO, 1978).

Community participation has been the subject of a number of subsequent WHO meetings and studies, none of which has seriously questioned the validity of the idea. It continues to receive ritual obeisance within the organization, in spite of the fact that this approach—as with community development—usually has produced meager results in the Third World.

Constraints Imposed by Western Ideologies

In international health agencies, basic policies, program priorities, and doctrines are presumed to reflect the considered judgment of objective and dispassionate health professionals. Often they do. Yet there are always supraorganizational influences underlying the policy-determining process, the impact of which is not always appreciated. Stone suggests that the "cultural imprint of the West" is manifest and expressed in "the rhetoric and the fads," and in the style and approach of development. "It is as though the world of international development, although ostensibly geared toward maximizing its relevance to the poor of the Third World, has become like a mirror in which the values, interests and philosophies of the West are found reflected" (Stone, 1989:206). Community participation, which "now stands as an established development strategy," is an example: the concept entails the Western values of self-reliance, equality, and individualism, values to which most of us subscribe. Yet, she points out, it is a mistake to assume that these values equally characterize Third World communities.

Contemporary international concerns with nutrition and interest in "women in development" also reflect a contemporary Western ideology, Stone believes:

> Nutrition is now a major and growing focus in development programs. And regardless of the scientific soundness of this focus, the fact remains that nutrition loomed as a major thrust in international development circles at the same time as "nutrition" became a subject of great popular fascination in the United States. Nutrition programs multiplied in the Third World around the time that the Americans began to criticize their junk food, measure their cholesterol, and to perceive sound nutrition as a solution to *their* problems.
>
> Another, perhaps more pointed, case is "Women in Development" (WID), now a major concern within virtually every development agency in the world. Again, regardless of the value or soundness of WID programs, they did not arise from the expressed interests and felt needs of the masses of the Third World poor. Rather, a development focus on women grew from the fact that the status of women, and attendant questions of sexual equality, became burning issues in the West. (Stone, 1989:206)

Of course, the cultural ideology of the West as reflected in the international health agencies goes far beyond community participation, nutrition, and "women in development." It constitutes a basic statement about a sociopolitical and economic system, the correctness of which is self-evident to its leaders and most of its people. The bilateral health agencies must operate within the constraints of this ideology. They must be cautious in advocating policies such as major land reform and wealth redistribution, even though sociopolitical and economic changes in much of the world are seen by program planners as necessary to achieve higher health levels. The multilateral organizations are somewhat more flexible on these points; they can advocate socialist as well as capitalist responses to health needs. Yet they, too, can go only so far, since withdrawal of the financial support of the West would render them impotent; they must walk a fine line indeed.

Constraints Imposed by Professional and Personal Characteristics of Agency Personnel

Bureaucrats do not, and cannot be expected to, function with formalistic impersonality. They have likes and dislikes, prejudices, friendships, and enmities. These, and many other personal characteristics, influence their role performances, and hence the functioning of their organizations. Personality traits like these are individual. Other personality traits may be thought of as group-based, characterizing the members of professions, and professionals as a class. They also affect the performance of individuals and, consequently, organizational activities. Competent professionals have a positive self-image; they have confidence in their ability and they take pride in their work. Some professionals can work quietly, satisfied with the knowledge that they are doing a good job. But many more exhibit—or conceal with varying degrees of success—a need for ego gratification, which comes from recognition by their peers. Hence they like to promote activities in which they can demonstrate their professional skills. Sometimes this leads to confusion of personal and organizational needs.

Pride in performance and a positive self-image obviously are important elements in stimulating the best possible work. But when present in excess, in projects where cooperative efforts and intersectoral policies are desirable, these personal-professional factors can jeopardize planning and program operations. For, carried away with enthusiasm, some professionals readily believe that their contributions are the key to program success and that they should have first call on resources. In primary health care, for example, lip service is paid to the importance of integrated programs that include agriculture, education, access roads, and the like. Yet few whose primary field is health doubt that health activities— and particularly their own specialties—should receive first attention.

The policies, programs, and priorities of large organizations, including those concerned with international health, reflect a pair of processes: a public and explicit planning mechanism, *and* the often private professional concerns and enthusiasms of powerful individuals and groups within the organization.

Competition for Clients

Bureaucracies, international health agencies included, need clients to justify their existence. The worst thing that can happen to such a bureaucracy is to solve the problems it was set up to solve, and thus to be left without clients. At least two groups of clients of international health agencies can be identified. The first is the individual community member, a human being in need of health protection and care. There are adequate numbers of these clients, enough for everyone searching for a client, and the supply will not dry up. But help to community members is filtered through intermediate clients, the health ministries and services of the countries receiving developmental aid. In contrast to community members, these clients *are* limited in number; there are not always enough of them to satisfy the needs of all organizations involved in international health work. This leads to competition among donor agencies, with results sometimes inimical to the host country's best interests.

Sterling gives a vivid picture of such competition in Kathmandu in the mid-1970s:

> At last count when I was there, about 700 missionaries of progress were racketing around town in their Land Rovers and Toyota jeeps, representing some fifty donor-states and agencies, all urging assorted projects on a nation the size of Arkansas. Among the foreign benefactors are USAID, the Indian Cooperation Mission, the Chinese, Russians, British, Canadians, Australians, New Zealanders, Pakistanis, and Swiss, the Japanese Overseas Cooperation Volunteers, the German Volunteer service, the Ford Foundation, the Rockefeller Foundation, the Dooley Foundation (using volunteer airline hostesses who take six months off for good works), Anglia University, Cornell University, [and] the World Bank. (Sterling, 1976:14)

And these are only a few examples. Such an abundance of foreign aid stresses the capacity of many Third World governments to provide the counterpart services and personnel expected by most development agencies.

The Workshop Syndrome

Meetings are the lifeblood of bureaucracies. The simplest form is that well-known bureaucratic phenomenon, the staff meeting. At higher levels meetings take the form of longer regional and international conferences and workshops. The numbers, varieties, and frequencies of such meetings in international health organizations are quite dazzling: USAID meetings in Washington, UNICEF meetings in New York, WHO meetings at headquarters in Geneva and in the regional offices.

One is led to speculate as to their raison d'être. Some justifications are obvious: it is important that world leaders in various health fields meet and discuss common concerns, that they assess the gravity of health threats (such as AIDS), that they take stock of progress in controlling diarrheal diseases, and that they plan future activities. Major workshops can play another important role, that of validating organization policies and programs. For example, Justice writes of Nepal that "Kathmandu officials place great importance on high-level conferences because they are a visible activity that extends legitimacy to programs such as ICHP [Integrated Community Health Program]" (Justice, 1986:78).

Beyond these obvious justifications there are latent reasons why the pattern is so popular, particularly in multilateral organizations. This has to do with the nature of professional employment in Third World countries, and with the attraction of a career in the United Nations agencies. In developed countries employment in international health organizations can be challenging and interesting, and professionally desirable. But whether the agency is public or private, compensation is comparable to that in many other lines of work. To land a job with USAID is not, for an American, a particular financial plum and if, for any reason, a technical specialist leaves the organization, comparable employment elsewhere is a reasonable expectation.

But the picture is quite different in WHO, for example, where a majority of the professional jobs are now held by physicians and other health specialists from Third World countries. For them a WHO (or UNICEF, or World Bank) appointment *is* a financial plum. At international salary levels they enjoy a standard of living far above what they might otherwise expect, in addition to early retirement, a generous pension, international travel, and association with colleagues on a regional and worldwide basis. Consequently, such appointments are eagerly sought after. In comparison to professional colleagues in their home countries, Third World UN staff members are a highly privileged group. They are, however, vulnerable: to dismissal because of poor performance, or performance deemed dangerous to the well-being of the organization; and to the envy of their less fortunate national colleagues.

Vulnerability, of course, leads to cautious behavior. Tendler illustrates this point in her analysis of USAID, where she found that "outpost-level" employees responding to the uncertainties of Washington political and interagency constraints opted for "a kind of safe-for-all-occasions, problem-avoiding" approach to their jobs (Tendler, 1975:25). But what is safe behavior? Talk and discussion, rather more than vigorous action. I believe that multilateral health organization meetings, many on the same topic, repeating similar general recommendations (always calling for further study of the problem), at least to some extent fulfill the role of providing visible evidence of concern with health problems, in an activity that carries minimal risk to participants.

I have noted, particularly in the regional offices of WHO, that, in addition to providing safe-for-all-occasions activities for permanent staff members, conferences and workshops also fulfill an envy-reducing role vis-à-vis national colleagues who would like to, but do not, hold similar appointments. For the latter group, occasional participation in WHO regional meetings is attractive for financial and prestige reasons. Temporary appointees receive both a daily honorarium for services rendered and a per diem to cover away-from-home expenses. These payments are very attractive to health personnel in many Third World countries, where salary scales are low by international standards. Especially when participants stay with local friends (often the case), thus saving most of the per diem, payment for a two-week meeting may equal several months of regular salary. National participants of regional meetings also have the satisfaction of feeling that they are a part of the international action and that, although they lack the status and salary of permanent WHO employees, at least they share peripherally in the good life provided by the organization.

Unfortunately, this pattern of sharing may reflect patronage behavior not consistent with the highest levels of professional practice. Since regional conference participants usually are nominated by national health authorities rather than the meeting organizers, administrators often appoint faithful staff members whose turn to travel has come, rather than individuals whose qualifications best fit the conference specifications. Consequently, workshop participants often have little notion as to the goals of the meeting; at best they are dead weight, and at worst they squander valuable time with extraneous talk.

Poor Quality of Behavioral Research

A good deal of the behavioral research carried out by international health organizations has been of poor quality. I have described (Foster, 1987) how in WHO in the early 1980s bureaucratic constraints and the research assumptions of the medical profession significantly inhibited first-class investigations. I suggested that "even the most comprehensive statements on the importance of behavioral research stress communities, not health services. Health bureaucracies operate on the assumption that the purpose of behavioral research is to find out how to persuade target populations to change their behavior more nearly to conform to what health projects call for" (Foster, 1987:711). It is taken for granted that health care delivery programs, in spite of minor shortcomings, are the appropriate vehicle for raising health levels.

Probably it is unrealistic to expect that behavioral analysis will ever play much of a role in policy and planning activities. One part of the problem is that behavioral research rarely is concerned with administrative organizations. To illustrate, the concept of "community participation," an often-enunciated international health doctrine, sounds attractive as a basic policy. What could be more democratic than inviting villagers to join government administrators and planners in deciding how best to meet local health needs? Yet experience shows that those in positions of power in centralized governmental systems are rarely willing to surrender authority in the interest of democratic participation. More often than not the concept of community participation is diametrically opposed to administrative policies, which do not change easily.

A second part of the problem is how to incorporate behavioral information into the planning process. Time constraints inherent in the bureaucratic process place a premium on rapid decisions. Although good behavioral research can be done more rapidly than is sometimes thought, it takes time for this information to work its way up the ladder. In any event, high-level officials often doubt the utility of behavioral information. To illustrate, in Nepal Justice found that officials in donor agencies and in government "generally agreed that cultural information is rarely used in planning." Among the reasons given was the belief that such information was not available, and "when it was available, it was not very useful" (Justice, 1986:111). In the case of USAID's project paper outlining its Nepal health and family planning programs, Justice found that the "social soundness analysis" was condensed to three pages (plus eight in the appendix). "Agency representatives whom I interviewed implied that it was included primarily as a formality to fulfill the requirements specified by Congress" (p. 116).

For reasons such as these, behavioral research in international health organizations probably will continue to play a minor role, largely limited to the identification of social and cultural factors that are relevant to community acceptance or rejection of health programs decided upon by distant planners, programs in which the community has had little input.

Rebuilding Agencies for International Health

This chapter raises a number of questions that must be addressed by international health agencies if they are significantly to improve their performances. They include, but by no means are limited to, the following:

1. Can the reflexive bureaucratic model be institutionalized so that more realistic premises will underlie the definition of problems in health program planning?
2. How can corporate memories be strengthened? How can the necessary resources be built into large organizations so that they are better able to profit from their own past experience, and from relevant experiences of other organizations?
3. How can the dangers of the early enunciation of policy doctrines restricting innovative thinking in international health organizations be avoided?
4. How can the threat of attempting to satisfy Western ideological concerns by incorporating them into international health planning be controlled?
5. To what extent do professional-personality factors impinge on planning processes? Does overall balance in projects suffer because of the influ-

ence of powerful personalities? Or is an occasionally adversarial process the appropriate way to determine organizational policies?

6. How serious is the "competition for clients" syndrome in development assistance programs? Can, or should, anything be done about this problem?

7. Does the "workshop syndrome" divert international health agencies' personnel from other activities to the extent that overall goals of the institutions are compromised? Should the number of meetings be limited?

8. How can the scope of behavioral research in international health agencies be broadened to include not only client groups but also the agencies that plan and carry out assistance programs? What can be done to ensure greater use of such research in setting policy and in program operations?

Acknowledgment

This is a revision of an article first published in *Social Science and Medicine* 25 (1987):1039–1048.

References

Ashby E (1966) Universities: British, Indian, African. A Study in the Ecology of Higher Education. Cambridge, Mass: Harvard University Press.

Basch PH (1978) International Health. New York: Oxford University Press.

Bichmann W (1983) Primary health care: a new strategy? Lessons to learn from community participation. Paper presented at the workshop "Primary Health Care in the Developing World," 10th International Congress of Preventive and Social Medicine, Heidelberg/Mannheim, September 27–October 1.

Cipolla CM (1976) Public Health and the Medical Profession in the Renaissance. Cambridge: Cambridge University Press.

Djukanovic V, Mach EP (1975) Alternative Approaches to Meeting Basic Health Needs in Developing Countries. Geneva: World Health Organization.

Foster GM, ed. (1951) A cross-cultural anthropological analysis of a technical aid program. Washington, DC: Smithsonian Institution, July 25. [Mimeo]

Foster GM (1952) Relationships between theoretical and applied anthropology: a public health program analysis. *Human Organization* 11:5–16.

Foster GM (1953) Use of anthropological methods and data in planning and operation (10-year evaluation of the bilateral health programs of the Institute of Inter-American Affairs). *Public Health Reports* 68:841–857.

Foster GM (1982a) Applied anthropology and international health: retrospect and prospect. *Human Organization* 41:189–197.

Foster GM (1982b) Community development and primary health care: their conceptual similarities. *Medical Anthropology* 6:183–195.

Foster GM (1987) World Health Organization behavioral science research: problems and prospects. *Social Science and Medicine* 24:709–717.

Justice J (1986) Policies, Plans and People. Culture and Health Development in Nepal. Berkeley: University of California Press.

Korten DC, Alfonso FB (1981) Bureaucracy and the Poor. Closing the Gap. Singapore: McGraw-Hill.

Muhondwa EPY (1986) Rural development and primary health care in less developed countries. *Social Science and Medicine* 22:1237–1256.

Newell KW (1975) Health by the People. Geneva: World Health Organization.

Philips J (1955) "The Hookworm Campaign in Ceylon." In: Hands across Frontiers. HM Teaf Jr, PG Franck, eds. Ithaca, NY: Cornell University Press, pp. 265–305.

Ramalingaswami V (1986) The art of the possible. *Social Science and Medicine* 22:1097–1103.

Simmons O (1955) "The Clinical Team in a Chilean Health Center." In: Health, Culture and Community. B Paul, ed. New York: Russell Sage Foundation, pp. 325–348.

Sterling C (1976) Nepal. *Atlantic Monthly*, October: 14–25.

Stone L (1989) Cultural crossroads of community participation in development: a case from Nepal. *Human Organization* 48:206–213.

Tendler J (1975) Inside Foreign Aid. Baltimore: Johns Hopkins Press.

WHO (1977) Community Involvement in Primary Health Care. A Study of the Process of Community Motivation and Continued Participation. Report for the 1977 UNICEF-WHO Joint Committee on Health Policy. Geneva: World Health Organization. JC21/UNICEF–WHO/77.2.

WHO (1978) Primary Health Care. Report of International Conference on Primary Health Care, Alma-Ata, USSR, September 6–12. Geneva: World Health Organization.

WHO (1979) Formulating Strategies for Health for All by the Year 2000. Geneva: World Health Organization.

APPENDIX

Resources in Anthropology

Medical Anthropology

General

American Anthropological Association. Graduate Programs in Medical Anthropology. A Directory, 1993–94. Washington, DC: American Anthropological Association.

Anderson R (1996) Magic, Science, and Health. Philadelphia: Harcourt Brace.

Brown PJ, ed. (1998) Understanding and Applying Medical Anthropology. Mountain View, Calif: Mayfield Publishing Co.

Hahn RA (1995) Sickness and Healing. An Anthropological Perspective. New Haven: Yale University Press.

Helman C (1994) Culture, Health and Illness. An Introduction for Health Professionals. Stoneham, Mass: Butterworth-Heinemann.

Hill CE, ed. (1994) Training Manual in Medical Anthropology. Washington, DC: American Anthropological Association.

McElroy A, Townsend PK (1996) Medical Anthropology in Ecological Perspective. Boulder, Colo: Westview Press.

Sargent CF, Johnson TM (1996) Medical Anthropology. Contemporary Theory and Method. Westport, Conn: Praeger.

Specific to topic or region

Inhorn M, Brown PJ (1997) The Anthropology of Infectious Disease. Amsterdam: Gordon and Breach.

Nichter M, Nichter M (1996) Anthropology and International Health. Asian Case Studies. Amsterdam: Gordon and Breach.

Journals
Culture, Medicine and Psychiatry
Human Organization
Medical Anthropology
Medical Anthropology Quarterly
Practicing Anthropology
Social Science and Medicine

Methods of Anthropology and Medical Anthropology

Agar MH (1980) The Professional Stranger. An Informal Introduction to Ethnography. San Diego, Calif: Academic Press.
Bernard HR (1994) Research Methods in Anthropology. Qualitative and Quantitative Approaches. Thousand Oaks, Calif: Sage Publications.
Devereux S, Hoddinott J (1993) Fieldwork in Developing Countries. Boulder, Colo: Lynne Reinner Publishers.
Fetterman DM (1998) Ethnography. Step by Step. Newbury Park, Calif: Sage Publications.
Jorgensen DL (1989) Participant Observation. A Methodology for Human Studies. Newbury Park, Calif: Sage Publications.
Krueger R (1994) Focus Groups. A Practical Guide for Applied Research. Newbury Park, Calif: Sage Publications.
Kutsche P (1998) Field Ethnography. A Manual for Doing Cultural Anthropology. Upper Saddle River, NJ: Prentice Hall.
Manderson L, ed. (1996) Handbooks and manuals in applied research. *Practicing Anthropology* 18:3–36.
Miles MB, Huberman AM (1994) Qualitative Data Analysis. Newbury Park, Calif: Sage Publications.
Scrimshaw SCM, Hurtado E (1988) Rapid Assessment Procedures for Nutrition and Primary Health Care. Anthropological Approaches to Improving Programme Effectiveness. Tokyo: United Nations University.

Anthropological Organizations

American Anthropological Association (AAA): 4350 North Fairfax Drive, Suite 640, Arlington, VA 22203; Telephone: 703–528–1902; FAX 703–528–3546; Internet: www.ameranthassn.org.
Society for Medical Anthropology: Contact through American Anthropological Association.
Society for Applied Anthropology: P.O. Box 24083, Oklahoma City, OK 73124; Telephone: 405–843–5113; FAX 405–843–8553; e-mail: sfaa@telepath.com.

Glossary

Allopathic medicine A medical system in which therapies are designed to be antagonistic to the disease. It is a principal therapeutic modality in biomedicine.

Back translation To confirm the correctness of a translation, translated material is translated back into the original language and compared with the original material to assess the correctness of the first translation.

Biomedicine The predominant medical system of Western societies in which sickness is viewed as rooted principally in biological causes and treatment is designed to respond to these causes.

Case-control study A study design in epidemiology in which persons with and without a particular outcome of interest (e.g., an infectious disease) are compared in terms of some characteristic thought to be associated with this outcome.

Cluster sampling The selection of population units, called clusters (e.g., schools or villages), and of individuals within those units, for study.

Emic and etic Anthropologists describe initial approaches to a new culture—from the outside—as "etic," and later approaches that are meaningful to participants of that culture—from the inside—as "emic." Borrowed from "phonetics" and "phonemics" in linguistics, etics refers to a universal system for transcribing sounds, and emics to the description of sound distinctions that are meaningful in particular languages.

Ethnography The systematic and in-depth description of a culture and society.

FES Acronym for focused ethnographic study, a systematic procedure for collecting anthropological information on specified health conditions.

Focus group A research method in which an interview guide is used in interviewing individuals in a group to quickly assess their ideas and attitudes about a topic.

Formative research Investigations conducted for program design and planning.

Free listing An anthropological technique for exploring local concepts, in which informants are asked to list all the examples known to them of a subject under study, such as childhood diseases or climatic conditions.

Homeopathic medicine A medical theory and practice in which healing is thought to occur by administration of minuscule amounts of substances that, in larger doses, produce symptoms similar to those of the disease. (Contrasts with allopathic medicine.)

Participant observation A basic approach of social and cultural anthropology in which the anthropologist participates in events of the research setting while at the same time making observations; participation is a means of observation.

Participatory research Research in which the "subjects" of the study play a prominent role in some or all phases of the research.

RAP Acronym for rapid assessment procedure, a systematic method for collecting anthropological information following a standardized protocol which combines quantitative and qualitative approaches. RAP is designed to require one to two months of research, in contrast to traditional ethnographic studies, which often require years of research to complete.

Semistructured interviews Interviews in which the interviewer has an objective (e.g., assessment of the informant's beliefs or attitudes on a topic) and guides the informant in certain directions, while also allowing conversation to flow. Questions in semistructured interviews are referred to as "open-ended," meaning that the respondent is not limited to a fixed set of response options.

Snowball sampling Sampling in which one person selected for participation in a study recommends for inclusion others who, in turn, indicate others, and so on.

Structured interviews Interviews in which the interviewer has an objective (e.g., assessment of the informant's beliefs or attitudes on a topic) and pursues this objective by posing a fixed set of questions. Structured interviews may also have a fixed set of response options.

Unstructured interviews Interviews in which the interviewer has an objective (e.g., assessment of the informant's beliefs) but does not attempt to rigidly follow a fixed set of questions. Conversation on the topic is allowed to "flow."

Index

Acute respiratory infection. *See* ARI
Aid, technical
  benefit of sociocultural research, 351
  models of delivery, 349–52
  organizational dynamics in, 351–52
AIDS. *See also* STD
  chapter topic, 63–80
  prevention of, 77–79
Allopathic
  medicine, 306, 309, 313
    defined, 367
  practitioners. *See also* Physicians; Health
    care providers
    unlicensed (chota) doctors, in Pakistan,
      86–87, 90, 93–94, 103, 106
American Indians (Northwest)
  chapter topic, 142–59
  political and economic environment,
    143–45
Analysis
  content, 239–40
  cultural consensus, 121, 131
  qualitative content, 121
Anemia, 45, 51. *See also* Iron deficiency;
    Malaria
  malarial, 46

Anglo, defined, 119
Anthropological approach and methods
  in childhood pneumonia study (Pakistan),
    98
  in health planning, 342
  integrating with epidemiology, 98, 159
  integrating with public health, 21–23
  in mosquito net intervention (Tanzania),
    44–60
  in Nepal, to study international planners,
    328, 330
  in public health, 12–21, 42
  qualitative-quantitative "dispute", 13, 118
  to study driving behaviors (Niue Island),
    212
  to study pharmaceutical use (Nigeria), 177
  teaching to lay investigators, 307
  in Therapist-Spiritist project (Puerto
    Rico), 288
  in tobacco policy change study (US), 142,
    149, 158, 159
Anthropological research
  computers in, 19, 20
  misconceptions about, 338–39
  process of, 89
  steps in, 13

Anthropology
    general principles of, 6–12
    in public health, scope of, xvii–xviii
Anthropology, medical, 6, 22
    resources, 365–66
Antibiotic therapy, inappropriate, 85, 87, 94, 106, 108
ARI (acute respiratory infection), 84, 190, 320
Assessment
    baseline
        data, in Hausa pharmaceutical use study (Nigeria), 167
        study, in tobacco policy change study (US), 148–49
    in child nutrition project (Indonesia), 186–93, 203
    in tobacco policy change study (US), 150, 152–54, 155
Assistant Nurse-Midwife Program (Nepal)
    Assistant nurse-midwives' role in maternal and child health, 327, 337, 338, 341
    changes needed, 337–38
        increase cultural appropriateness, 338
    chapter topic, 327–42
    ignoring cultural information, 335, 336, 340
    problems faced by assistant nurse-midwives, 332–35, 342
    problems in planning, 335–337
    successful aspects, 337
Ayurvedic medicine, 306, 309, 313

Back translation
    in breast cancer control study (US), 119
    defined, 367
    described, 18
    in family planning study (Côte D'Ivoire), 262
Behavior change
    Bandura's theory of, 133
    in breast cancer risk factor intervention, 133, table 134
    in child nutrition project (Indonesia), 187–88
    in road user behavior study (Niue Island), 231
    in tobacco policy change study (US), 156, 157
Beliefs, cultural. See also Cultural values
    and biomedical guidelines, 118
    about cancer, 124. See also Breast cancer
    effect on use of health services in Southern California, 117
    effect on use of therapeutic drugs, chapter topic, 165–179
    fatalistic beliefs

about illness or disease, 27, 41, 107, 174–78
    in Africa, 77
    in breast cancer control study (US), 133, 137
    in Indonesia, 185
    in road user behavior study (Niue Island), 224
illness, causes of
    among Hausa of Nigeria, 174
    among Shona of Mozambique, 68–71
    God, 123
    hot-cold, described, 110 n.5
    hot-cold, in pneumonia, 92
    in southern Africa, 77
    spirits, 49, 50, 51, 53, 54, 70, 77, 86
    witchcraft and/or sorcery, 49, 50, 53, 70, 71, 77, 174, 175
    impact on planning intervention (breast cancer control study (US)), 133
    impact on pneumonia treatment in Pakistan, 85
    importance of understanding, 64
    investigation of, 38
    magico-religious beliefs, 72, 185
    pollution beliefs, 70, 77
    popular or folk beliefs, 28, 30
    role in disease transmission, 29, 30
Biomedical model, 27, 28, 38, 41
    explanatory models, 27–28, 38, 41, 167
Biomedicine
    acceptance of, in Côte D'Ivoire, 270
    compared with other ethnomedicines, 7, 167, 169, 283, 284, 286
    compared with public health, 28
    defined, 80 n.1, 367
    linking with other ethnomedicines, 279, 280
Birth
    rate, in Côte D'Ivoire, 258
        need to limit, 265, 266, 267, 271–73
    rate, in Nepal, 331
    spacing, 257, 262, 269–70, 273
Breast cancer
    attitudes about prevention and treatment, table 125
    beliefs about risk factors, 123–31, table 126, models of 131–33, 138
    chapter topic, 117–139

Cancer risk from tobacco, 143, 159
    reducing, chapter topic, 142–59
Cancer, breast. See Breast cancer
Case definition, described, 28
Case finding, described, 34
Case histories. See Illness histories

Case study, 212, 232
Case-control study
    defined, 367
    of mothers' ability to recognize
        pneumonia, 98–101
Chicana, defined, 119
Child feeding practices. *See* Nutrition
Christian(s), 58
    clergy, in Mozambique, 78
    in India, 311
Classification systems, 48. *See also*
        Ethnomedicine; Disease
        classification
Clinical practitioners. *See* Physicians
Clinics. *See* Health centers
Cohort study, 135, 198, 201
Collaborative programs. *See* Programs,
        collaborative
Communication. *See also* Education
    between researchers and local residents,
        51
    bridging gap between communities and
        health services (India), 302
    building on local beliefs in Mozambique,
        75
    child nutrition improvement efforts
        (Indonesia), 184, 186, 193–206
        effective messages, 203–5
        traditional sources of information, in
            Indonesia, 192–93
        materials, 196–97, 198
        media, use of, 195–97, 202
    of concept of AIDS in Mozambique, 73–
        74
    of correct pneumonia diagnosis, 109
    role in contraceptive use, 274
    in tobacco policy change study (US),
        materials, 150
        posters, 155, 157, 158
Community
    hard-to-reach populations, xviii, 42, 67,
        120, 138
    participation in program development, 13
        in breast cancer control study (US),
            119, 121
        chapter topic, 300–320
        importance of, xvi–xvii, xviii
        in tobacco policy change study (US),
            147, 149
Community health programs, 341
    chapter topic, 44–60, 300–320
    Community Health Committees (India),
        table 314, 315–16
    in Nepal, 329
Côte D'Ivoire, site of study, 257–75

Cultural adaptation (of program to target
        population)
    in child nutrition project (Indonesia),
        chapter topic, 182–206
    failure of, in assistant nurse-midwife
        program (Nepal), 328, 330, 334, 342
    in health programs, 12, 250
    lack of, in international health agencies,
        350–51
Cultural relativity, 7–9
Cultural sensitivity
    in addressing causes of road traffic
        crashes, 230
    development of, in AIDS prevention
        study (Mozambique), 65–66
    in developing health programs in Nepal,
        330
    importance in anthropology, 8–9, 10, 11,
        13, 22–23
    in intervention. *See* Intervention,
        culturally sensitive
    in surveys, 305
    in understanding tribal culture (US), 159
Cultural values
    among Javanese of Indonesia, 185
    in child nutrition project (Indonesia),
        188–89
    in family planning study (Côte D'Ivoire),
        274
    in health agencies, 336, 351–53
    in pesticide protective equipment study
        (Mexico), 245, 249
    in road user behavior study (Niue Island),
        212, 216, 217, 218–19, 220, 224,
        225–27, 230, 231
    in tobacco policy change study (US), 145,
        146–47, 148, 151, 156, 157
Culture, defined, 7

Diarrhea and diarrheal diseases, 33, 93,
        107, 190, 331
Disease beliefs, 27. *See also* Beliefs, cultural
Disease classification
    among Hausa in Nigeria, 167
    of influenza, 31
    among Shona in Mozambique, 69, 71
    of "viral syndrome," 35
Disease, communicable, 28, 29, 32
    AIDS prevention, chapter topic, 63–80
    control of, 30, 41
    folk flu, chapter topic, 27–42
    obstacles to investigating, 32–35, 37
    obstacles to control, 38–40, 41
    reportable, 30
        diagnosis of, *table* 36, 38

Economics
in child nutrition project (Indonesia), 189, 202
effect on family (Côte D'Ivoire), 265, 266, 268, 269, 272–75 mentioned
effect on health, 4, 51, 64, 107, 109, 167
effect on health policy and programs, 11, 258, 339
effect on road traffic crashes, 214, 230. *See also* Road traffic crashes
effect on safety in pesticide usage, 246, 249, 251 n.4
element of social organization, 19
in mosquito net intervention (Tanzania), 51, 55, 57
Education. *See also* Communication; Literacy
of community and family, to improve health and nutrition, 183
effect on health care seeking, 95, 104, 109
health education, 27, 29
as responsibility of assistant nurse-midwives, Nepal, 331
culturally appropriate, 307
enhancing, 135
improving cultural appropriateness through participatory research, 320
inhibiting, 133
improving family life, 267
including anthropology in public health curriculum, 22
in mosquito net intervention (Tanzania), 52, 54, 55
pneumonia education campaigns, 108
effects on risk factor knowledge
importance of including cultural beliefs, 138
low education levels, 236
positive, 136–37
teaching populations with low education levels, 134–35
Epidemiological data, in folk flu study (US), 29
Epidemiology and epidemiologists, 31–35
approach to disease outbreak, 28
described, 28
"folk epidemiology," 309, 310
limitations of, 109
Ethnicity, effect on health, 101, 109, 202
in assistant nurse-midwife program (Nepal), 334
in breast cancer control study (US), chapter topic, 117–39
in child nutrition project (Indonesia), 186, 189, 191, 199, 202

in mosquito net intervention (Tanzania), 58–59
in pesticide protective equipment study (Mexico), 245
in Therapist-Spiritist project (Puerto Rico), 282
in tobacco policy change study (US), chapter topic, 142–59
Ethnobotany
chapter topic, 165–79
Ethnographic findings
in breast cancer control study (US), 121–33; *tables* 122, 124 (Demographics); *table* 123 (Health-related characteristics); *table* 125 (Attitudes); *tables* 126, 132 (Risk factors)
in Community Diagnosis project (India), 307
in folk flu study (US), 29
in pesticide protective equipment study (Mexico), 239–40
Ethnographic interviews. *See* Interviews, ethnographic
Ethnographic methods, 304
combined with survey, 118, 239, 248
in Community Diagnosis project (India), 307
in designing interventions, 107, 108
in pesticide protective equipment study (Mexico), 239–43
"rapid," 65, 107, 108
in road user behavior study (Niue Island), 215
Ethnography
in breast cancer control study (US), chapter topic, 117–39
concept of, 7
defined, 368
described, 118
in family planning study (Côte D'Ivoire), chapter topic, 257–75
in Therapist-Spiritist project (Puerto Rico), 282–84, 286
perspective of, 7, 106–7
policy ethnography
chapter topic, 327–43, 345–63
described, 275 n.1
in understanding pneumonia in Pakistan, 108–10
Ethnomedicine, 51
and biomedicine, 7, 75, 167, 169
chapter topic, 165–79
linking with biomedicine, 280
defined, 7
internal logic of, 60

in mosquito net intervention (Tanzania), *table* 47, 48–49
Shona healers (Mozambique), 68–71, 77
Evaluation
  of AIDS prevention workshop (Mozambique), 79–80
  in breast cancer control study (US), 136–37
  in child nutrition project (Indonesia), 186, 198–203, *table* 201
  of mosquito net intervention (Tanzania), 56–59
  of Therapist-Spiritist project (Puerto Rico), 287, 292–94
  of tobacco policy change (US), 148

Factionalism, effect on health in mosquito net intervention (Tanzania), 59
Family. *See also* Patriliny; Matriliny
  effect of economy on, 272
  effect on health care seeking, in Pakistan, 96, 97, 100–101, 103–4, 107, 111 n.7
  fathers
    in child nutrition project (Indonesia), role in child rearing, 189, 193
    in family planning study (Côte D'Ivoire), in decision-making, 272
    responsibilities of, 268
  structure, in Côte D'Ivoire, 259, 264–65, 269, 271–72
    as interview topic, 262
  structure, in Indonesia, 185
  structure, in Pakistan, 86
Family planning, 183, 320
  in Côte D'Ivoire, chapter topic, 257–75
    desire for, 258
  in Nepal, 327, 331, 334
  media messages, 272
  need to expand scope of services, 271–75
  program, 186, 259
Family, extended
  in Côte D'Ivoire, 264–65, 271–73, 275
  effect on health care, 101
  in Indonesia, 185
  in Pakistan, 86, 87, 97, 101
Fatalism. *See* Beliefs, cultural
Feeding practices, child. *See* Nutrition
FES. *See* Focused Ethnographic Study
Field notes, 19. *See also* Observation
  in pesticide protective equipment study (Mexico), 239
  in road user behavior study (Niue Island), 211, 215, 228, 229
  in tobacco policy change study (US), 153, 156

Fieldwork. *See also* Observation
  in folk flu study (US), 30
  general aspects of, 15–20
Flu, defined, 31
Focus groups
  in AIDS prevention study (Mozambique), 66, 68
  in breast cancer control study (US), 119
  in child nutrition project (Indonesia), 187, 188
  in Community Diagnosis project (India), 307, 310
  defined, 368
  described, 18, 107
  in family planning study (Côte D'Ivoire), 259–60, 261–62
  in mosquito net intervention (Tanzania), 49
Focused Ethnographic Study (FES)
  of acute respiratory infection, 85, 107–8
  in AIDS prevention study (Mozambique), 66
  defined, 368
  described, 20
Folk beliefs. *See* Beliefs, cultural
Folk flu, chapter topic, 27–42
Folk healing. *See* Healing, traditional
Folk model, 28. *See also* Models
Formative research, 203
  aims of, 301
  in Community Diagnosis project (India), 301, 303, 318
  defined, 368
Free listing
  in breast cancer control study (US), 120
  in Community Diagnosis project (India), 308–9
  defined, 368
  described, 17, 48
  of risk factors for (breast) cancer, 124–31

Gender, effects on health care
  in assistant nurse-midwife program (Nepal), 327, 328, 332, 333, 336, 338, 341, 342
  in Pakistan, 95, 101, 102
  in Tanzania, 55
Government and politics, role of. *See also* Program failings or demise
  in AIDS prevention study (Mozambique), 66, 73, 74, 78
  in child nutrition project (Indonesia), 182, 183, 184, 187, 193, 197, 205, 206
  effect on health planning, 11, 339
  effect on health, 4, 107
  element of social organization, 19

Government and politics, role of (*continued*)
  in family planning study (Côte D'Ivoire), 257, 258, 259, 262, 267, 274, 275
  increasing number of village health workers, Pakistan, 109
  in maternal and child health, 268, 269, 273
  in mosquito net intervention (Tanzania), 58, 59, 60
  and pesticide usage, 237–38, 249–50
  on Niue Island, 220

Healers, indigenous. *See* Healers, traditional
Healers, traditional. *See also* Healing, traditional; Spiritism
  ability to cure STDs in Mozambique, 76–77
  belief systems, similarities to biomedicine, 69, 72, 75, 78
  beliefs, change in as result of project, 80
  chapter topic, 63–80
  in collaborative programs in Mozambique, 64–65, 73–74, 75–76, 79, 80
  as community mental health resources in Puerto Rico, 286, 288
  in Hausa pharmaceutical use study (Nigeria), 167
  in India, 306
  in Pakistan, 86, 96, 109
  sexually transmitted illness-related beliefs and practices, in Mozambique, 66–73
  success in treating sexually transmitted disease, 76–77
  in Tanzania, 49, 50, 51–52
  understanding of AIDS, in Mozambique, 71–73
Healing, traditional. *See also* Spiritism; Healers, traditional
  characteristics in ethnic minority communities, 282
  in Puerto Rico, integrating with mental health care, chapter topic, 279–96
Health bureaucracies. *See also* Health planners and planning; International health agencies
  and anthropologists, need for mutual understanding, 340
  chapter topic, 345–63
  culture of, 336, 351–53
  resistance to change, 303
  understanding approaches of, 328–29, 337, 339

Health care
  in childhood pneumonia study (Pakistan), 84, 100, 103, 104
  primary. *See* Primary health care
  problems with access to, 64, 122, 128, 268, 341
Health care providers. *See also* Allopathic practitioners; Healers, traditional; Midwives; Physicians
  health workers, as study participants key informant, in Pakistan, 89
  health workers, community (CHW) in Community
    Diagnosis project (India), 300
    duties of, 302, 312–13, *table* 313
    history of, 302–3
    preferred characteristics, 311–312, *table* 312
    problems with programs, 301, 302
    selection of, 314, *table* 314
  health workers, community volunteer in Indonesia (kaders), 183, 193
    as community educators, 194, 195, 196, 200, 202, 204–5
    evaluation after training, 202
    improved knowledge of child feeding, 199
    as study participants, 187, 199
    training of, to educate others, 197, 198, 204
  health workers, village
    in Tanzania, 48, 49, 50, 51
    as participants in family planning study (Côte D'Ivoire), 260–62 mentioned, 264–69 mentioned, 271, 272, 273–75
    as participants in Therapist-Spiritist project (Puerto Rico), 285, 286, 288–96 mentioned
    as public educators, 268–69
    role in maternal and child health, 273
Health centers, government-run
  in Côte D'Ivoire, 259, 268, 269, 270
  in India, 302, 306
  infrequent use of, in Pakistan, 90, 93, 95, 105
  mental health, in Puerto Rico, 282, 286
  rural, in Nepal, 329, 331, 332, 333, 334, 341
Health committees, community
  in Community Diagnosis project (India), 300
Health culture, 27, 41, 311, 318. *See also* Ethnomedicine
Health education. *See* Education; *See also* Communication

Health planners and planning. *See also* Health bureaucracies; International health agencies; Policymakers
  consideration of community priorities, 300, 309
  contributions of anthropology, 330, 338–40
  failure to use results, 339
  difference in community and planners' views, 319
  distance from recipient population, problems caused by, 304, 330, 350
  effects of regional differences, 319
  importance of cultural information in, chapter
    topic, 327–42, 340, 342
  lessons from child nutrition project (Indonesia), 203
  in Mozambique, 78–79, 80, 81
  objections to using anthropological data, 5, 339
  sociocultural information, importance of, 338–40
Health workers. *See* Health care providers
Health, maternal and child
  in Côte D'Ivoire, 257
    as interview topic, 262
    services, use of, in Côte D'Ivoire, 270
  improving in Indonesia, 183, 184
  need for in Nepal, 331
Hepatitis
  transmission of, 40
  viral, 30, 33, 34, 40
Hindu(s), 185, 332
Homeopath, homeopathy
  defined, 368
  in India, 313
  in Pakistan, 86
Hot-cold. *See* Beliefs, cultural; Illness, treatment.

Illness histories, 107
  in childhood pneumonia study (Pakistan), 89, 90, 94, 95, 96, 101–6
  in folk flu study (US), 35–37, 40
  patient records, 87
Illness perceptions, 27, 33–34, 41, 45
Illness, causes of. *See* Beliefs, cultural
Illness, local definition of. *See* Disease classification; Ethnomedicine
Illness, treatment. *See also* Mental health care; Pneumonia, treatment
  among Hausa (Nigeria), 174, 176
  "balance of opposites," 175–76
  hot-cold, 175–76
  use of pharmaceuticals, *table* 170–73

hot-cold, in pneumonia, 92, 102
inappropriate antibiotics, 38–39, 87, 94, 108
inappropriate for pneumonia, 96, 106
misdiagnosis, 37, 38
Immigrants
  in Indonesia, 185
  migration to city, 55
  in Southern California, 121
  in Tanzania, 58
India, site of study, 300–320
Indians, American. *See* American Indians
Indigenous healers. *See* Healers, traditional
Indonesia, site of study, 182–206
Infectious disease control. *See* Disease, communicable
Influenza, defined, 31
Informant
  defined, 15
  in Hausa pharmaceutical use study (Nigeria), 169
  key, in AIDS prevention study (Mozambique), 67
  key, in Community Diagnosis project (India), 307, 310
  key, in family planning study (Côte D'Ivoire), 260, 261, 263
  key, in mosquito net intervention (Tanzania), 56
  key, in childhood pneumonia study (Pakistan), 88, 89, 90, 102
Injury, traffic. *See* Road traffic crashes
Injury, unintentional. *See also* Road traffic crashes
  as cause of death in Nepal, 331
  as cause of morbidity and mortality, 228
  causes of, on Niue Island
    alcohol, 226–27
    condition of vehicle, 218
    driver behavior, 222–23, 230
    infrastructure, 217
    other, 224
    spirits (aitu), 224–25
  medical care for, on Niue Island, 228–29
Insecticide. *See* Pesticides
International health
  agencies. *See also* Health bureaucracies; Health
    evaluating, 353–54
    failure to recognize cultures of recipient populations, 350–51
    planners and planning, 327–344, 345–364
    problems in, 354–63
    role of organizational characteristics, 346
    types of, 348–49
    value of studying, xvii

International health (*continued*)
  importance of sociocultural values in,
    345–46
  policy, 336
    selective use of research findings, 356
  programs, chapter topic, 345–63
Intervention, culturally sensitive, 41, 165, 179
  in AIDS prevention program
    (Mozambique), 75–77
  in breast cancer control study (US), 133–
    37, 138
  in child nutrition project (Indonesia),
    197–98
  community-based mosquito net
    (Tanzania), chapter topic, 45–60
  factors in road traffic crash reduction,
    232, 230
  in tobacco policy change study (US), 142,
    145–52
    obstacles to, 150–51
Interview guide, 89
  in family planning study (Côte D'Ivoire),
    262
Interviews, ethnographic, 138
  in breast cancer control study (US), 118,
    119–21
  in pesticide protective equipment study
    (Mexico), 239
  in tobacco policy change study (US), 148–49
Interviews, focused
  in folk flu study (US), 30
Interviews, in-depth
  in AIDS prevention study (Mozambique),
    66, 67, 68
  in child nutrition project (Indonesia), 187
  in childhood pneumonia study (Pakistan),
    89
  in Community Diagnosis project (India), 307
Interviews, phone
  in tobacco policy change study (US), 154
Interviews, semistructured
  in AIDS prevention study (Mozambique),
    67
  defined, 368
  described, 18
  in family planning study (Côte D'Ivoire),
    260
  in Hausa pharmaceutical use study
    (Nigeria), 169
  in mosquito net intervention (Tanzania),
    56, 57
  in pesticide protective equipment study
    (Mexico), 247
  in Therapist-Spiritist project (Puerto
    Rico), 284

Interviews, structured
  defined, 369
  described, 17
  in Nepal, 328
Interviews, types of, 16–18
Interviews, unstructured
  defined, 369
  described, 16
  in mosquito net intervention (Tanzania),
    49, 50, 56
  in Nepal, 328
  in Therapist-Spiritist project (Puerto
    Rico), 283
Iron deficiency, 46. *See also* Anemia
Islam. *See* Religion; Leaders, religious

KAP surveys (Knowledge, attitude, and
    practice), 305
  in AIDS prevention, 63
  in breast cancer control study (US),
    135
Knowledge, attitude, and practice surveys.
    See KAP surveys

Language, use of local
  in breast cancer control study (US), 120,
    133, 135
  in child nutrition project (Indonesia),
    187
  in family planning study (Côte D'Ivoire),
    262
  importance of, 18
    in AIDS prevention study
      (Mozambique), 73
  with interpreters, 18, 102
    in childhood pneumonia study
      (Pakistan), 89, 99, 102
  in road user behavior study (Niue Island),
    215
Language, semantics
  chapter topic, 27–42
  as epidemiological issue, 32
  terms for malaria and other illnesses
    (Tanzania), 48, 49–51
Latina, defined, 119
Leaders and leadership
  local or community
    in child nutrition project (Indonesia),
      187, 196, 197
    in mosquito net intervention
      (Tanzania), 57, 59
  religious
    as healers, in Pakistan, 86
    in implementing child nutrition project
      (Indonesia), 187, 196, 197

influence of religious leaders in
Indonesia, 185, 193
in mosquito net intervention
(Tanzania), 48
Literacy, effect on health care, 54, 59, 109,
184–85

Malaria fever, 49, 50
Malaria transmission, 44, 48
control of, 54
effect of treated mosquito nets, 48
Malaria, 320, 331
chloroquine resistance to, 46
mortality, 54
in pregnancy, 50, 51
relationship to anemia, 50, 51
terms for malaria and other illnesses
(Tanzania), 48, 49–51
Malaria, cerebral, 46, 50, 51
Malaria, clinical, 45, 48, 49, 51
Malnutrition. See Nutrition
Maternal and child health. See Health,
maternal and child
Matriliny, 259, 264, 272, 306, 311. See also
Family
Media. See Communication
Medical knowledge, local. See
Ethnomedicine
Medical practitioners. See Physicians
Medicines. See also Pharmaceuticals
access to
of allopathic practitioners in Pakistan,
87
in Community Diagnosis project
(India), 316–18, table 317
in family planning study (Côte
D'Ivoire), 268
modern, in disease treatment, 58
Mental health care
integrating with Spiritism
difficulties, 290–92
successes, 292–94
integrating with traditional healing,
chapter topic, 279–96
balanced study of both systems, 288–
89
community mental health, 281–82
social, political, religious context, 280–
82
in relation to Spiritism, 290
Mexico, site of study, 235–50
Midwives. See also Assistant Nurse-Midwife
Program
in child nutrition project (Indonesia),
187, 193, 195, 197

as participants in family planning study
(Côte D'Ivoire), 260, 261, 264. See
also Health care providers
in Tanzania, 50
Migration. See Immigrants
Models. See also Pneumonia, folk model;
Biomedical model
of breast cancer risk, 131–33
cultural, 121
folk, 28
of international health programs, 349–52
Mortality
child, 45, 47, 48, 50, 52, 84, 182, 331
infant, 46, 86, 302, 306, 331, 341
in Côte D'Ivoire, 257–58
injury as cause, 213
malaria-related, 54
maternal, 331, 341
in Côte D'Ivoire, 257–58
pneumonia-related, 102, 109
from road traffic crashes, 214, 223
Mosquito nets
chapter topic, 44–60
impact on malaria transmission, 48, 57
insecticide-treated, 45, 48, 56–59, 60
Mosquitoes
anopheline, 48
as cause of malaria, 49
infected, 46, table 47, 51, 52, 54
Mozambique, site of study, 63–80
Muslim(s), 86
clergy, in Mozambique, 78
healing, in Nigeria, 167
in India, 311
in Indonesia, 185, 193
in Nepal, 333

National Cancer Institute (NCI), 145, 159
National Institute of Mental Health
(NIMH), 282, 285
Native Americans. See American Indians
Nepal, site of study, 327–42
Nigeria, site of study, 165–79
Niue Island, site of study, 211–32
Nutrition
child feeding practices
chapter topic, 182–206
communication strategy to improve,
194–205
educating mothers, benefits of, 199–203
malnutrition, 182, 184, 191
new practices, 187–88, 191
recommendations for improving, 192
results of nutrition project, 199–203,
table 201, 203

Nutrition, child feeding practices
(*continued*)
    scope of project, 194
    traditional, 189–91
deficiencies, as cause of death in Nepal, 331
during illness, 191, 309–10
improvement in Indonesia, chapter topic,
    182–206

Observation
    in child nutrition project (Indonesia), 187
    field observations
        in family planning study (Côte
            D'Ivoire), 260, 270
        in tobacco policy change study (US),
            152–53, 156–58
    in Hausa pharmaceutical use study
        (Nigeria), 167, 169
    of health-related practices, 107
    in pesticide protective equipment study
        (Mexico), 240, 247
    in Therapist-Spiritist project (Puerto
        Rico), 283
    role in anthropological research, 18–19, 89
Operational research, 44

Pakistan, site of study, 84–110
Participant observation
    benefit of, 305
    in Community Diagnosis project (India),
        307
    defined, 347, 368
    described, 15
    in folk flu study (US), 29, 30
    in mosquito net intervention (Tanzania),
        56
    in Nepal, 328
    in road user behavior study (Niue Island),
        215–16
    in study of international health agencies,
        347–48
Participatory research
    analysis of, 318–20
    as basis for health programs, 310–18
    benefits of, 305
    chapter topic, 300–320
    in community problem-solving, 306, 320
    defined, 368
    and social science, 303–5
    in Therapist-Spiritist project (Puerto
        Rico), 284
    to understand local health concerns, 308–
        10
Patriliny, 185, 259, 264, 272, 306, 311. *See
    also* Family

Pediatric clinic
    in childhood pneumonia study (Pakistan),
        94–97
    in folk flu study (US), *table* 36
Pesticides
    chapter topic, understanding usage
        behaviors, 235–51
    cultural impact on changing usage
        behaviors, 248–49
    health impacts, negative 235–36, 238,
        242–43
    improving handling practices, 248
    knowledge of danger and precautions,
        240–42, 245, 247–48
    mosquito nets, treating, 44, 45, 55, 56–58
    poisoning
        causes of worldwide, 236
        failure of educational campaigns, 248
        reducing health risks, 238
    risks in using. *See* Risk, perception of
    side effects of, 56
    special issues for women and children,
        247–48
    toxicity, 57, 58, 235, 249
Pharmaceuticals. *See also* Medicines
    in childhood pneumonia study (Pakistan),
        93, 94, 95, 96, 105
    compared with medicinal plants, 168
    in developing countries, chapter topic,
        165–79, *table* 170–73
    incorporation into existing culture, 174,
        178–79
    used with medicinal plants, 169, 177–79
Physicians. *See also* Healers, traditional;
        Health care providers
    in childhood pneumonia study (Pakistan),
        94, 95, 106
    in folk flu study (US), 35–38, 40, 41, 42
    as participants in breast cancer control
        study (US), 120, 122, 131
    as participants in family planning study
        (Côte D'Ivoire), 261, 264. *See also*
        Health care providers
Pile sorting, described, 17, 48–49
Planners and planning. *See* Health planners
        and planning
Pneumonia, childhood
    chapter topic, 84–110
    as cause of death in Nepal, 331
Pneumonia, diagnosis
    accuracy of, in Pakistan, 85, 105–106
    healers' ability to diagnose correctly, in
        Pakistan, 93–94
    mothers' understanding of, in Pakistan,
        84, 90, 92–97 (mentioned), 98–101

Pneumonia, folk model, 88, 100, *illus.*, 91
differences from biomedical model, 90
local concepts of, 89
mothers' understanding of, in Pakistan,
90–92
Pneumonia, treatment
accurate, effects of local knowledge, in
Pakistan, 85
delays in, 84, 96, 104
effects of family on, 100
hot-cold, 92–93, 102
inappropriate, 102, 106, 108
mothers' understanding of, in Pakistan, 97
in Pakistan, 92–94, 96
reducing mortality, 109
Policy change
in tobacco policy change study (US),
chapter topic, 142–59
Policy development
chapter topic, 345–63
family planning, 271
importance of local input, 60
Policymakers
in Côte D'Ivoire, 262, 275
as participants in family planning study,
260, 261, 263–66 mentioned, 268,
269, 272
importance of translating anthropological
concepts, xvii
need to study, 60, 328–29, 330
chapter topic, 345–63
Politics. *See* Government and politics
Pollution beliefs, 70, 77
Pollution
as cancer risk, 128, 129–30, 131
as cause of pneumonia, 84
Polygamy, 259, 264, 266, 267, 268
Popular beliefs. *See* Beliefs, cultural
Population policy
culturally appropriate in Côte D'Ivoire,
chapter topic, 257–75
culturally inappropriate, 271
policy implications, 270–75
Practitioners, traditional. *See* Healers,
traditional
Primary health care. *See also* Health centers
chapter topic, 300–320
community involvement in, 300, 302, 307
survey results, 311–18; *tables* 312, 313,
314, 317
community-based, 328, 332
in Community Diagnosis project (India),
300
in international health policy, 327
Primary health centers. *See* Health centers

Program failings or demise
in assistant nurse-midwife program
(Nepal), 328, 334–35, 342 n.1
efforts to improve, 338, 341–42
failures of planning agencies, 335–37
neglecting sociocultural knowledge,
332–33
role of sociocultural knowledge, 345–46
in child nutrition project (Indonesia), 204
ignoring culture of recipient population, 5
personnel change as cause, 80
politics, role of
in community health programs, 301
in Community Diagnosis project
(India), 318
in Therapist-Spiritist project (Puerto
Rico), 294, 296
reasons for, in Community Diagnosis
project (India), 318–19
in Therapist-Spiritist project (Puerto
Rico), 291–92, 295–96
Program successes
in AIDS prevention study (Mozambique),
79–80
in breast cancer control study (US), 136–
37
in child nutrition project (Indonesia),
197, 199–203
in tobacco policy change study (US), 155–
58, 159
in Therapist-Spiritist project (Puerto
Rico), 293–94
Programs, collaborative
in Côte D'Ivoire, for family planning, 257,
259
in Indonesia, for child nutrition
improvement, 183, 184
development of strategy 193–97
partnership, importance of, 205–6
training, 197–98, 204–5
in Mozambique, for AIDS prevention, 64,
65, 66–68, 73–74, 75
in Puerto Rico, Therapist-Spiritist
project, 282, 284–87, 294
program objectives, 285
in United States, for tobacco policy
change, 145, 158–59
Programs, community-based
in India, chapter topic, 300–320
in Indonesia, 183
Programs, national, adaptation for local use
in Indonesia, 184, 206
Project planning, participant involvement
in, 293, 295. *See also* Participatory
research

Public health. *See also* Epidemiology;
    Anthropological approach and
    methods
  benefits of using anthropological
    approach, xvi–xvii
  obstacles to improving, 4–5
Puerto Rico, site of study, 279–96

Qualitative research. *See* Research,
    qualitative
Qualitative-quantitative "dispute," 13, 118.
    See also Anthropological approach
    and methods
Questionnaire, semistructured
  in breast cancer control study (US), 119
  in pesticide protective equipment study
    (Mexico), 239
Questionnaires
  in Therapist-Spiritist project (Puerto
    Rico), 287, 293
  use in anthropology, 17
Questions, closed-ended
  in breast cancer control study (US), 119
  in childhood pneumonia study (Pakistan),
    89
Questions, open-ended. *See also* Interviews,
    semistructured
  in breast cancer control study (US), 119
  in childhood pneumonia study (Pakistan),
    89, 95, 99
  in family planning study (Côte D'Ivoire),
    262
  in Hausa pharmaceutical use study
    (Nigeria), 168, 169
  in pesticide protective equipment study
    (Mexico), 239, 247

Ranking
  in breast cancer control study (US), 120–
    21
  described, 17
Rapid Assessment Procedures (RAP)
  defined, 368
  described, 20, 305
  in study of acute respiratory infection,
    107, 108
  in tobacco policy change study (US), 152
Rapport, importance of, xviii, 15, 89, 188,
    307, 308, 311
Refugees, effects on residents, 63
Religion. *See also* Leaders, religious;
    Spiritism
  role of mosques in health promotion, 58
Research, ethnomedical, 79

Research, formative. *See* Formative research
Research, operational, 44
Research, participatory. *See* Participatory
    research
Research, qualitative
  in assistant nurse-midwife program
    (Nepal), 328
  in child nutrition project (Indonesia),
    187
  in Community Diagnosis project (India),
    307, 311
  in mosquito net intervention (Tanzania),
    52–53
Research setting
  of AIDS prevention study (Mozambique),
    65–66
  of assistant nurse-midwife program
    (Nepal), 330–33, 340–42
  of breast cancer control study (US), 119
  of child nutrition project (Indonesia),
    184–86
  of childhood pneumonia study (Pakistan),
    86, 87
  of Community Diagnosis project (India),
    305–8
  of family planning study (Côte D'Ivoire),
    259
  of folk flu study (US), 29
  of Hausa pharmaceutical use study
    (Nigeria), 165–67
  of mosquito net intervention (Tanzania),
    45
  of pesticide protective equipment study
    (Mexico), 237–38
  of road user behavior study (Niue Island),
    212–14, 216–17
  of Therapist-Spiritist project (Puerto
    Rico), 280–81
  of tobacco policy change study (US), 143–
    45, 146
Risk factors
  for breast cancer, beliefs about, 120–21,
    124–31, *table* 126, *table* 132
  in pesticide protective equipment study
    (Mexico), 242
  for road traffic crashes, 213, 231, 232
  role of culture in, 232
Risk, perception of
  in pesticide protective equipment study
    (Mexico), 242, 249
    effects of cultural factors on, 242–46
    effects of economics on, 245, 246
    effect of physical environment on, 245,
      246

in road user behavior study (Niue Island), 212, 225–27, 230–32
seasonal variations, 52–54
Road traffic crashes (RTC). *See also* Injury, unintentional
causes
alcohol, 225–27, 228
cultural values affecting, 230
spirits, 224–25
chapter topic, 211–32
cost of, to nation, 227–29
economic growth, role of, 214
injury, 213–14
medical care for, 228–29
mortality, 214, 223, 229
as public health issue, 229
prevention of, 230–31
failure to use protective gear, 224
interventions, 231
understanding cultural norms, 231
RTC. *See* Road traffic crashes

Sampling
cluster, 306
defined, 367
convenience, 89
organization-based, 119–20
random, 94
self-selected, 239
snowball
defined, 167, 369
in pesticide protective equipment study (Mexico), 239
systematic, 53, 54
Sexually transmitted disease. *See* STD
Sexually transmitted illness
defined, 80 n.1
sexually transmitted illness-related beliefs and practices among traditional healers in Mozambique, 66–73
Side effects
of insecticide usage, 56
of pharmaceuticals, 174, 175
Snowball sampling. *See* Sampling, snowball
Social organization
analysis of, 19
on Niue Island, in road user behavior study, 216, 218–19
Sorcery. *See* Beliefs, cultural
Spiritism
as community mental health resource in Puerto Rico, 286, 288
chapter topic, 281–96

community reactions to Therapist-Spiritist project (Puerto Rico), 289–90
compared with biomedicine, 283, 284, 288
as ethnomedical system, 284
integrating with biomedicine, 290–95
difficulties, 290–92, 295–96
successes, 292–94
in relation to mental health care, 290
Spiritists as participants in Therapist-Spiritist project (Puerto Rico), 286, 288–96 mentioned
Spirits. *See* Beliefs, cultural
STD, sexually transmitted disease, 320
chapter topic, 63–80
defined, 80 n.1
treatment of, 64
Surveillance (in epidemiology), 33, 35
Survey(s)
in breast cancer control study (US), 118, 119, 138
in Community Diagnosis project (India), 310–18
selected responses, *tables* 312, 313, 314, and 317
cross-sectional, in child nutrition project (Indonesia), 198
health, in Hausa pharmaceutical use study (Nigeria), 169
of mosquito net usage (Tanzania), 54–55
of pesticide usage (Mexico), 239–43
combined with ethnographic methods, 248, 250

Tanzania, site of study, 44–60
Tobacco, use of
chapter topic, 142–59
health impact, 145
ceremonial versus recreational use, 142, 143, 146–47, 157
Training. *See also* Communication; Education
as exchange of information
in Mozambique, 76
in Puerto Rico, 285–87
of lay investigators in Community Diagnosis project (India), 307
Translation. *See also* Back translate; Language
of anthropological concepts, xvi, xvii, 8, 21
failure to translate, 21
need for, in health planning (Nepal), 339
of public health knowledge into local terms (Mozambique), 74
Treatment. *See* Illness, treatment

UNICEF (United Nations Childrens Fund)
  as multilateral international health
      agency, 348
  in nutrition project (Indonesia), 184, 193,
      205, 206
  as sponsor of AIDS prevention workshop
      (Mozambique), 79
  staff members as study participants,
      family planning (Côte D'Ivoire), 263
  in support of assistant nurse-midwife
      programs (Nepal), 328, 329
United States, site of study
  breast cancer control study, 117–39
  folk flu study, 27–42
  tobacco policy change study, 142–59
United States Agency for International
      Development. See USAID
USAID (United States Agency for
      International Development)
  as bilateral international health agency,
      348, 360
  Community Health Program, 329

in nutrition project (Indonesia), 184, 193,
    205
in population policy development (Côte
    D'Ivoire), 257
staff members as study participants,
    family planning (Côte D'Ivoire), 263

Vehicle safety. See also Road traffic crashes
  in road user behavior study (Niue Island),
      221
Viral syndrome, 27–42 mentioned

WHO (World Health Organization)
  and assistant nurse-midwife program
      (Nepal), 328, 329, 336
  diagnostic criteria, 95
  efforts to reduce pneumonia mortality,
      85, 110 n.1, 110 n.3, 107
  as multilateral international health
      agency, 348, 353, 354, 360, 361
Witchcraft. See Beliefs, cultural
World Health Organization. See WHO